Speech-Language Pathology and Early Intervention:

From Theory to Evidence-Based Practice

Corey Herd Cassidy, PhD, CCC-SLP

Copyright © 2025 by Corey Cassidy

All rights, including that of translation, reserved. No part of this publication may be reproduced, stored in a retrieval system, or transmitted in any form or by any means, electronic, mechanical, recording, or otherwise, including photocopying, recording, taping, web distribution, or information storage and retrieval systems without the prior written consent of the publisher.

For permission to use material from this text, contact us by email: coreyherd@gmail.com

Every attempt has been made to contact the copyright holders for material originally printed in another source. If any have been inadvertently overlooked, the publisher will gladly make the necessary arrangements at the first opportunity.

Library of Congress Cataloging-in-Publication Data:

ISBN-13: 979-8-218-61976-3

Table of Contents

Foreword 4

Introduction..5

Acknowledgments 7

Contributor...9

Dedication..10

Part I
Foundations, Principles, and Evidence Supporting Early Intervention

Chapter 1 Introduction to Early Intervention and the Role of the Speech-Language Pathologist 12

Chapter 2 Guiding Principles of Early Intervention..41

Chapter 3 Evidence-Based Approaches and Practices in Early Intervention 66

Part II
Early Intervention in Practice

Chapter 4 Considerations for Early Intervention Services in the Natural Environment 89

Chapter 5 Current Levels of Functioning 119

Chapter 6 Screening, Evaluation, and Assessment in Early Intervention 164

Chapter 7 Eligibility Determination and Development of the Individualized Family Service Plan 200

Chapter 8 Culturally and Linguistically Responsive Practices in Early Intervention 232

Chapter 9 Treatment in the Natural Environment 260

Chapter 10 Best Practices for Assessment and Treatment of Speech Sound Development 290

Chapter 11 Feeding and Swallowing Assessment and Intervention 315

Chapter 12 Special Populations 359

Appendix A...408

Appendix B...414

Appendix C...427

Appendix D...439

Appendix E...440

Foreword

Speech-language pathologists (SLPs) providing early intervention services know firsthand that the earlier children receive services, the more likely they are to achieve successful learning outcomes in communication and swallowing skills. Effective services are family-centered, evidence-based, and designed to meet the needs of infants and toddlers from birth to age 3 years who have or could be at risk for developmental delays or disabilities.

This book is a must-read for anyone who is considering or engaged in early intervention practice. In Part I, the reader will study the foundations and principles of early intervention and the role of the SLP while exploring the highest quality of evidence supporting early intervention service delivery. Part II takes the reader deep into the essential elements of practice, including considerations for services in the natural environment, screening, evaluation and assessment, feeding assessment and intervention, and determining and writing functional outcomes.

The author has also included a chapter on culturally and linguistically responsive practices, a particularly important addition as Individuals with Disabilities Education Act (IDEA) Part C Regulations state that families of infants and toddlers with a disability must have access to culturally responsive services.

Dr. Cassidy's comprehensive work in early intervention has laid the groundwork for state guidelines in this practice area. In addition, her widely respected knowledge and expertise continue to provide the guiding principles for SLPs providing services based on the integration of the highest quality research, informed professional judgment and expertise, and family preferences and values for the birth-to-3 population. This timely book is sure to be a comprehensive and valuable addition to your professional bookshelf.

Melanie W. Hudson, MA, CCC-SLP, F-ASHA, F-NAP, BCS-CL

Introduction

I first joined the world of early intervention (EI) as an SLP at the turn of the 21st century. Even though I had earned my undergraduate and graduate degrees in communication sciences and disorders and spent more than 5 years as a licensed SLP in several public school systems across the country, I had no idea how to address the developmental needs of infants or toddlers. I had no training in adult learning strategies and no knowledge about coaching, communicating, and collaborating with parents, caregivers, and colleagues. What I did have was an interest in all things regarding early childhood, an open mind, and extraordinary mentors who were excited to teach me everything they knew about EI.

Now, with more than 25 years of experience working with young children and their families, I love serving as an SLP in EI! Through this arena, I am able to pay it forward every day by sharing my experiences, knowledge, and skills by teaching—empowering infants and toddlers to get their needs and wants met, sharing the strategies I have learned with families to support their children's development, connecting and collaborating with early childhood educators and childcare providers to ensure best practices in all-natural settings, and communicating with colleagues to serve on interprofessional teams and engage with one another to best support the whole child and every child.

In addition to my work as an SLP, I have had the honor to teach and serve as a faculty member in higher education institutions for more than two decades. I have taught thousands of undergraduate and graduate students across multiple disciplines. I love this form of teaching as well. I love sharing my knowledge. I love watching students light up when they learn something new … something I have taught them!

There are no secrets in EI. To succeed, we must share our knowledge, perspectives, strategies, and skills. We need to share with children, parents and caregivers, colleagues, and each other. Through this textbook, I want to share all the secrets. I want the reader to recognize how amazing, fulfilling, and empowering EI is for us as the providers and the families we serve.

I want to make it clear that we need passionate and engaged clinicians who care about and want to work with the families who need us most. In addition to my perspective, experience, and joy in EI, I want to share the best the research and literature have to offer. I want the reader to be empowered to provide effective, outstanding services and feel confident and competent in their choices with and for children and their families. I want this textbook to pull SLP students into this world and give faculty a clear, simple, yet comprehensive context from which to teach the material.

Many textbooks, even the most outstanding ones, provide so much information that the reader often struggles or is unwilling to spend the time it takes to read the content. The knowledge I share in this textbook is intended to serve as a starting point for students and providers on the path to a position in EI. My purpose is to provide students with information they recognize, can relate to, and can apply immediately as new SLPs in EI and to provide instructors with material that is accessible, applicable, and offers a direct connection between teaching and practice. I hope instructors and students will take the time to read the content without becoming overwhelmed.

Critical thinking questions are included at the end of each chapter to facilitate discussion or incorporate into independent student activities. Additional materials, including glossary, comprehensive list of references, and links to online resources, references, videos, and webinars, are provided for consideration and use by both instructors and students. A set of 10 case studies with corresponding reflection questions, all of which can be connected to each chapter, support in-class engagement and discussion of the material or can be incorporated into course assignments. Microsoft PowerPoint slides connected to each chapter are also available upon request for instructors to incorporate into classroom lectures.

Finally, I have written this text in first-person plural tense (we/us) to set the tone and convey the message that this is about *our* journey into the world of EI. We are learning together, and this is our path. I hope this material feels warm, enriching, and passionate. Ultimately, my goal is to establish a foundation of and support the knowledge and skills of practicing and future SLPs in EI; by ensuring our own confidence and competence, we can and will empower and build upon the capacities of the children and families with whom we work.

Just as I consistently share with the parents and caregivers with whom I work daily, we each play a crucial role in serving infants and toddlers and empowering them to communicate. We should never underestimate our contribution when we walk into a child's home and begin to build our relationship with a family.

As we arm ourselves with the knowledge gained from this textbook, we prepare to teach and share our knowledge, skills, and experiences with those who need it most. We are learning the secrets of EI to inform and coach parents and caregivers who will then teach and empower their own children.

Acknowledgments

Writing a textbook was as hard as I thought it might be and more rewarding than I could ever have imagined. This process and product would not have been possible without the love, commitment, and unwavering support of my husband, Jim Cassidy. Thank you for encouraging me when I needed it the most, consistently showing up and leaning in as my partner for our family, and always being your authentic self. You are exactly who I need in my life every day, even when I don't want to admit it!

I would be remiss if I did not acknowledge and share my appreciation for my mother, Carol Herd. My mom has been an SLP for more than 50 years and has served in a variety of settings and across multiple populations. Early on, she knew I was meant to follow in her footsteps, mentioned it multiple times when I was young, waited patiently until I realized my own path and future in the field, and offered me my first professional opportunity to step into a related role. Since that summer of 1992, my commitment to the field and passion for our discipline has never wavered. Mom, you were right all along!

Corinne (Cori) Hill was my first mentor and true friend in the early intervention arena. More than 20 years ago, she took a chance and hired me to work with infants, toddlers, and families through what is now the Infant and Toddler Connection of Harrisonburg-Rockingham County, Virginia. Cori continues to serve as an amazing role model and a beautifully bright light in the world of EI for those who practice in the Commonwealth of Virginia and across the country. As an early childhood educator and professional development expert with more than 30 years of knowledge, perspective, and experience, Cori continues to teach, mentor, and inspire EI providers who are just starting out, as well as those of us who are seasoned and continue to have so much to learn. Cori is also the author and genius behind the true-to-life case studies presented in this textbook and companion website.

I must also give sincere thanks to Emily Guill. Emily was a student at Radford University when I first moved to Virginia; she continues to be one of my closest friends while serving as one of the most creative, committed, and outstanding speech-language pathologists I know. Emily provided me with the initial feedback and suggestions necessary to mold this textbook into what it has become. She kept the encouragement coming with each chapter she reviewed and ensured I did not miss a beat in both voice and content.

I need to share a special thank you and shout-out to my dear friend and colleague, Rebecca Epperly. Rebecca has been by my side personally and professionally, offering her sage advice for almost 18 years. Each time she offers me her wise wisdom, I roll my eyes and pretend to ignore it, only to put it in my "vault," where it has eventually and inevitably been dragged back out and put to good use…every time. Rebecca is also an SLP with an enormous heart; she has had a significant clinical impact on and touched the lives of countless individuals and families over the years.

Dr. Vicki Pitstick provided fresh eyes and kept me going, offering and following through to create the initial outlines for the PowerPoint slides now available on the companion website. As an expert in student-faculty connections and student belonging in higher education, Vicki's authenticity and genuine love for her friends, family, and colleagues is evident in every encounter and interaction in which she engages.

I must thank Ms. Melanie Hudson for her beautiful foreword and the professional impact she has had on me over the past 15 years. Melanie is one of my speech-language pathology role models, mentors, and heroes. She is an inspiration to many of us, and I can only hope to have the positive influence she has had and will continue to have in our field. Her light shines brightly.

Finally, my deepest appreciation goes to the infants and toddlers and their families who have had the biggest impact on my life and who never cease to amaze me with their grit, determination, compassion, and vision.

Contributor

Corinne Foley Hill, MEd

Virginia Early Intervention Professional Development Center Director
Professional Development Specialist
Partnership for People with Disabilities
Virginia Commonwealth University
Waynesboro, Virginia

This work is dedicated to my son, August (Auggie) James, who helps me remember what I love most in my life; my daughter, Olivia (Olive) Kathleen, who inspires me to play more often every day; my husband, Jim, who reminds me who I really am and how to love with all my heart; and our dog, Brownie, the clear leader of the family (according to Auggie) and the one who kept me company each and every day while I worked on and wrote this textbook.

Part I
Foundations, Principles, and Evidence Supporting Early Intervention

Chapter 1

Introduction to Early Intervention and the Role of the Speech-Language Pathologist

Learning Outcomes

When we have completed this chapter, we will be able to:

- Present a detailed history of legislative support for the birth–age 3 population.
- Discuss the most current Individuals with Disabilities Education Act (IDEA) regulatory requirements focused on early intervention (EI) policies, procedures, and practices.
- Describe the range of EI services that support families through IDEA Part C.
- Provide an overview of the speech-language pathologist (SLP) scope of practice, roles, and responsibilities in EI.
- Share an overview of the American Speech-Language-Hearing Association (ASHA) guiding principles in providing EI services.
- Outline the Recommended Practices in Early Intervention as developed by the Division of Early Childhood (DEC) of the Council for Exceptional Children.

What Will We Learn and How Can We Apply It?

Welcome to the world of early intervention (EI)! This chapter presents the detailed history of EI in the birth–age 3 population and the most current Individuals with Disabilities Education Act (IDEA) regulatory requirements regarding EI policies, procedures, and practices that affect infants and toddlers with disabilities and their families. The range of EI services that support families through IDEA will also be presented. Additionally, we explore current content addressing the speech-language pathologist (SLP) scope of practice, roles, and responsibilities in EI; an introduction and overview of the American Speech-Language-Hearing Association (ASHA) guiding principles in providing EI services; EI-related Council of Academic Accreditation (CAA) standards and implementation procedures for the Certificate of Clinical Competence in Speech-Language Pathology; and the Division of Early Childhood (DEC) recommended practices in EI. Although we dive deeper into the empirical data in Chapter 3, this chapter wraps up with a presentation of the key theories and evidence-based practices we implement to effectively deliver EI services.

Why does it matter that we learn about the regulatory requirements, policies, principles, and evidence that supports our practice? Although the information in this chapter might be a bit dry, knowing the EI history and foundation for our practices provides us with the knowledge and evidence we need to be most effective with our families and ensures we are providing best practices to the precious children and families who believe in and trust us. Let's get started!

Introduction to Early Intervention

Early intervention refers to evidence-based, specialized services designed to meet the needs of families with infants and toddlers from birth to age 3 who have or could be at risk for developmental delays or disabilities. The primary goal of EI services is to lessen the effects of a disability or delay by addressing the identified needs of young children across five developmental areas: cognitive development, communication development, physical development (including vision, hearing, and sensory integration), social and emotional development, and adaptive development (IDEA, 2004). These services are designed to provide resources and support for the child and family to ensure that the child has every opportunity to develop and learn.

IDEA is a federally mandated system originally introduced in 1975 as Public Law 94-142 and known as the Education for All Handicapped Children Act. It was enacted to ensure equitable educational opportunities for children age 5 to 21. Over time, the system has been restructured and renamed to ensure services delivered to young children and their families are effective, engaging, and evidence based. In 1997, the Act was revised to include the Program for Infants and Toddlers with Disabilities, also called Part C, to serve children from birth to age 3 and their families. The most current act, the Individuals with Disabilities Education Improvement Act, was authorized in 2004 with additional IDEA Part C Final Regulations confirmed in 2011 (IDEA, 2011); all of these documents are referred to by the acronym *IDEA*. The 2004 and 2011 documents present and reflect empirically based EI policies and practices.

In 2007 and 2008, ASHA presented a series of documents intended to guide SLPs working in the EI arena, with a clear scope of practice and our roles and responsibilities (ASHA, 2007, 2008a, 2008b, 2008c). In 2008, ASHA also presented five guiding principles that reflect evidence-based best practices for SLPs and audiologists who are providing Part C EI services to young children and their families. These documents served as the foundation for practice in EI until recently, when ASHA rescinded them in lieu of the Early Intervention Practice Portal on the ASHA website. The scope of the Practice Portal page in EI is focused on the process as a holistic practice and gives us updated information, references, and resources (ASHA, 2023). Updates addressing ASHA's five EI principles, as well information for implementation and best practice, are now also available through the ASHA Early Intervention Practice Portal (ASHA, 2023).

Broadly speaking, EI services are specialized educational, health, and therapy-based services designed to meet the needs of infants and toddlers (and their families) from birth to age 3 who have or could be at risk for developmental delays or disabilities. EI services bring families and service providers from many aspects of the community together, including public and private agencies, childcare centers, local school districts, and private practitioners.

Supports and services are intended to work together to meet children's unique needs and those of their family in their natural environments. Depending on each child's needs, EI services can range from simple to complex. They may involve processes considered less complicated, such as prescribing glasses for a 2-year-old, to those significantly more complex, such as developing and implementing a multifaceted, comprehensive approach with a variety of services and team members. Depending on the child's needs, EI services can also include a variety of services. Table 1–1 illustrates a sample of the many services that may be provided to young children and their families in EI.

Table 1–1. Early Intervention Services Provided Under IDEA Part C Final Regulations

- Assistive technology devices and assistive technology services
- Counseling and home visits
- Early identification, screening, and assessment services
- Family training
- Health services necessary to enable the infant or toddler to benefit from the other early intervention services
- Medical services only for diagnostic or evaluation purposes
- Occupational therapy
- Physical therapy
- Psychological services
- Service coordination services
- Sign language and cued language services.
- Social work services
- Special instruction
- Speech-language pathology and audiology services
- Transportation and related costs that are necessary to enable an infant or toddler and the infant's or toddler's family to receive another service described in this paragraph
- Vision services

Note. From "Part C Final Regulations," by Individuals with Disabilities Education Improvement Act (2011; https://www.gpo.gov/fdsys/pkg/FR-2011-09-28/pdf/2011-22783.pdf).

Legislative History of Early Intervention

In 1964, the Mental Retardation Facilities and Community Mental Health Centers Construction Act of 1963 (Pub. L. 88-164) was enacted. According to Allen (1984), this legislative act was "the first major landmark for the participation of the federal government in service, training, and research activities focused specifically on mental retardation and related developmental problems" (p. 11). In 1968, the U.S. Congress created the Handicapped

Children's Early Education Program (HCEEP) under the Handicapped Children's Early Assistance Act (Pub. L. 91-230). The purpose of this act for the preschool-age child was to "demonstrate the feasibility of early education to the American public" (Ackerman & Moore, 1976, p. 669). Ackerman and Moore (1976) noted, "the act provided monies for demonstration programs, insisted that such programs be geographically dispersed, mandated the involvement of parents, and ordered dissemination of the results to the communities that surrounded the preschool programs" (p. 669).

Prior to 1975, however, approximately 1 million children with disabilities were granted only minimal education in separate facilities and institutions and continued to be denied pertinent services. Public Law 94-142, also known as the Education for All Handicapped Children Act (EHA; Pub. L. 94-142) was enacted in 1975, and the eventual impact was enormous. This act mandated a free appropriate public education (FAPE) for all children with disabilities from 5 to 21 years of age. The law provided states with incentives for serving preschool-age children, and it required that services be delivered in the least restrictive environment (LRE). During this time, the federal government also began offering a commitment to support the development of personnel preparation programs focused on young children with disabilities. EHA is considered by many to be the most significant act in the history of education with regard to children with disabilities.

In 1986, IDEA was passed, and the law was revised to create the Infant and Toddlers with Disabilities Program (Part H). This legislation provided new funding for children from birth through age 2 years with disabilities and created additional financial incentives for states to provide services once a child turns 3 years old. The 1986 amendment required participating states to develop statewide interagency infant and toddler programs for children with disabilities and their families. This amendment to the original EHA served the federal mandate for special education services in each state for children with disabilities from birth to 21 years of age. It outlined the system of funding employed for special education and related services. Provisions were put in place through Part H of IDEA that provide incentives to states to ensure children from birth to age 3 receive services. Congress established the Part H (EI) program of IDEA in recognition of an immediate need to:

- Augment the development of infants and toddlers with disabilities.
- Decrease costs by minimizing the need for special education through EI.
- Maximize independent living while minimizing the likelihood of institutionalization.
- Increase the capacity of families to meet their children's needs.

Individuals with Disabilities Education Act Part C

In 1997, IDEA (Pub. L. 105-17) was restructured and Part H became Part C—the Program for Infants and Toddlers with Disabilities. IDEA was modified once again in 2004 as the Individuals with Disabilities Education Improvement Act (IDEA, 2004). Federal Part C regulations now require that a statewide policy and system of EI services are in effect to ensure that appropriate EI services are available to all infants and toddlers with disabilities or significant developmental delays and their families. For a state to participate in the program, it must ensure that EI will be available to all eligible children and their families. Each state's governor must designate a lead agency to receive the funding and to administer the program. The governor must also appoint an Interagency Coordinating Council (ICC), including parents of young children with disabilities, to advise and assist the lead agency. Currently, all states and eligible territories are participating in the Part C program. Annual funding to each state is based on census figures for the number of children from birth to 3 years of age in the general population. Part C requires that states deliver services in natural environments. Under Section 303.26 of Part C, natural environments are defined as "settings that are natural or normal for the child's same age peers who have no disabilities" (IDEA, 2004). Additionally, EI services are determined based on individualized, functional outcomes developed in partnership with the family that reflect the children and family's strengths, priorities, and needs. These functional outcomes are developmental in nature, rather than medical, and focus on supporting the child's development and participation in family and community activities, as well as the family's needs and priorities. As providers, we base plans for service delivery in EI on the unique needs of each child and family and a focus on the coordination of capacity-building, developmental activities that promote the child's optimal development, in addition to the facilitation of the child's participation in family and community activities.

In 2011, the IDEA Part C Final Regulations (IDEA, 2011) were presented. The Final Regulations reflected changes made to the IDEA, as amended by the Individuals with Disabilities Education Improvement Act of 2004, and made other necessary changes needed to implement the EI Program for Infants and Toddlers with Disabilities. One of the most significant changes in these regulations supported states in using their discretion and extending eligibility for Part C services through age 5 to children with disabilities who are eligible for services under Part B, Section 619 (Preschool Grants), and who previously received services under Part C (ASHA, 2023).

Each state's Part C system presents a distinct funding structure. Part C programs coordinate EI funding through a combination of federal, state, local, and private sources. Annual federal funding to each Part C program varies, based on the census figures for the number of children between the ages of birth and 2 years in the general population in each state, and the majority of Part C funding tends to come from the state (ASHA, 2023; Hebbeler et al., 2009). Part C federal funds cover EI administrative costs, and services are supported by state funding, third-party payers (e.g., Medicaid and private insurance), and families who pay fees for services (Searcy, 2018; Vail et al., 2018). Evaluations, assessments, development of the Individualized Family Service Plan, and service coordination are provided at no cost to families (IDEA, 2004). Some programs also offer additional EI services on a sliding scale or free of charge, although specific policies vary from state to state. Some private insurance and Medicaid plans cover EI services. When a child is not eligible for EI services, or transitions out of a Part C program, families can choose to pay for services themselves or use their medical insurance to seek private services beyond what an EI program or school district offers (ASHA, n.d.; ASHA, 2023; Vail et al., 2018).

Scope of Practice in Speech-Language Pathology

The ASHA Scope of Practice in Speech-Language Pathology (2016b) includes a statement of purpose, definitions of the SLP and speech-language pathology, a framework for speech-language pathology practice, a description of the domains of speech-language pathology service delivery, delineation of speech-language pathology service delivery areas, domains of professional practice, references, and resources. According to ASHA (2016b), the SLP is defined as a professional who addresses the areas of communication and swallowing across the life span. These two terms, *communication* and *swallowing*, are broad and encompass many components within the SLP scope of practice. Communication includes speech production, fluency, language, cognition, voice, resonance, and hearing. Swallowing includes all aspects of swallowing as well as related feeding behaviors. This document is a guide for SLPs across all clinical and educational settings to promote best practices and it states that the practice of speech-language pathology includes the provision of EI services for infants and toddlers with communication needs.

According to the Scope of Practice (ASHA, 2016b), the overall objective of speech-language pathology services is to optimize our clients' abilities to communicate and to swallow to improve their quality of life, based on the best available evidence. The SLP scope of practice is comprised of five domains of professional practice and eight domains of service delivery. We provide services to individuals with a wide variety of speech, language, and swallowing differences and disorders that range in function from completely intact to completely compromised. The diagnostic categories in our scope of practice are consistent with relevant diagnostic categories under the World Health Organization's (WHO, 2014) ICF, the American Psychiatric Association's (2013) *Diagnostic and Statistical Manual of Mental Disorders*, the categories of disability under the IDEA of 2004, and those defined by two semiautonomous bodies of ASHA, including the Council on Academic Accreditation in Audiology and Speech-Language Pathology and the Council for Clinical Certification in Audiology and Speech-Language Pathology (ASHA, 2016b).

As SLPs, our professional practice domains include administration and leadership, advocacy and outreach, education, research, and supervision. The eight domains of speech-language pathology service delivery are assessment; collaboration; counseling; modalities, technology, and instrumentation; population and systems; prevention and wellness; screening; and treatment. Table 1–2 presents an overview of the roles and responsibilities of the SLP within each service delivery domain.

Table 1–2. Domains of Speech-Language Pathology Service Delivery

Assessment
• SLPs are experts in the differential diagnosis of communication, speech, language, feeding, and swallowing disorders. Based on the International Classification of Functioning, Disability, and Health, the SLP assessment process includes evaluation of body function, structure, activity, and participation within the context of environment and personal factors. The process also includes culturally and

linguistically appropriate behavioral observation and standardized and/or criterion-referenced tools; use of instrumentation; interview of the child and family; and review of records, case history, and prior test results. The assessment process in early intervention is typically conducted in collaboration with other service providers through an interprofessional team approach.

Collaboration
- Collaboration involves communication and shared decision-making among all members of a team, including the client and family members, to provide strong service delivery and functional outcomes. Collaboration occurs across all SLP practice domains.
- Within early intervention, SLPs collaborate with other professionals and service providers to assist with the development and implementation of individualized family service plans.

Counseling
- Counseling by the SLP involves educating, guiding, and supporting clients and their families throughout their early intervention journey. Counseling may address acceptance, adaptation, and decision-making about communication, feeding and swallowing, and/or related disorders. The SLP may need to focus on interactions with family members as they process emotional reactions, thoughts, feelings, and behaviors related to or in response to the child's communication, feeding and swallowing, and/or related disorders.

Modalities, technology, and instrumentation
- SLPs use advanced instrumentation and technologies to evaluate, provide intervention, and support the clients and their families in our care. We are also involved in the research and development of emerging technologies and apply our knowledge in using these technologies to provide and enhance the quality of the services we provide.

Population and systems
- In addition to direct services, SLPs engage in the management of populations to improve overall health and education as well as the experience of the children and families they serve; in some situations, we also have a role in reducing the cost of care by improving the efficiency and effectiveness of service delivery. We need to be aware of the changes, internal and external, to the work environment to be flexible and effective with our clients and their families. Our awareness carries over into multiple roles, including:
  - Using plain language to facilitate clear communication.
  - Collaborating with other professionals to improve communication with individuals who have communication challenges.
  - Reducing the cost of care by designing and implementing strategies that focus on function and outcomes through a combination of direct intervention, collaboration with other service providers, and education provided to the families to engage in strategies within their everyday activities and routines.

- Coaching families and other providers about strategies and supports that facilitate prelinguistic and linguistic communication skills of infants and toddlers.

Prevention and wellness
- Prevention and wellness activities are an integral domain of early intervention. These may include engagement that addresses the reduction of the incidence of a new disorder, the identification of disorders at an early age or stage, and the opportunity to decrease the severity or impact of a disability associated with an existing disorder or disease.

Screening
- SLPs are experts in the screening of individuals for possible communication, hearing, feeding, and swallowing disorders. In early intervention, SLPs are also trained to screen, monitor, and support young children's development in all development domains, as well as the needs and priorities of families. These screenings support holistic service delivery and facilitate referrals for appropriate follow-up in a cost-effective and timely manner for both the child and their family.

Treatment
- The ultimate goal of SLP intervention is to improve an individual's functional outcomes related to communication, speech, language, feeding, and swallowing. Early intervention includes the outcomes of the family unit. SLPs collaborate with other service providers and family members to establish treatment outcomes and design, implement, and document the delivery of services based on best available practices. We provide culturally and linguistically appropriate services; deliver the appropriate frequency and intensity of treatment based on evidence-based practices; engage in treatment activities that are within the scope of our professional competence; and use performance data to guide clinical decisions and determine the effectiveness of treatment.

Note. Adapted from the "Scope of practice in speech-language pathology" by the American Speech-Language and Hearing Association, 2016 (www.asha.org/policy/).

Clinical Competence Standards for Speech-Language Pathologists

The Council for Clinical Certification in Audiology and Speech-Language Pathology (CFCC) is the semiautonomous credentialing body of ASHA that defines the standards for clinical certification in speech-language pathology and audiology, determines the application of these standards in granting certification to individuals, has the authority to withdraw an individual's certification, and administers the certification maintenance program. The CFCC frequently surveys and analyzes evidence-based practices and current services in the field of speech-language pathology and updates the standards and implementation procedures as needed. The most recent Standards and Implementation Procedures for the Certificate of Clinical Competence, developed to fit current practice models better, were implemented in 2020. They include revisions that were approved in January 2023. These standards relate directly to our roles and responsibilities in the EI arena (CFCC, 2018, 2023).

In addition to the certification standards, each state has the right to establish additional requirements that we must follow to work in the EI setting. ASHA maintains a comprehensive state-by-state website with information collected from state licensure boards and regulatory agencies responsible for developing these requirements.

Roles and Responsibilities of Speech-Language Pathologists in Early Intervention

Once we have demonstrated we are prepared to practice, based on the Standards and Implementation Procedures for the Certificate of Clinical Competence, we are qualified to administer direct services to families and young children who demonstrate or are at risk of developing disabilities or delays in the areas of communication, speech, language, cognition, emergent literacy, and feeding and swallowing difficulties (ASHA, 2016b). As SLPs in EI, our roles are vast and include a wide range of responsibilities. According to ASHA (2008b, 2023), we are expected to engage in the following roles when serving young children and their families:

- Serve as an expert regarding norms and expectations of children between birth to 5 years across all developmental domains; policies and procedures related to screening, evaluating, and assessing infants and toddlers with, or at risk for disabilities at the federal, state, agency, and professional levels; and current evidence-based practice in early intervention.

- Participate in ongoing continuing education and professional development related to the nature, assessment, and treatment of speech, language, communication, cognition, and swallowing development and disorders in infants and young children.

- Conduct prevention, early identification, screening, evaluation, and assessment practices to identify infants and toddlers with, or who could be at risk for, a delay or disorder.

- Establish eligibility for services and develop an Individualized Family Service Plan for the implementation of services and supports based on evidence-based SLP approaches and practices.

- Maintain and report documentation regarding treatment outcomes and progress; use data to support changes in and transitions to services; as needed and per eligibility requirements, revise intervention plans and determine appropriate discharge criteria.

- Collaborate with other service providers and related disciplines to ensure appropriate service delivery is provided to each child and family; consult with and refer to team members and colleagues in other disciplines, as and when appropriate.

- Implement inclusive practices with and support families based on their cultural beliefs, values, and priorities.

- Participate in transition planning to ensure seamless transition and timely access to services for families moving from one program to another.

- Raise awareness and serve as an advocate for the profession of speech-language pathology in EI through activities that support public policy, funding, and infrastructure.

In addition to those responsibilities focused on direct care of families and young children, we engage in additional roles to provide effective support in EI (ASHA, 2016b). These roles address the needs and experience of the individuals served, and, in some circumstances, may address how we work with families to reduce the cost of care. We also engage in improving the efficiency and effectiveness of service delivery in natural settings beyond the home environment. According to the ASHA (2016b) Scope of Practice in Speech-Language Pathology, we, as SLPs, need to engage in the following practices:

- Facilitate clear communication by using family-friendly language.
- Coach families and EI providers about strategies and supports that facilitate the development of prelinguistic and linguistic communication skills of infants and toddlers.
- Decrease the cost of EI services by designing and implementing strategies that are functional and by helping young children and families reach their goals through direct intervention, supervision of and collaboration with other service providers, and engagement of the child and family within natural, everyday activities and routines.
- Support and collaborate with classroom teachers, for those children engaged in childcare, to implement strategies for supporting communication and using appropriate, engaging strategies.

Within our practice, we must also consider the ASHA Code of Ethics (ASHA, 2016a), which states SLPs must only participate in roles within the professional scopes of practice. EI SLPs must demonstrate documented high levels of competence evidenced by level of education, discipline-specific training, and experience. Additionally, our roles and responsibilities in EI are guided by both state licensure regulations and service delivery models as implemented by local agencies.

The American Speech-Language and Hearing Association Guiding Principles of Early Intervention

In 2007 and 2008, ASHA presented a series of documents intended to guide SLPs working in the EI arena, with a clear scope of practice and our roles and responsibilities (ASHA, 2007, 2008a, 2008b, 2008c). In 2008, ASHA also presented five guiding principles that reflect evidence-based best practices for SLPs and audiologists who are providing Part C EI services to young children and their families. These documents served as the foundation for practice in EI until recently, when ASHA rescinded them in lieu of the Early Intervention Practice Portal on the ASHA website. The scope of the Practice Portal page in EI is focused on the process as a holistic practice and gives us updated information, references, and resources (ASHA, 2023). Updates addressing ASHA's five EI principles, as well information for implementation and best practices, are now also available through the ASHA Early

Intervention Practice Portal (ASHA, 2023). Providing us with a guide for implementation of practice in EI, these principles are as follows:

- Services are family centered. Families are presented with every opportunity to be involved in all aspects of a child's EI services. It is not just the individual child, but the family as a whole, who receives services based on their capacity and that builds on their strengths (Crawford & Weber, 2014; DEC, 2014; Dunst, 2002, 2017; Dunst & Trivette, 2007; McWilliam, 2010a; National Resource Center for Family Centered Practice [NRCFCP], 2023; Ross, 2018).

- Services are culturally and linguistically responsive. Families of young children with disabilities must have access to culturally responsive services and EI services presented in the language(s) most likely to result in an accurate picture of the child's skills (IDEA, 2011). SLPs providing EI services must work with families and caregivers to ensure they are able to implement strategies in their home language (Peredo, 2016).

- Services are developmentally supportive and engage children in their natural environments. SLPs provide these services by engaging in authentic experiences, active exploration, and interactions consistent with a child's age, cognitive and communication skills, strengths, and interests to address the family's routines, concerns, and priorities (DEC, 2014).

- Services are comprehensive, coordinated, and team-based. To ensure the SLP and other providers are maximizing service delivery and family and child outcomes, we are all expected to consult and communicate with one another and coordinate our approaches and services. All members of the team must work together to recognize shared competencies across disciplines and ensure evidence-based interventions complement one another (Early Childhood Personnel Center, 2017).

- Services are based on the integration of the most recent and highest quality research, informed professional judgment and expertise, and the preferences and values of the family.

Additional details and discussion regarding each of these principles, as well as the evidence that supports implementing each within our practice, are presented in detail in Chapter 2.

Division for Early Childhood Recommended Practices in Early Intervention

In addition to ASHA, the DEC of the Council for Exceptional Children developed a set of recommended practices that address best practices for all EI service providers (DEC, 2014). The Recommended Practices in EI/Early Childhood Special Education are based on the DEC's belief that when providers and families have the knowledge, skills, and disposition to implement these practices, young children who have or are at risk for developmental delays and disabilities and their families are more likely to achieve positive outcomes. Additionally, families and practitioners are more likely to help children achieve their highest potential. They were developed to guide providers and families regarding the most effective ways to address learning outcomes and promote the development of young children, birth through 5 years of age, who have or are at risk for developmental delays and disabilities. The document was created to help bridge the gap between research and implementation by highlighting the best available empirical evidence and evidence-based practice in the EI and early childhood arenas. The DEC Recommended Practices support access and participation by children in inclusive settings and natural environments, address diversity of culture, language, and ability, and offer guidance for providers in the areas of leadership, assessment, environment, family, instruction, interaction, teaming and collaboration, and transition (DEC, 2014). Table 1–3 presents additional details about each of these areas and the recommended practices that support each on

Table 1–3. DEC Recommended Practices in Early Intervention

Leadership	• Leaders create a culture and a climate in which practitioners feel a sense of belonging and want to support the organization's mission and goals. • Leaders promote adherence to and model the DEC Code of Ethics, DEC Position Statements and Papers, and the DEC Recommended Practices. • Leaders develop and implement policies, structures, and practices that promote shared decision-making with practitioners and families. • Leaders belong to a professional association(s) and engage in ongoing evidence-based professional development. • Leaders advocate for policies and resources that promote the implementation of the DEC Position Statements and Papers and the DEC Recommended Practices. • Leaders establish partnerships across levels (state to local) and with their counterparts in other systems and agencies to create coordinated and inclusive systems of services and supports. • Leaders develop, refine, and implement policies and procedures that create the conditions for practitioners to implement the DEC Recommended Practices. • Leaders work across levels and sectors to secure fiscal and human resources and maximize the use of these resources to successfully implement the DEC Recommended Practices. • Leaders develop and implement an evidence-based professional development system or approach that provides practitioners with a variety of supports to ensure they have the knowledge and skills needed to implement the DEC Recommended Practices.

	- Leaders ensure practitioners know and follow professional standards and all applicable laws and regulations governing service provision.
- Leaders collaborate with higher education, state licensing and certification agencies, practitioners, professional associations, and other stakeholders to develop or revise state competencies that align with DEC, the Council for Exceptional Children (CEC), and other national professional standards.
- Leaders collaborate with stakeholders to collect and use data for program management and continuous program improvement and to examine the effectiveness of services and supports in improving child and family outcomes.
- Leaders promote efficient and coordinated service delivery for children and families by creating conditions for practitioners from multiple disciplines and the family to work together as a team.
- Leaders collaborate with other agencies and programs to develop and implement ongoing community-wide screening procedures to identify and refer children who may need additional evaluation and services.
Assessment	- Practitioners work with the family to identify family preferences for assessment processes.
- Practitioners work as a team with the family and other professionals to gather assessment information.
- Practitioners use assessment materials and strategies that are appropriate for the child's age and level of development and accommodate the child's sensory, physical, communication, cultural, linguistic, social, and emotional characteristics.
- Practitioners conduct assessments that include all areas of development and behavior to learn about the child's strengths, needs, preferences, and interests.
- Practitioners conduct assessments in the child's dominant language and in additional languages if the child is learning more than one language.
- Practitioners use a variety of methods, including observation and interviews, to gather assessment information from multiple sources, including the child's family and other significant individuals in the child's life.
- Practitioners obtain information about the child's skills in daily activities, routines, and environments such as home, center, and community. Practitioners use clinical reasoning in addition to assessment results to identify the child's current levels of

	functioning and to determine the child's eligibility and plan for instruction. • Practitioners must implement a systematic, ongoing assessment to identify learning targets, plan activities, and monitor the child's progress to revise instruction as needed. • Practitioners use assessment tools with sufficient sensitivity to detect child progress, especially for the child with significant support needs. • Practitioners report assessment results so that they are understandable and useful to families.
Environment	• Practitioners provide services and supports in natural and inclusive environments during daily routines and activities to promote the child's access to and participation in learning experiences. • Practitioners consider Universal Design for Learning principles to create accessible environments. • Practitioners work with the family and other adults to modify and adapt the physical, social, and temporal environments to promote each child's access to and participation in learning experiences. • Practitioners work with families and other adults to identify each child's needs for assistive technology to promote access to and participation in learning experiences. • Practitioners work with families and other adults to acquire or create appropriate assistive technology to promote each child's access to and participation in learning experiences. • Practitioners create environments that provide opportunities for movement and regular physical activity to maintain or improve fitness, wellness, and development across domains.
Family	• Practitioners build trusting and respectful partnerships with the family through interactions that are sensitive and responsive to cultural, linguistic, and socioeconomic diversity. • Practitioners provide the family with up-to-date, comprehensive, and unbiased information in a way that the family can understand and use to make informed choices and decisions. • Practitioners are responsive to the family's concerns, priorities, and changing life circumstances. • Practitioners and the family work together to create outcomes or goals, develop individualized plans, and implement practices that address the family's priorities and concerns and the child's strengths and needs. Practitioners support family functioning, promote family confidence and competence, and strengthen

	family–child relationships by acting in ways that recognize and build on family strengths and capacities. • Practitioners engage the family in opportunities that support and strengthen parenting knowledge and skills and parenting competence and confidence in ways that are flexible, individualized, and tailored to the family's preferences. • Practitioners work with the family to identify, access, and use formal and informal resources and supports to achieve family-identified outcomes or goals. • Practitioners provide the family of a young child who has or is at risk for developmental delay or disability and is a dual-language learner with information about the benefits of learning in multiple languages for the child's growth and development. • Practitioners help families know and understand their rights. • Practitioners inform families about leadership and advocacy skill-building opportunities and encourage those interested in participating.
Instruction	• Practitioners, with the family, identify each child's strengths, preferences, and interests to engage the child in active learning. • Practitioners, with the family, identify skills to target for instruction that help a child become adaptive, competent, socially connected, and engaged and that promote learning in natural and inclusive environments. • Practitioners gather and use data to inform decisions about individualized instruction. • Practitioners plan for and provide the level of support, accommodations, and adaptations needed for the child to access, participate, and learn within and across activities and routines. • Practitioners embed instruction within and across routines, activities, and environments to provide contextually relevant learning opportunities. • Practitioners use systematic instructional strategies with fidelity to teach skills and to promote child engagement and learning. • Practitioners use explicit feedback and consequences to increase child engagement, play, and skills. • Practitioners use peer-mediated intervention to teach skills and to promote child engagement and learning. • Practitioners use functional assessment and related prevention, promotion, and intervention strategies across environments to prevent and address challenging behavior. • Practitioners implement the frequency, intensity, and duration of instruction needed to address the child's phase and pace of

	learning or the level of support needed by the family to achieve the child's outcomes or goals. • Practitioners provide instructional support for young children with disabilities who are dual-language learners to assist them in learning English and in continuing to develop skills through the use of their home language. • Practitioners use and adapt specific instructional strategies effective for dual-language learners when teaching English to children with disabilities. • Practitioners use coaching or consultation strategies with primary caregivers or other adults to facilitate positive adult–child interactions and instruction intentionally designed to promote child learning and development.
Interaction	• Practitioners promote the child's social-emotional development by observing, interpreting, and responding contingently to the range of the child's emotional expressions. • Practitioners promote the child's social development by encouraging the child to initiate or sustain positive interactions with other children and adults during routines and activities through modeling, teaching, feedback, or other types of guided support. • Practitioners promote the child's communication development by observing, interpreting, responding contingently, providing natural consequences for the child's verbal and nonverbal communication and using language to label and expand on the child's requests, needs, preferences, or interests. Practitioners promote the child's cognitive development by observing, interpreting, and responding intentionally to the child's exploration, play, and social activity by joining in and expanding on the child's focus, actions, and intent. • Practitioners promote the child's problem-solving behavior by observing, interpreting, and scaffolding in response to the child's growing level of autonomy and self-regulation.
Teaming and collaboration	• Practitioners representing multiple disciplines and families work together as a team to plan and implement supports and services to meet the unique needs of each child and family. • Practitioners and families work together as a team to systematically and regularly exchange expertise, knowledge, and information to build team capacity and jointly solve problems, plan, and implement interventions.

	• Practitioners use communication and group facilitation strategies to enhance team functioning and interpersonal relationships with and among team members. • Team members assist each other to discover and access community-based services and other informal and formal resources to meet family-identified child or family needs. • Practitioners and families may collaborate with each other to identify one practitioner from the team who serves as the primary liaison between the family and other team members based on child and family priorities and needs.
Transition	• Practitioners in sending and receiving programs exchange information before, during, and after transition about practices most likely to support the child's successful adjustment and positive outcomes. • Practitioners use a variety of planned and timely strategies with the child and family before, during, and after the transition to support successful adjustment and positive outcomes for both the child and family.

Note. From the "DEC recommended practices in early intervention/early childhood special education 2014," by the Division for Early Childhood, 2014 (http://www.dec-sped.org/recommendedpractices). Printed with permission.

Introduction to the Evidence Supporting Early Intervention

We are now aware that Part C services under IDEA are intended to enhance the development of infants and toddlers with disabilities, to minimize potential developmental delay, and to reduce educational costs to society by minimizing the need for continuing special education services as children with disabilities reach school age (IDEA, 2004, §1400[20]). As SLPs, we strive to provide the most effective services to the infants, toddlers, and families with whom we work. To ensure this is the case, we must use methods that have been demonstrated to be effective through scientific evidence, clinical experience, and client needs. The combination of these variables gives us the evidence on which we base our practices. There are several areas of practice that have been the focus of empirical research and support the foundations, practices, and approaches currently used in EI. These practices are based on the integration of current high-quality research, informed professional expertise and perspective, and family preferences and values (DEC, 2014). The foundation of support for practice includes both internal and external evidence. Internal evidence is based on policy, informed clinical opinion, values and perspectives of professionals and consumers, and professional consensus; external evidence is drawn from empirical research published in peer-reviewed journals. All of these considerations are evaluated in the delivery of EI services to realize positive outcomes for infants, toddlers, and their families (DEC, 2014). Although we will explore the current research thoroughly in Chapter 3, the following sections provide an overview of the most widely accepted evidence-based practices implemented in EI today.

The Earlier Served, the Better

Children grow and develop differently and at their own pace. Decades of research support the fact that the period from birth to age 3 is a critical time in a child's development and an important time for parents to have access to accurate information and consistent support (Center on the Developing Child at Harvard University [CDCHU], 2008, 2010). Research has shown that a child's earliest experiences play a critical role in brain development. It is, therefore, crucial that services are provided during these early years (CDCHU, 2008). According to the CDCHU (2008, 2010), neural circuits, including those that create the foundation for learning, behavior, and health, are the most flexible during the first 3 years of life. Findings also indicate that early social and emotional development and physical health support the foundation for both cognitive and language skills to develop. Positive early experiences that involve stable relationships with responsive adults within safe and supportive environments and appropriate nutritional opportunities are all key elements of healthy brain development (CDCHU, 2010). According to Guralnick (2011), the earlier we intervene with supports and services (e.g., swallowing and feeding consultations with a newborn in the neonatal intensive care unit; as the family transitions from the medical center to home with a medically fragile infant; addressing prelinguistic skills with an infant with Down syndrome), the more likely children who have disabilities or developmental delays are to achieve successful learning outcomes related to the development of effective communication, language, and swallowing skills. EI services have been shown to positively influence outcomes across developmental domains, including health, language and communication, cognition, and social and emotional well-being of infants and toddlers who have disabilities or are at risk for developmental delays (ASHA, 2008b; Branson & Demchak, 2009; CDCHU, 2010; Guralnick, 2011; Hebbeler et al., 2007; Joint Committee on Infant Hearing, 2007; Landa et al., 2011).

Natural Environments

As presented earlier, IDEA (2004, 2011) states that services for infants and toddlers are to be implemented "to the maximum extent possible, in the *natural environments* including home and community settings in which children without disabilities participate." Natural environments, however, are not just places; they are also those places where children and their families spend a typical day. They include those locations where all young children, regardless of ability, spend their time. For most families, natural environments include the family home and day care, but they might also include a family member's house, a park, the library, a grocery store, a restaurant, or even a favorite place in the backyard. Clinical settings are not a natural part of a child's day. The evidence-based literature demonstrates that natural environments offer the best opportunities for EI activities and promote inclusion in both family and community activities. Our goal, as SLPs in EI, is to help families support their children's development within their natural environments and through their everyday routines and activities. The research indicates young children learn best, and tend to generalize the skills they acquire, when they are engaged in everyday, natural learning opportunities in familiar places and with familiar people (Chiarello, 2017; Dunst et al., 2006; Hwang et al., 2013; Rush & Shelden, 2020; Trivette et al., 2004).

Family-Centered Practices

ASHA's (2008a) first guiding principle that reflects current best practices in EI addresses the delivery of *family-centered services*. This practice involves working collaboratively with families in all aspects of EI and is based on a strong foundation of research. A family-centered approach recognizes the importance of all family members and involves the awareness and inclusion of the beliefs, values, principles, and practices that strengthen the family's capacity to enhance their child's development and learning (IDEA, 2004).

Effective family-centered practices are responsive to the unique circumstances of each family and ensure families are presented with unbiased and comprehensive information with which to make informed decisions (DEC, 2014). Family-centered practice refers to a way of working with families across service systems to build their capacity to care for and optimize their child's development. The approach focuses on the important influence of the family on the child's development and acknowledges the impact that only families can have on their child's outcomes. When family-centered practices are used, we build on the strengths of the family, meet the family's changing needs, collaborate with the family, and support the family's ability to build partnerships with other people and organizations (Crawford & Weber, 2014; Rush & Shelden, 2020). According to the NRCFCP (2023), family-centered practice is based on the belief that the best way to meet a child's needs is within their families and to engage in services that involve, strengthen, and support families; the empirical research supports this belief (Bernheimer & Weisner, 2007; Cole et al., 2019; Crawford & Weber, 2014; Heidlage et al., 2019; McWilliam, 2010a, 2010b; Raver & Childress, 2015; Roberts & Kaiser, 2011, 2015; Rush & Shelden, 2011, 2020; Stredler-Brown, 2017).

Routines-Based Intervention

As we have learned, best practice in EI focuses on the delivery of family-centered services (ASHA, 2008a). This practice involves working collaboratively with families in all aspects of EI and recognizes the importance of awareness and inclusion of the beliefs, values, principles, and practices that strengthen the family's capacity to enhance their child's development and learning (IDEA, 2004). *Routines-based intervention* (RBI) is an approach that builds the capacity of the family to address the child's strengths and needs by embedding instruction within the context of a family's everyday activities and routines (McWilliam, 2010b). According to McWilliam (2010b), daily routines are defined as "naturally occurring activities happening with some regularity, including caregiving events and simply hanging-out times" (p. 69). When we practice RBI and collaborate with other providers, family members, caregivers, and teachers, we develop child-specific strategies practiced within the family's natural environment (McWilliam, 2010a, 2010b; Raver & Childress, 2015). According to Bernheimer and Weisner (2007), "no intervention, no matter how well designed or implemented, will have an impact if it cannot find a slot in the daily routines of an organization, family, or individual" (p. 199).

The research is clear that children learn and develop best when they participate in natural learning opportunities that occur in everyday routines and activities within the lives of their family and/or community (Bernheimer & Weisner, 2007; Crawford & Weber, 2014; McWilliam, 2010a, 2010b; Rush & Shelden, 2020). Embedding skills and implementing strategies within everyday activities and daily routines helps parents and caregivers equip their children with support that encourages development, increases children's participation in activities with their families, and supports carryover of skills when we are not there (Crawford & Weber, 2014). Learning occurs between intervention visits, through play initiated by the child during everyday routines and activities, with multiple repetitions, and lots of practice. Children are more likely to master functional skills that occur through high-frequency activities embedded in their own routines (Bernheimer & Weisner, 2007; Crawford & Weber, 2014; Dunst et al., 2012; McWilliam, 2010a, 2010b; Rush & Shelden, 2020).

Strengths-Based Practices

Young children learn in different ways, and identifying family strengths is integral to the implementation of effective EI practices. Considering this, we need to furnish opportunities for children and their families to engage in meaningful and varied learning experiences to ensure infants and toddlers can show us what they know. A *strengths-based approach* in EI focuses on identifying what works for the child instead of focusing on what is "wrong" with the child and on their deficits. A strengths-based approach to EI, therefore, focuses on identifying what works for the infant or toddler, and their parents or caregivers, rather than on the child's delays or deficits (Fenton et al., 2015).

Research has shown that affirming family strengths increases parents' sense of confidence and competence (Dunst, 2020; Fox et al., 2015; Schertz & Horn, 2017; Trivette et al., 2010). Positive self-efficacy, in turn, has been found to correlate to child learning outcomes and parent–child interaction (Albanese et al., 2019; Boyce et al., 2017; Dunst, 2020; Dunst et al., 2012; Mas et al., 2019). Due to their child's unique learning needs, families in EI might feel less confident and competent in promoting their child's development (Innocenti et al., 2013). Using existing family strengths ensures strategies are embedded in the family's way of life, perspectives, and beliefs. The foundation of the strengths-based approach to practice in EI also supports the acknowledgment of the family's language(s) and culture(s) as positive contributors to a child's development. Particularly because of our unique role in addressing a child's communication and language development, this practice also encourages us to view multilingualism as an asset and to support children in maintaining their first language while learning English as a second or additional language (Fenton et al., 2015).

Practice-Based Coaching

Practice-based coaching is a well-established, evidence-based approach used in EI to build the capacities of the families with whom we work by supporting them to learn, develop, and use knowledge and skills to enhance their child's development in a wide range of areas. Rush and Shelden (2020) defined practice-based coaching as an "adult learning strategy used to support the [parent or caregiver] in identifying, obtaining, and mobilizing the knowledge and skills necessary to achieve an intended outcome" (p. 13). As effective EI providers, we empower families when we coach the caregivers to support their children in their natural environments (Hanft et al., 2004; Rush & Shelden, 2020). Following the first guiding practice of family-centered services in EI (ASHA, 2008a), we support families during visits by joining the family in their routines and activities and coaching caregivers as they practice using intervention strategies with their children (Rush & Shelden, 2020). A key to the practice of coaching with families in EI is the belief that all families are both competent and capable of supporting their children.

Rush and Shelden (2011, 2020) contributed empirical data to support five key practices in providing effective practice-based coaching with families: joint planning, observation, action/practice, reflection, and feedback. The research indicates that, when used in combination, these practices result in positive outcomes between families and their children's development and generalization of knowledge and skills (Rush & Shelden, 2020). The Teach-Model-Coach-Review (TMCR) approach (Roberts et al., 2019) is a second evidence-based coaching practice that incorporates coaching to teach families and caregivers support strategies, particularly within the context of play, to facilitate and expand their children's language skills (Roberts & Kaiser, 2015; Roberts et al., 2019). This approach is rooted in adult learning principles and incorporates the five key strategies of the coaching model presented by Rush and Shelden (2011, 2020).

Primary Service Provider Approach

We know effective EI is maintained when a team of providers and the family work collaboratively to support the needs of the child and family. The *transdisciplinary team model*, in which a group of professionals work in a collaborative model to share the responsibilities of evaluating, planning for, and implementing EI services for infants and toddlers, is widely accepted as a best practice in EI (ASHA, 2008a). The *primary service provider* (PSP) approach to teaming is considered an advancement of the transdisciplinary teaching model and has become common practice in EI within the last decade (Lineberger, 2022). This evidence-based approach is defined as a process for supporting families of young children engaged in EI services, in which one provider, often the SLP, is identified as the PSP for each family. The PSP then receives support from other team members through consulting and coaching of strategies to specifically include during dynamic assessment and intervention with the child to promote and address a range of child and family priorities (Shelden & Rush, 2022).

When a PSP approach is implemented according to the evidence-based guidelines, their impact is intended to increase the capacity of caregivers and providers. The research indicates the inclusion of PSP teams promotes increased family and caregiver participation and control of the EI process, also resulting in an increase in competence and confidence of the provider members of the team when supporting children, families, and caregivers during daily routines and activities (Bell et al., 2010; Boyer & Thompson, 2014; Moore et al., 2012; Rausch et al., 2021; Shelden & Rush, 2022; Yang et al., 2013).

Collaborative Practice

Regardless of the approach we take, best practices in EI include coordinated intervention through collaborative practice among and between the service providers and family. To effectively support the family within the child's natural environment and to support the child's relationship with the family, teamwork is essential. The most current and collaborative approach in EI, and a combination of the layers of teamwork as presented thus far, is *interprofessional education (IPE) and interprofessional collaborative practice (IPP)*. Consistent with the WHO definitions, ASHA defines IPE as an "activity that occurs when two or more professions learn about, from, and with each other to enable effective collaboration and improve outcomes for individuals and families we serve" (ASHA, 2023). ASHA defines IPP as service that occurs when multiple providers from different professional backgrounds administer comprehensive health care or educational services by "working with individuals and their families, caregivers, and communities to deliver the highest quality of care across settings" (ASHA, 2023).

IPP is the recommended approach in EI to ensure providers are working in a coordinated effort and families are actively engaged (ASHA, 2023; Coufal & Woods, 2018). As an interdisciplinary field with a history of collaborative teamwork, EI outcomes are often attributed to IPP. We need to engage with other service providers and family members within the EI system through interprofessional collaboration to ensure effective and meaningful service delivery. As members of interprofessional teams, our contributions might vary depending on the knowledge and skills we possess, as well as those represented by other service providers and professionals on the team. The Interprofessional Education Collaborative (2016) presented guiding principles and core competencies that intersect with the collaborative team approach required within EI services to implement the highest quality of services. The Interprofessional Education Collaborative core competencies define the goals and outcomes for both preprofessional preparation and professional practice across disciplines. To ensure effective services in EI, we must embrace and demonstrate services defined and delivered by the framework of these competencies (Bell et al., 2010; Boyer & Thompson, 2014; Hong & Reynolds-Keefer, 2013; Moore et al., 2012; Shelden & Rush, 2022).

Summary

EI is a federally mandated system that operates under Part C of IDEA. The system, which has been restructured multiple times since its inception in 1997, authorizes services to meet the needs of infants and toddlers, and their families, from birth to age 3 who have been or could be at risk for developmental delays or disabilities. In addition to the history and evolution of, as well as range of services supported within IDEA Part C, we explored our SLP scope of practice and the EI-related CAA standards and implementation procedures in which we must engage to earn and maintain the Certificate of Clinical Competence in Speech-Language Pathology. The roles and responsibilities in which we engage, as SLPs, are often integral to the successful outcomes of infants, toddlers, and their families who receive EI services. Therefore, we examined an introduction to and overview of the ASHA guiding principles in providing EI services and DEC recommended practices in EI. Although we will dive deeper into the empirical evidence supporting EI in Chapter 3, we also introduced an overview of the primary approaches we implement to effectively serve children and families in EI.

Critical Thinking Questions

1. Why is the history of legislative support for the birth–age 3 population important for us to know when providing these services to young children and their families?

2. Provide an outline of the current Individuals with Disabilities Education Act (IDEA) regulatory requirements focused on EI policies, procedures, and practices.

3. How might you describe the range of services presented under IDEA Part C to parents and caregivers who are just getting involved in the EI system?

4. Provide an overview of the speech-language pathologist (SLP) scope of practice, roles, and responsibilities in EI.

5. Name the American Speech-Language-Hearing Association (ASHA) guiding principles for providing EI services.

6. What are the Recommended Practices in Early Intervention as developed by the Division of Early Childhood (DEC) of The Council for Exceptional Children? Why is it important we understand and consider these practices when discussing our roles and responsibilities in EI with our colleagues and the families we serve?

References

Ackerman, P., & Moore, M. (1976). Delivery of educational services to preschool handicapped children. In T. D. Tjossem (Ed.), *Intervention strategies for high risk infants and young children* (pp. 669–688). University Park Press.

Albanese, A. M., Russo, G. R., & Geller, P. A. (2019). The role of parental self-efficacy in parent and child well-being: A systematic review of associated outcomes. *Child Care, Health and Development, 45*(3), 333–363. https://doi.org/10.1111/cch.12661

Allen, K. E. (1984). Federal legislation and young handicapped children. *Topics in Early Childhood Special Education, 4*(1), 9–18.

American Speech-Language-Hearing Association. (2007). *ASHA SLP health care survey 2007: Caseload characteristics.* https://www.asha.org/uploadedFiles/research/memberdata/HC07CaseloadRprt.pdf

American Speech-Language-Hearing Association. (2008a). *Core knowledge and skills in early intervention speech-language pathology practice.* https://doi.org/10.1044/policy.KS2008-00292

American Speech-Language-Hearing Association. (2008b). *Roles and responsibilities of speech-language pathologists in early intervention: Guidelines.* https://doi.org/10.1044/policy.GL2008-00293

American Speech-Language-Hearing Association. (2008c). *Roles and responsibilities of speech-language pathologists in early intervention: Technical report.*

https://doi.org/10.1044/policy.TR2008-00290

American Speech-Language-Hearing Association. (2016a). *Code of ethics*. https://www.asha.org/policy/et2016-00342/

American Speech-Language-Hearing Association. (2016b). *Scope of practice in speech-language pathology*. https://www.asha.org/policy/sp2016-00343/

American Speech-Language-Hearing Association. (2023). *Early intervention* [Practice portal]. https://www.asha.org/practice-portal/professional-issues/early-intervention/

American Speech-Language-Hearing Association. (n.d.). *State-by-state*. https://www.asha.org/advocacy/state/

Bell, A., Corfield, M., Davies, J., & Richardson, N. (2010). Collaborative transdisciplinary intervention in early years—Putting theory into practice. *Child: Care, Health and Development, 36*(1), 142–148. https://doi.org/10.1111/j.1365-2214.2009.01027.x

Bernheimer, L. B., & Weisner, T. S. (2007). "Let me just tell you what I do all day" … The family story at the center of intervention research and practice. *Infants and Young Children, 20*(3), 192–201.

Boyce, L. K., Seedall, R. B., Innocenti, M. S., Roggman, L. A., Cook, G. A., Hagman, A. M., & Jump Norma, V. K. (2017). Influence of a parent-child interaction focused bookmaking approach on maternal parenting self-efficacy. *Infants and Young Children, 30*(1), 76-93. https://doi.org/10.1097

Boyer, V. E., & Thompson, S. D. (2014). Transdisciplinary model and early intervention: Building collaborative relationships. *Young Exceptional Children, 17*(3), 19–32. https://doi.org/10.1177%2F1096250613493446

Branson, D., & Demchak, M. (2009). The use of augmentative and alternative communication methods with infants and toddlers with disabilities: A research review. *Augmentative & Alternative Communication, 25*, 274–286.

Center on the Developing Child at Harvard University. (2008). *In brief: The science of early childhood development*. https://harvardcenter.wpenginepowered.com/wp-content/uploads/2007/03/InBrief-The-Science-of-Early-Childhood-Development2.pdf

Center on the Developing Child at Harvard University. (2010). *The foundations of lifelong health are built in early childhood*. https://developingchild.harvard.edu/wp-content/uploads/2010/05/Foundations-of-Lifelong-Health.pdf

Chiarello, L. A. (2017). Excellence in promoting participation: Striving for the 10 Cs—Client-centered care, consideration of complexity, collaboration, coaching, capacity building, contextualization, creativity, community, curricular changes, and curiosity. *Pediatric Physical Therapy, 29*(3), 16–22.

Cole, B., Pickard, K., & Stredler-Brown, A. (2019). Report on the use of telehealth in early intervention in Colorado: Strengths and challenges with telehealth as a service delivery model. *International Journal of Telerehabilitation, 11*(1), 33–40. https://doi.org/10.5195/ijt.2019.6273

Coufal, K., & Woods, J. (2018). Interprofessional collaborative practice in early intervention. *Pediatric Clinics of North America, 65*, 143–155. https://doi.org/10.1016/j.pcl.2017.08.027

Council for Clinical Certification in Audiology and Speech-Language Pathology of the American Speech-Language-Hearing Association. (2023). *2023 standards revisions.* https://caa.asha.org/reporting/standards/2023-standards-revisions/

Council for Clinical Certification in Audiology and Speech-Language Pathology of the American Speech-Language-Hearing Association. (2018). *2020 standards for the certificate of clinical competence in speech-language pathology.* https://www.asha.org/certification/2020-slp-certification-standards/

Crawford, M. J., & Weber, B. (2014). *Early intervention every day! Embedding activities in daily routines for young children and their families.* Brookes.

Division for Early Childhood. (2014). *DEC recommended practices in early intervention/early childhood special education 2014.* http://www.dec-sped.org/recommendedpractices

Dunst, C. J. (2002). Family-centered practices: Birth through high school. *Journal of Special Education, 36*(3), 139–147. https://doi.org/10.1177/00224669020360030401

Dunst, C. J. (2017). Family systems early childhood intervention. In H. Sukkar, J. Kirby, & C. J. Dunst (Eds.), *Early childhood intervention: Working with families of young children with special needs* (pp. 36–58). Routledge.

Dunst, C. J. (2020). Modeling the relationships between parent strengths, parenting efficacy beliefs, and child social-emotional behavior: Shared activities and child well-being. *International Journal of Child Development and Mental Health, 8*(2), 11–18.

Dunst, C. J., Bruder, M. B., Trivette, C. M., & Hamby, D. W. (2006). Everyday activity settings, natural learning environments, and early intervention practices. *Journal of Policy and Practice in Intellectual Disabilities, 3*, 3–10. https://doi.org/10.1111/j.741-1130.2006.00047.x

Dunst, C. J., Raab, M., & Trivette, C. M. (2012). Characteristics of naturalistic language intervention strategies. *Journal of Speech-Language Pathology & Applied Behavior Analysis, 5*, 8–16. https://www.thefreelibrary.com/Characteristics+of+naturalistic+language+intervention+strategies.-a0299887454

Dunst, C. J., & Trivette, C. M. (2007). Capacity-building family-centered intervention practices. *Journal of Family Social Work, 12*, 119–143. https://www.researchgate.net/profile/Carl-Dunst/publication/248920565_Capacity-Building_Family-Systems_Intervention_Practices/links/5fbbcf38299bf104cf6e61ca/Capacity-Building-Family-Systems-Intervention-Practices.pdf

Early Childhood Personnel Center. (2017). *Cross-disciplinary personnel competencies alignment.* https://ecpcta.org/cross-disciplinary-alignment

Fox, G. L., Nordquist, V. M., Billen, R., & Savoca, E. F. (2015). Father involvement and early intervention: Effects of empowerment and father role identity. *Family Relations, 64*(4), 461-475. https://doi.10.111/fare.12156

Fenton, A., Walsh, K., Wong, S., & Cumming, T. (2015). Using strengths-based approaches in early years practice and research. *International Journal of Early Childhood, 47*(1), 27–52.

Guralnick, M. J. (2011). Why early intervention works: A systems perspective. *Infants & Young Children, 24*, 6–28. https://doi.org/10.1097/IYC.0b013e3182002cfe

Hanft, B. E., Rush, D. D., & Shelden, M. L. (2004). *Coaching families and colleagues in early childhood.* Brookes.

Hebbeler, K. (2009, June 11). *First five years fund briefing; Education that works: The impact of early childhood intervention on reducing the need for special education services* [Presentation]. https://files.eric.ed.gov/fulltext/ED522123.pdf

Hebbeler, K., Spiker, D., Bailey, D., Scarborough, A., Mallik, S., Simeonsoon, R., … Nelson, L. (2007). *Early intervention for infants & toddlers with disabilities and their families: Participants, services, and outcomes. Final report of the National EI Longitudinal Study (NEILS).* https://www.sri.com/wp-content/uploads/2021/12/neils_finalreport_200702.pdf

Heidlage, J. K., Cunningham, J. E., Kaiser, A. P., Trivette, C. M., Barton, E. E., Frey, J. R., & Roberts, M. Y. (2019). The effects of parent-implemented language interventions on child linguistic outcomes: A meta-analysis. *Early Childhood Research Quarterly, 50*, 6–23. https://doi.org/10.1016/j.ecresq.2018.12.006

Hong, B. S., & Reynolds-Keefer, L. (2013). Transdisciplinary team building: Strategies in creating early childhood educator and health care teams. *International Journal of Early Childhood Special Education, 5*(1), 30–44.

Hwang, A. W., Chao, M. Y., & Liu, S. W. (2013). A randomized controlled trial of routines-based early intervention for children with or at risk for developmental delays. *Research in Developmental Disabilities, 34*(10), 3112–3123. https://doi.org/10.1016/j.ridd.2013.06.037

Individuals With Disabilities Education Improvement Act of 2004, Pub. L. No. 108-446, §

632, 118 Stat. 2744 (2004). http://idea.ed.gov/

Individuals With Disabilities Education Improvement Act. (2011). Part C Final Regulations. 34 C.F.R. §§ 303 (2011). https://www.gpo.gov/fdsys/pkg/FR-2011-09-28/pdf/2011-22783.pdf

Innocenti, M. S., Roggman, L. A., & Cook, G. A. (2013). Using the PICCOLO with parents of children with a disability. *Infant Mental Health Journal, 34*, 307–318. https://doi.org/10.1002/imhj.21394

Interprofessional Education Collaborative. (2016). *Core competencies for interprofessional collaborative practice: 2016 update.* https://ipec.memberclicks.net/assets/2016-Update.pdf

Joint Committee on Infant Hearing. (2007). Year 2007 position statement: Principles and guidelines for early hearing detection and intervention programs. *Pediatrics, 120*(4), 898–921. https://pediatrics.aappublications.org/content/120/4/898

Landa, R., Holman, K., O'Neill, A., & Stuart, E. (2011). Intervention targeting development of socially synchronous engagement in toddlers with autism spectrum disorder: A randomized controlled trial. *Journal of Child Psychology and Psychiatry, 52*(1), 13–21. https://doi.org/10.1111/j.1469-7610.2010.02288.x

Lineberger, A. (2022). Characteristics and consequences of a primary service provider approach to teaming in early intervention. *CASEmakers, 9*(1), 1–5. https://fipp.ncdhhs.gov/wp-content/uploads/CASEmaker-Characteristics-and-Consequences-of-a-Primary-Service-Provider-Approach-to-Teaming-in-Early-Intervention-5.5.pdf

Ludwig, J., & Phillips, D. A. (2008). Long-term effects of Head Start on low-income children. *Annals of the New York Academy of Science, 1136*, 257–268.

McWilliam, R. A. (2010a). Assessing families' needs with the routines-based interview. In R. A. McWilliam (Ed.), *Working with families of young children with special needs* (pp. 27–60). Guilford.

McWilliam, R. A. (2010b). *Routines-based early intervention: Supporting young children and their families.* Brookes.

Mental Retardation Facilities and Community Mental Health Centers Construction Act of 1963, Pub. L. No. 88-164, 1576 (1963).

Moore, L., Koger, D., Blomberg, S., Legg, L., McConahy, R., Wit, S., & Gatmaitan, M. (2012). Making best practice our practice: Reflections on our journey into natural environments. *Infants & Young Children, 25*(1), 95–105. https://doi.org/10.1097/IYC.0b013e31823d0592

National Resource Center for Family Centered Practice. (2023). *What is family centered practice?* https://nrcfcp.uiowa.edu/what-is-family-centered-practice

Peredo, T. N. (2016). Supporting culturally and linguistically diverse families in early intervention. *Perspectives of the ASHA Special Interest Groups, 1*(1), 154–167. https://doi.org/10.1044/persp1.SIG1.154

Rausch, A., Bold, E., & Strain, P. (2021). The more the merrier: Using collaborative transdisciplinary services to maximize inclusion and child outcomes. *Young Exceptional Children, 24*(2), 59–69. https://doi.org/10.1177%2F1096250620922206

Raver, S. A., & Childress, D. C. (2015). *Family-centered early intervention: Supporting infants and toddlers in natural environments.* Brookes.

Roberts, M. Y., & Kaiser, A. P. (2011). The effectiveness of parent-implemented language interventions: A meta-analysis. *American Journal of Speech-Language Pathology, 20,* 180–199.

Roberts, M. Y., & Kaiser, A. P. (2015). Early intervention for toddlers with language delays: A randomized controlled trial. *Pediatrics, 135*(4), 686–693. https://doi.org/10.1542/peds.2014-2134

Roberts, M. Y., Curtis, P. R., Sone, B. J., & Hampton, L. H. (2019). Association of parent training with child language development: A systematic review and meta-analysis. *Journal of the American Medical Association Pediatrics, 173*(7), 671–680. https://doi.org/10.1001/jamapediatrics.2019.1197

Ross, K. D. (2018). *SLPs in early childhood intervention: Working with infants, toddlers, families, and other care providers.* Plural Publishing.

Rush, D. D., & Shelden, M. L. (2011). *The early childhood coaching handbook.* Brookes.

Rush, D. D., & Shelden, M. L. (2020). *The early childhood coaching handbook* (2nd ed.). Brookes.

Schertz, H. H., & Horn, K. (2017). Family capacity-building: Mediating parent learning through guided video reflection. In C. Trivette & B. Keilty (Eds.), *Recommended practices monograph series no. 3: Families: Knowing families, tailoring practices, building capacity* (pp. 125-134). Division for Early Childhood.

Searcy, K. L. (2018). Funding and documentation for early intervention (0 to 3 years). In N. Swigert (Ed.), *Documentation and reimbursement for speech-language pathologists: Principles and practice* (pp. 251–291). Slack Incorporated.

Shelden, M. L., & Rush, D. D. (2022). *The early intervention teaming handbook: The primary service provider approach* (2nd ed.). Brookes.

Stredler-Brown, A. (2017). Examination of coaching behaviors used by providers when delivering early intervention via telehealth to families of children who are deaf or hard of hearing. *Perspectives of the ASHA Special Interest Groups, 2*(9), 25–42.

Trivette, C. M., Dunst, C. J., & Hamby, D. (2004). Sources of variation in consequences of everyday activity settings on child and parenting functioning. *Perspectives in Education, 22*(2), 17–36. https://eric.ed.gov/?id=EJ687912

Trivette, C. M., Dunst, C. J., & Hamby, D. W. (2010). Influences of family-systems intervention practices on parent-child interactions and child development. *Topics in Early Childhood Special Education, 30*(1), 3–19. https://doi.org/10.1177/0271121410364250

Vail, C. O., Lieberman-Betz, R. G., & McCorkle, L. S. (2018). The impact of funding on Part C systems: Is the tail wagging the dog? *Journal of Early Intervention, 40*, 229–245.

Yang, C. H., Hossain, S. Z., & Sithartham, G. (2013). Collaborative practice in early childhood intervention from the perspectives of service providers. *Infants & Young Children, 26*(1), 57–73. https://doi.org/10.1097/IYC.0b013e3182736cbf

Chapter 2
Guiding Principles of Early Intervention

Learning Outcomes

When we have completed this chapter, we will be able to:

- Present the ASHA key principles that guide SLPs in providing EI services.

- Discuss family-centered services and the importance of building rapport with infants, toddlers, and families.

- Describe the definitions and implementation of culturally and linguistically responsive services in EI.

- Explain the foundation for and importance of natural environments in the provision of EI services.

- Recount the comprehensive and coordinated steps in the EI process, including considerations regarding eligibility, the creation of the Individualized Family Service Plan (IFSP), the role of the service coordinator, and transition in services.

- Present the importance of the team approach in EI and the evidence-based approaches that support interprofessional practice.

What Will We Learn and How Can We Apply It?

In 2008, ASHA presented five key principles to guide SLPs in providing Part C EI services rooted in evidence-based practices to young children and their families. Updates addressing the five principles, as well as implementation for best practice, are now also available through the ASHA EI Practice Portal (ASHA, 2021). This chapter presents these principles and examines how we, as SLPs working in EI, can effectively implement each one, beginning with effective establishment and maintenance of rapport with children and their families through family-centered services. The concept of cultural responsiveness in the EI arena, including the definitions and the circumstances that influence the provision of effective and appropriate family-centered services and the implementation of culturally and linguistically responsive services, is defined and explored. The importance of considering and incorporating natural environments into the provision of EI services is presented and discussed. This chapter discusses the importance of comprehensive and coordinated services in EI, including each step of the processes and pathways. In addition, the chapter presents the concept of service coordination for those of us who work in the EI arena, and it introduces information about interprofessional collaboration and evidence-based collaborative practices in EI programs. Finally, we focus on the principle of the team in EI, including types of collaborative approaches and the evidence that supports interprofessional practices.

It is so important that families of infants and toddlers who are at risk for, or who have been diagnosed with, disabilities receive all the supports and services they need to thrive. EI services should be tailored to the individual child and the changing needs and priorities of each family. These ASHA principles provide us, as SLPs, with the guidance we need to best serve the infants, toddlers, and families in our care.

The ASHA Guiding Principles of Early Intervention

In 2008, ASHA presented five key principles to guide SLPs in providing Part C EI services rooted in evidence-based practices to young children and their families. Updates addressing the five principles, as well as information related to implementation, are now also available through the ASHA EI Practice Portal (ASHA, 2021) and reflect current best practices as we provide EI for young children and their families (ASHA, 2008a, 2023). These principles specifically note that supports and services must be (a) family-centered; (b) culturally and linguistically responsive; (c) developmentally supportive and promote children's participation in their natural environments; (d) comprehensive, coordinated, and team-based; and (e) based on the highest quality internal and external evidence available. Each one of these principles is discussed in greater detail in the following sections.

Family-Centered Services

The first guiding principle that reflects current best practices for us when we are working within the EI arena, focuses on the delivery of services that are *family-centered* (ASHA, 2008a). The principle of family-centered services is based on a family-systems model for implementing EI and family support assessment and intervention practices. According to Dunst and Trivette (2009), the family-systems model focuses on four evidence-based operational components. The model is implemented by first identifying the family's *concerns and priorities*. At this level, family aspirations and priorities are identified using needs-based assessment procedures and strategies to determine what the family considers important. The second step toward implementation of the family-systems model is identification of the *supports and resources* that can be used by the family to address their concerns and priorities. The family's personal social network and potential sources of information and assistance are identified, in addition to emphasizing the particular strengths of the family that increase their likelihood to use those resources needed to meet their needs. The third step in the model involves identifying family members' existing *abilities and interests* to obtain needed supports and resources. At this point, the family's strengths and capabilities are explored and considered as a basis for promoting their abilities to obtain and mobilize their resources. The fourth and final step in implementation of the family-systems model involves coaching the family to use *help-giving practices to build their capacity*. These practices are used by the family to carry out actions intended to obtain supports and resources to meet their identified priorities and concerns. This final step is intended to enhance a family's ability to become more self-sustaining with respect to acquiring, recognizing, and utilizing their own competencies and skills to effectively meet their needs and achieve their goals (Dunst, 2017;

Dunst & Trivette, 2009).

Effective family-centered practices involve working collaboratively with families in all aspects of service delivery. It means relating to family members as people, not "patients." A family-centered approach recognizes the importance of all family members, including brothers and sisters, grandparents, and extended family members. Furthermore, this approach involves the awareness and inclusion of the set of beliefs, values, principles, and practices that strengthen the family's capacity to enhance their child's development and learning (IDEA, 2004). Effective family-centered practices are responsive to the unique circumstances of each family and provide families with unbiased and comprehensive information to make informed decisions (DEC, 2014).

IDEA Part C requires that families are granted the opportunity to participate in all aspects of their child's services. To ensure the family, and not just the child, receives EI services that build on their strengths, collaboration between families and providers must be the foundation of family-centered services (Crawford & Weber, 2014; DEC 2014; Dunst, 2017; Dunst & Trivette, 2009; McWilliam, 2010a; Ross, 2018). Families collaborate with providers to design and implement services that align specifically with their own preferences, resources, concerns, and priorities (IDEA, 2011). This collaboration leads to a partnership that creates a learning environment supportive of both the child's and family's needs while achieving mutually agreed on outcomes and promoting family capacities (DEC, 2014; Roberts et al., 2016). To put the components of the family-centered model and effective collaboration into practice, families and providers must form a partnership. This partnership begins by determining our own definitions and roles as well as those of the family. The term *family* can have many different meanings. Families define themselves by who lives together, who makes decisions, what roles family members play, and how members support each other. Each family operates as a system, and for each child, the family system represents the group of individuals who have the most influence on that child's growth and development. Building rapport, collaborating with one another, and facilitating an individualized, supportive EI process are all critical components to working effectively with each family. By asking questions about routines, joining their activities, and communicating effectively, EI service providers learn about how each family works. Services can then be implemented that include opportunities for families and caregivers to actively participate in intervention (DEC, 2014). These steps also offer families an opportunity to see that identified family dynamic information is vitally important for individualized and meaningful services for their unique child and family (IDEA, 2011; SpecialQuest Multimedia Training Library, 2007).

As SLPs, we must learn to adapt our knowledge and expertise to fit the needs of each child and family, ensuring that the family's needs are being addressed and learning is supported. The unique needs of each child and family determine which skills we use, how knowledge is shared, and which strategies are developed. We should combine our professional expertise and activities with the child- and family-specific expertise that the parent brings to the table. Together, we can create intervention focused on how the family will encourage the growth, development, and participation of their child when we are not present (McWilliam, 2004). Raver and Childress (2015) reported that families need to be involved and responsive to their child's needs and development to ensure intervention is effective. Engagement and involvement by families is essential to strengthen their existing knowledge and skills to promote the child's development of new skills, and to enhance both child and family outcomes (DEC, 2014).

When we use a family-centered approach, we effectively collaborate with families to share information, strengthen family functioning, empower decision making, and facilitate family participation throughout the EI process. Establishing a positive relationship with a family is key to facilitating their participation throughout the EI process. We play an important role in developing the relationship and facilitating family participation. Building rapport and trust that lead to a true partnership begins with the first contact and continues through transition (Jung & Grisham-Brown, 2006). Meeting families where they are; practicing active listening; and helping them identify priorities, resources, strengths, and needs related to their child's development and their family provide the foundation for a supportive EI system.

In our role, we join the parents, through our relationship, in our common concerns about their infant or toddler. We both observe the child's growth and development and offer developmentally appropriate anticipatory guidance. We also identify the strengths that each parent brings to the relationship with his or her child and identify and support the parent's pleasure in the child.

Parents and family members spend the most time with their child and development at this stage moves rapidly; there is no doubt encouraging parents and families to take the lead in the EI experience is essential. We must take our knowledge and learn to adapt and apply it with each family in each intervention visit as young children's development occurs within the context of their family and community (Dunst et al., 2001). Just as the guiding principles of Part C recognize that infant and toddler development unfolds during family routines and activities, supports and services that focus on these routines and activities provide family members with useful, meaningful strategies that can be used daily within the context of those activities unique to each individual family (Raver & Childress, 2015; Woods et al., 2004).

Establishing and Maintaining Rapport

Building *rapport* with a family begins with the first contact and affects the relationship throughout the process of intervention. Strong rapport takes time to establish and effort to maintain, but it can be a means of encouraging open communication and learning for everyone involved. We are able to build strong relationships with the families we serve by establishing a positive foundation through a family-centered perspective. By recognizing the family's strengths and perspectives in the first stages of the EI process, we can consider the demands of intervention in relation to the benefits at each subsequent stage. Keeping an open dialogue with family members and discussing both demands and benefits on a consistent basis are key to maintaining rapport among the team members. Suggestions for building positive relationships with families include the following (Cassidy, 2023; IDEA, 2011; SpecialQuest Multimedia Training Library, 2007):

- Demonstrate genuine interest in the family's life, routines, activities, interests and in the child's needs and achievements.

- Be sensitive to each family's readiness to share information and to receive feedback.

- Encourage and support a family member's participation at a level that is comfortable for them.

- Encourage family members to be active participants in all aspects of the EI process.

- Respect the family's time by being punctual for visits and offering flexible scheduling.

- Acknowledge the complexities of raising a child with developmental delays or disabilities and helping as needed.

- Provide complete, unbiased information and allow family members time to make informed decisions, even when their decisions differ from choices we might make.

- Respect the family's rights throughout the EI process.

Culturally and Linguistically Responsive Services

The second guiding principle that reflects current best practices for those of us in the EI arena states that families of infants and toddlers with a disability or developmental delay must have access to *culturally and linguistically competent* services (IDEA, 2011). The descriptor *'culturally and linguistically diverse'* refers to children and families who reside in the United States but who come from homes in which a language other than English is spoken and whose cultural identity differs from mainstream U.S. culture (Puig, 2012).

Using the family systems approach, we deliver EI services by supplying knowledge and training to families as they navigate the world of raising their children with disabilities (Dunst & Trivette, 2009). A 2007 ASHA survey of SLPs indicated that, in all settings, approximately 29 percent of caseloads consist of culturally and linguistically diverse clients (ASHA, 2007). In a 2013 survey of SLPs who work in EI programs, only 7% reported being able to effectively communicate with a family without an interpreter in a language other than English; while less than half thought they had received enough knowledge in their coursework to work effectively with culturally and linguistically diverse families, and only about a quarter had engaged in practical experiences with culturally and linguistically diverse families (Caesar, 2013). It is not surprising that results from the National EI Longitudinal Study indicated that families from diverse ethnic and racial backgrounds and families at lower income levels who had participated in EI services were less satisfied with services than White families and those families at higher income levels (Hebbeler et al., 2007; Raspa et al., 2010; Turnbull et al., 2009). To effectively support families, it is therefore necessary to develop a heightened level of sensitivity to the influences of cultural values, customs, and beliefs as well as to the strengths that cultural and linguistic identity bring to the family system (Peredo, 2016; Segal & Beyer, 2006).

We interact with families of many different cultures. *Culture* is defined as "people's values, religion, ideals, language, artistic expressions, patterns of social and interpersonal relationships and ways of perceiving, behaving and thinking" (Balthrop & Coleman, 2003). Different cultural dimensions can have an influence on a family's decisions regarding EI services and supports. *Cultural responsivity* is the ability to interact effectively with all people, regardless of their culture, and to recognize how their cultural dimensions could affect a family's approach to services for their child. By becoming more culturally sensitive, we will be able to reduce our own cultural biases and recognize the cultural issues important to each family.

Cultural responsiveness is necessary to ensure success in every step of the process when providing EI supports and services. The components of the family system are strongly influenced by culture as it influences how a family defines and structures itself (Wayman & Lynch, 1991). Culture influences family functions, the family life cycle, and events viewed by the family as stressors. Cultural perspectives that might relate directly to services within EI include views of (a) children and child-rearing, (b) disability and causation, (c) intervention, (d) medical treatment and healing, (e) family and family roles, and (f) language and communication styles (Hanson & Lynch, 1990; Peredo, 2016). Additionally, according to Hanson and Lynch (1990), several factors regarding the nature of EI itself should be considered to impart effective EI services to families from culturally and linguistically diverse backgrounds. These factors include (a) attitudes regarding intervention, (b) methods used and location of services, (c) qualifications of the service providers, and (d) styles of interaction and communication in the provision of services.

When providing services to families from diverse cultural backgrounds, we should consider those factors that affect families' perspectives as well as those considerations that might relate directly to such services. By listening to the family and learning about their family system, we can better promote effective intervention. During the initial assessment of the program planning process, we have the opportunity to ask questions and listen to the family members discuss their needs and concerns. Based on their feedback and by collaborating with family members, we should align outcomes with family culture, values, needs, and priorities. Additionally, using a routines-based approach to goal selection and intervention may be optimal (Kashinath et al., 2006; Woods et al., 2004). Because intervention activities are built directly into family routines that already exist, this approach builds on the strengths inherent to individual family systems while eliminating cultural mismatches. By determining optimal routines and empowering parents to incorporate opportunities into their own everyday activities, we are able to provide effective services while respecting and considering every family's culture and value system (Peña & Fiestas, 2009).

With regard to providing linguistically responsive services, we must consider both the home language(s) as well as acquisition of the language needed for the child's academic success. This consideration will look different depending on the services and supports given. IDEA regulations define *native language* as the language typically used by an individual. In the case of a child receiving services, native language is the language typically used by the parents or caregivers (IDEA, 2011). Prior written notice regarding EI services must be provided to families in their native language. Beyond the prior written notice, we deliver EI supports and services in the language(s) most likely to result in an accurate representation of the child's skills (ASHA, 2023; DEC, 2014; IDEA, 2011). We want to teach families and caregivers how to implement strategies in their home language to ensure their capacity to both comprehend and carry over knowledge and skills (Peredo, 2016). Service providers often work with families and interpreters to support both the home language(s) and acquisition of the language needed by the child for academic success. Chapter 8 further explores how we can effectively collaborate with families and interpreters to ensure our practices are inclusive and considerate of the family's home language.

Ultimately, we can build strong relationships with families and address their individualized needs by recognizing that each family is a whole unit with its own unique set of values. By respecting the choices that families make about child-rearing, serving the family's functional needs, and viewing the culture and the home language of the family as a strength, we can implement the principles of family-centered practice effectively to support culturally and linguistically diverse families in EI (Peredo, 2016).

Services Provided in the Natural Environment

Effective EI services meet the family where they are, at the level of their needs, and in the environments in which they find themselves. Each family exists within a system that includes the people with whom they interact, the supports and resources they have, and the places they go. The primary purpose of EI is to support family efforts and to build their confidence and competence in meeting the needs of their children. With that purpose in mind, intervention visits provided within each family's support system and natural environment should be best suited to positive developmental outcomes for children and families (ASHA, 2008b). Furthermore, services that address family routines, concerns, and priorities through authentic experiences, active exploration, and interactions with both people and the environment consistent with the child's age, cognitive skills, communication skills, strengths, and interests are considered developmentally supportive (DEC, 2014).

IDEA Part C (2004) requires that we engage in EI services, to the maximum extent appropriate, in natural environments. According to IDEA (2011), *natural environments* are defined as "settings that are natural or typical for a same-aged infant or toddler without a disability [and] may include the home or community settings." Natural environments include the home as well as other settings in which children without delays and disabilities participate in their communities. Natural environments are not locations where children go because of their disabilities, for our own convenience, or because of access to a special place or equipment. Natural environments are, instead, those settings and activities in which each individual child's family participates or in which they would like to participate.

When considering the provision of EI services in natural environments, we must determine not only 'where' we will provide the supports but also 'how' we will provide them. Children learn best when they learn in context and have multiple opportunities to practice skills and abilities throughout the day. It is much easier for infants and toddlers to generalize their newly learned skills when they have learned them during meaningful, functional activities as they happen naturally, rather than learning them in contrived situations in a clinical setting. It is our job to present parents with this perspective.

We must learn to think beyond the traditional home visit. We must consider the multitude of activities in which children and their family engage beyond our scheduled block of time (Hanft et al., 2004). Thinking beyond the typical home visit requires a shift in how EI has been delivered in many localities. Therefore, to help our teams move forward, we need to understand the similarities and differences between traditional home visiting and intervention provided when incorporating each family's priorities, routines, and activities. Services presented through traditional home visits tend to be limited to what can be accomplished during the span of time allotted for the visit. Specific skills can be addressed in isolation, and activities might be discussed but not practiced because they do not coincide with the scheduled time. In contrast, supports and services that consider the concept of natural environments use that allotted home visit time much differently. The time is used to explore a variety of family routines and activities to find out how they can be enhanced to address Individualized Family Service Plan (IFSP) outcomes, both during and between EI visits. Because we might join the family in those activities, the intervention visit should be scheduled in response to the activities being explored, and is therefore flexible with regard to day and time.

Engaging in intervention in the home or other natural settings and environments gives us the opportunity to see what daily life is like for the family. Familiar everyday experiences, events, and places should be incorporated as opportunities to promote incidental teaching and natural learning throughout each day (McWilliam, 2010a; Raver & Childress, 2015; Ross, 2018; Rush & Shelden, 2011). These interactions could include learning what goes well for each family in each scenario and determining what assistance the family might need. By becoming familiar with the specifics of each family's routine and activities, we can help parents develop individualized outcomes and intervention strategies based on those activities that are meaningful and useful to the family during their routine daily life.

Comprehensive and Coordinated Services

The fourth of the five guiding principles (ASHA, 2008a) states that EI services should be "comprehensive, coordinated, and team-based." Regardless of state or local programming methods, all young children and their families follow the same basic steps as they enter into and move through the EI system. These sequential steps, often called the *supports and services pathway,* involve a coordinated process that begins with a referral for assessment, and follows the child and family while they receive services through the Part C program.

Supports and Services Pathway

The supports and services pathway assists in the identification of eligible families to maximize family and child outcomes through the delivery of EI services. It consists of seven distinct components of service delivery: Referral, intake, eligibility determination, assessment for service planning, IFSP development, implementation and reviews of the IFSP, and transition activities. Embedded in each of these processes is the legal acknowledgment of the family's and child's procedural rights and safeguards. Each of the following elements within the typical sequence a family follows while involved in Part C services will subsequently be discussed in detail (IDEA, 2011):

- Referral
- Intake
- Eligibility determination
- Assessment for service planning
- Development of the Individualized Family Service Plan
- Implementation and review of the Individualized Family Service Plan
- Transition

Referral

A primary referral source, such as a parent, pediatrician, or health department representative, identifies a child who could have a developmental delay or might need further assessment. Referral sources often have concerns based on results of developmental screenings, observations, or a diagnosis indicating a potential developmental delay. Anyone in the community can make a referral of a child who might be eligible for Part C services as long as parent or guardian permission is secured. The referral is made to the Part C local Central Point of Entry at the lead agency. The Central Point of Entry collects the referral information and assigns a service coordinator to meet with the family. During the referral process, information regarding the local or statewide EI process is shared with the family, and initial information regarding the child and family is gathered. Each local lead agency develops policies and procedures in the community to ensure quick response from the Central Point of Entry and to move quickly toward the next step in the EI process. The IDEA (2011) requires that providers make referrals within 7 days after the infant or toddler is identified as having a possible disability or delay. Following receipt of a referral, the lead agency has 45 days to complete the intake or screening, initial evaluation, initial assessments, and initial team meeting to develop the initial IFSP for the child and the family (IDEA, 2011).

Intake

Intake involves meetings with the family, either in person or via telephone, to continue gathering information to determine eligibility. Such information includes developmental history, medical history and medical home information, family routines, schedules, and activities of interest, as well as the completion of a developmental screening, if needed. In-depth information is shared with the family regarding the Part C system, including eligibility criteria, IFSP development if the child is eligible, family cost share participation, and child and family procedural rights and safeguards. At this point, the Central Point of Entry, or a service coordinator who has been assigned to the family, begins the process of eligibility determination.

Eligibility Determination

Eligibility determination is the process of establishing whether a child meets the system's eligibility criteria to receive EI services. This process includes the evaluation of the child's skills and needs through a review of information, including medical and developmental reports, assessment reports, observations, and parent report. According to IDEA §303.321(a)(2)(i), evaluation is defined as "the procedures used by qualified personnel to determine a child's initial and continuing eligibility" (IDEA, 2011). Eligibility determination is based on the child's needs within his or her natural environment, which could include the home or any community setting in which children without disabilities participate (e.g., child-care centers, public playgrounds). All areas of a child's development are considered to determine whether the child has a delay or differences in development that might make him or her eligible for Part C services. As such, "no single procedure may be used as the sole criterion for determining a child's eligibility" (IDEA 2011, §303.321(b)); these procedures must include administration of an evaluation instrument, an interview with the parent to gather the child's history, identification of the child's level of functioning in each of the developmental areas, a gathering of information from a variety of sources to understand the full scope of the child's individual strengths and needs, and a review of the child's medical, educational, and other records. As needed, informed clinical opinion must also be considered in the process of determining eligibility (IDEA, 2011). This information is reviewed by a multidisciplinary team (identified later). This team determines whether a child meets one or more of the criteria for eligibility. Part C of IDEA (2004) states that systems must serve any child "under 3 years of age who needs EI services" (IDEA, 2004, §632(5)(A)) because the child "(i) is experiencing developmental delays, as measured by appropriate diagnostic instruments and procedures in one or more of the areas of cognitive development, physical development, communication development, social or emotional development, and adaptive development; or (ii) has a diagnosed physical or mental condition which has a high probability of resulting in developmental delay" (IDEA, 2004, §632(5)(A)).

Each state also has the option of serving children who show no delay but who are considered "at risk" for developmental challenges because of biological or environmental factors. IDEA Part C defines an at-risk infant or toddler as "an individual under 3 years of age who would be at risk of experiencing a substantial developmental delay if EI services were not provided to the individual" (IDEA, 2004). States have some discretion in setting the criteria for each of these variables. As a result, definitions of eligibility differ significantly from state to state.

Additionally, if a child is not found eligible for Part C services, families might choose to seek EI services through private or community resources and other federal or state-funded early childhood programs (e.g., Early Head Start). If a family continues to have any concerns about the need for EI, they can request a re-evaluation through their Part C program at a later time.

Assessment for Service Planning

Assessment, as defined by Part C of IDEA, includes "the ongoing procedures used by qualified personnel to identify the child's unique strengths and needs and the EI services appropriate to meet those needs throughout the period of the child's eligibility" (IDEA, 2011, §303.321(a)(2)). This is a multistep process that includes identification of the family's resources, priorities, and concerns through family-centered assessment, multidisciplinary team observations, and assessment of eligible children. In addition to assessing the family, assessment is also an opportunity to determine the child's strengths and needs in all areas of development. The assessment process provides the IFSP team with an opportunity to identify EI supports and services that might be necessary to address the child's unique needs. Although assessment tools may vary, ASHA (2008b) recommended combining formal and informal assessment tools that include both standardized and nonstandardized measures to ensure the most comprehensive picture of the child is obtained. This combination of assessment tools provides information regarding the skills of the child in comparison to same-age peers. Conducting an assessment with a comprehensive battery is more conducive to encouraging family and team member participation and collaboration and guiding the IFSP development. Some local and statewide systems have implemented specific requirements regarding the choice and use of assessment tools for the purposes of both eligibility determination and assessment for service planning.

Development of the Individualized Family Service Plan

Based on the assessment for service planning, the IFSP is developed. The IFSP is a written plan for providing EI services to eligible children and their families. The plan is developed jointly by the family, the service coordinator, SLPs, and others (e.g., an audiologist, physical therapist, nurse, social worker) who may be providing EI services to the child and family. The IFSP is based on the multidisciplinary evaluation and assessment of the child and the assessment of the resources, priorities, and concerns of the child's family. The plan includes outcomes, strategies, and the services necessary to enhance the development of the child and the capacity of the family to meet the special needs of the child (IDEA, 2004, §303.340(2)). Part C of IDEA mandates that the IFSP meeting must be conducted in settings as well as at times convenient for the family. The meeting and the documents must also be in the native language of the family. An interpreter must be involved if the native language of the family is not English. We must work collaboratively with the interpreter to ensure that families fully understand their rights and role in the EI system.

There are eight required components of the IFSP:

1. A statement of the infant's or toddler's present levels of physical development (including fine motor, gross motor, vision, hearing, and health status), cognitive development, communication development, social or emotional development, and adaptive (self-help) development based on objective criteria.

2. A statement (with the family's permission) of the family's resources, priorities, and concerns related to enhancing the development of the family's infant or

toddler with a disability.

3. A statement of the measurable results or outcomes expected to be achieved for the infant or toddler and the family. The statement should include emergent literacy and language skills developmentally appropriate for the child. Outcomes should be relevant to the family and focused on the whole child and their participation in activity settings important to the family (Infant & Toddler Connection of Virginia, 2003).

4. A statement of specific EI services based on peer-reviewed research, to the extent possible, necessary to meet the unique needs of the infant or toddler and the family. The statement should include the frequency, intensity, and method of delivering services.

5. A statement of the natural environments in which EI services will appropriately be provided. If the services are not furnished in a natural environment, a justification must be presented.

6. The projected dates of initiation of services and the anticipated length, duration, and frequency of the services.

7. The identification of the service coordinator from the profession most immediately relevant to the child's or family's needs (or who is otherwise qualified to carry out all applicable responsibilities under this part).

8. The steps to be taken to support the transition of the toddler with a disability to preschool or other appropriate services. This transition plan must be individualized for each child (Pub. L. 108-446, §636(d)).

According to IDEA §303.344(d)(4), when addressing the needs of children who are at least 3 years of age and receiving services through the provisions provided in the 2011 IDEA Part C Final Regulations, the IFSP must also include "an educational component that promotes school readiness and incorporates pre-literacy, language, and numeracy skills" (IDEA, 2011). Additional details and discussion about each of the IFSP components is presented in Chapter 7.

IFSP Implementation and Review

Implementation and review of the IFSP involves the coordination and monitoring of the delivery of IFSP supports and services. The IFSP must be developed within 45 days of the referral. EI services must begin within 30 days of the IFSP being written and agreed on by the multidisciplinary team. Periodic reviews are held to facilitate IFSP changes as necessary. These changes can reflect the child's development and any changes, including those that might be medical in nature, that occur regarding a family's priorities and concerns. IFSP reviews must take place at least once every 6 months or each time a child has either achieved a documented outcome or presents a new area of need (IDEA, 2004). Annual reviews must be completed within 365 days of the initial or previous annual IFSP meeting.

Transition

Transition includes a family's experience from provider to provider (e.g., SLP to occupational therapist) or from hospital or home-based programs to community-based programs (i.e., the entry and exit of children and families to and from EI services). This is an ongoing process that begins with the child and family as they enter the system and ends when they transition from the EI program under Part C to the next program or any other appropriate services identified for the child who is no longer eligible to receive Part C or Part B services. As the child approaches age 3, the IFSP team begins a formal transition process and develops a plan to ease the shift from EI to preschool special education (if applicable) or to another community-based service option (if the child is not eligible for preschool services). The service coordinator tends to be the provider who is primarily responsible for assisting families through the transition process. All service providers, including those of us who serve in this role, must be knowledgeable about the transition process. Transition should be discussed at every IFSP meeting. As the child approaches 30 months of age, the service coordinator should increase the level of detail of these discussions in preparation for the child "aging out" of the EI system at age 3. Under the Final Regulations (IDEA, 2011), notice of transition must occur no fewer than 90 days before the toddler's third birthday. Children transitioning from EI include those who no longer qualify for Part C supports and services prior to age 3, children who are turning 3 and whose parents do not want to pursue Part B services (essentially preschool services), and children who are between 2 and 3 years of age and are preparing to transition to Part B services.

Under the Final Regulations of IDEA (2011), each state has the option to choose to extend Part C services to those children who are eligible for preschool services beyond the age of 3 until they enter or are eligible under state law to enter kindergarten. The state could choose to implement this option for children beyond 3 years of age until the beginning of the school year following their third, fourth, or fifth birthday. An extended IFSP must contain an educational component that promotes school readiness and includes preliteracy, language, and numeracy skills (IDEA, 2011). Currently, very few states implement this option.

Regardless of their choice, each state must include a description of the policies and procedures in place to ensure an effective and seamless transition for young children from receiving EI services under Part C of IDEA to preschool or other appropriate services or for those who are exiting the Part C program altogether. Transition plans look different for each child and are dependent on the child's and family's needs. Regardless of where the child transitions, there might be an adjustment for the child and family when leaving the Part C system. We might be able to help the family with this adjustment by discussing the process and being prepared to answer any questions about the transition from Part C services to preschool services (IDEA Part B).

Service Coordination

Under IDEA 2004 Part C, *service coordination* is defined as an active, ongoing process that assists and enables families to access services and ensures their rights and procedural safeguards. Part C mandates that every family in the EI system receives service coordination at no cost.

In some states, the SLP, as a member of the IFSP team, may assume the functions of the service coordinator. When we are not responsible for the service coordination role, it is still imperative that we understand this role within the system to effectively collaborate with the service coordinator.

The service coordinator's primary function is to serve as the single point of contact for the family throughout the EI process. Service coordinators help the family identify and obtain necessary services and assistance. Often, the service coordinator also acts as the initial point of contact and could therefore play the important role of assisting the family as they begin to understand and process the nature of their child's disability and needs. The family's first interactions with the service coordinator could have a significant influence on their level of trust and expectations of the EI system overall (Dunst, 2002).

Once a referral has been made for EI services, a service coordinator is assigned to the family as quickly as possible and becomes actively involved in the IFSP process. According to ASHA (2023), IDEA (2011), and the Workgroup on Recommended Knowledge and Skills for Service Coordinators (2020), the tasks a service coordinator must accomplish efficiently and effectively include the following:

- Informing the family of their rights and procedural safeguards as well as the various timelines specified by Part C of IDEA 2004 and the final regulations implemented in 2011.

- Establishing a collaborative relationship with the family.

- Collecting information about family priorities, resources, and concerns, as well as daily routines and activities.

- Supporting the family's problem-solving skills as a course of action begins to develop.

- Planning the developmental evaluation/assessment, formulating questions that reflect the family's concerns, and addressing state eligibility standards with the family and the team members.

- Compiling and integrating information from various sources to develop a comprehensive developmental profile of the child.

- Facilitating communication among and between the various team members and the family to develop functional, meaningful outcomes based on the family and child's daily routines and activities.

- Ensuring that intervention services are provided in a timely manner and are directly related to functional outcomes, and they maintain communication and collaboration among team members in order to ensure that outcomes are being addressed.

- Coordinating EI and other services for the family (including educational, social, and medical supports and services that are not provided for diagnostic and evaluation purposes).

- Conducting referral and other activities to assist the family in identifying available providers.

- Overseeing the evaluation and review of the IFSP and subsequently monitoring the services specified in the IFSP.

- Conducting follow-up activities with the family and the team members.

- Coordinating and frequently reviewing the child's plan for transitioning from the EI system with the family.

The service coordinator supports the family members as they develop, implement, and monitor their intervention plan based on the IFSP. Service coordinators help families develop the knowledge and skills necessary to advocate for their children in the future. Service coordinators also access and coordinate resources and services for families. Ultimately, the service coordinator must ensure that the EI services are family-centered and collaborative among the multidisciplinary team members. When service coordination is not effective, families might not have a clear understanding of their child's strengths or needs. They could be left to coordinate information and services from multiple sources on their own. In this case, intervention and transition are likely to be fragmented, and the family may be unaware of all available resources (ASHA, 2008b). All service providers must communicate regularly with assigned service coordinators to ensure cohesion between their services and the needs of the children and families.

As members of the IFSP team, we assist the child, their family, and other professionals throughout the transition planning process (Searcy, 2018). In some cases, we might visit the new classroom or service provider with the family and take part in the initial individualized education program (IEP) meeting. When we serve in the role of service coordinator, we engage with the family through the following activities:

- Have direct responsibility for oversight of transition activities.

- Share knowledge regarding a wide range of resources in the community with the families.

- Ensure families have available information regarding the transition process.

- Ensure families know their opt-out rights, which vary by state; these rights allow parents and/or primary caregivers a specified window of time to refuse disclosure of information to state or local education agencies when the child is potentially eligible for preschool special education services.

The Team Approach

The EI system relies heavily on a team approach to service delivery. Regardless of the level of severity of a child's or family's needs, services in EI include all types of resources or supports that the child needs and is eligible to receive (ASHA, 2008b). When team members communicate well with one another, all participants reap the benefits from comprehensive services. Access to all necessary supports and services, the provision of skills and resources from multiple agencies, and the sharing of information and opinions across areas of expertise are just a few of the benefits of teams collaborating within the system.

The integration of services, including the coordination of the team members, is critical to the effective nature of EI. Additionally, they are essential elements of family-centered and best practices to support young children and their families (Early Childhood Personnel Center, 2017). Collaboration among team members ensures that opportunities for the development and coordination of interventions that complement one another are available. Team members who communicate well and collaborate across areas of expertise, including family members, benefit from joint professional development and consultation that results in enhanced knowledge and skills (Boyer & Thompson, 2014; Coufal & Woods, 2018). As discussed earlier, the roles and responsibilities of the service coordinator are central to successful communication among the EI team members. Part C of IDEA 2004 requires that members of the IFSP team coordinate their approaches, consult with one another, and recognize that the child and family outcomes are a responsibility to be shared by the entire team. Collaboration is dependent on the type of team model used, the lead agency's program guidelines, and the knowledge and skills of the individual team members (ASHA, 2008b). Although collaboration among team members may vary, professional communication with the family is essential.

Types of Teams in Early Intervention

Part C of IDEA 2004 uses the term *multidisciplinary* to describe the EI team approach, although other team models may be applied depending on the needs of the child and family. Three team models are commonly used within EI. In addition to multidisciplinary teams, interdisciplinary and transdisciplinary team models may be options within the local or state service delivery systems. Each one of these teams is different regarding the amount of communication and coordination required among team members (Paul-Brown & Caperton, 2001). Regardless of the model chosen, as SLPs, we often serve as members of the EI team.

Multidisciplinary Teams

In a multidisciplinary approach, service providers from different disciplines (i.e., physical therapy, occupational therapy, and audiology) assess or impart intervention to the family and child separately. Each provider completes an evaluation or assessment and makes recommendations independently of the other disciplines. Although several providers might be involved with the family, each professional works distinctly and separately in providing services. Team members therefore focus on their own disciplines and subsequent perspectives and do not tend to engage in collaborative planning or service provision. The service coordinator is typically a designated position within this type of team. Unfortunately, because collaboration among team members is often limited, cohesion of services could be affected (Paul & Roth, 2010). As stated earlier, Part C of IDEA (2011) requires a multidisciplinary composition of the IFSP team, including the parent and two or more individuals from separate disciplines or professions, with one of the individuals being the service coordinator.

Interdisciplinary Teams

Interdisciplinary teams have a greater focus on collaboration and communication. Typically, providers from various disciplines conduct the evaluation or assessment with the child and family individually; occasionally, an "arena" method of evaluation, in which multiple team members are present during the evaluation or assessment, may also be conducted. The team members then communicate with one another and integrate the findings to determine the needs, recommendations, and services for the child and his or her family (Paul & Roth, 2010).

Transdisciplinary Teams

The transdisciplinary team model involves a greater degree of collaboration among team members than the other service models. This approach is often more difficult to implement because of the need for increased collaboration and communication. It is the model, however, expected by IDEA (2011) to be used to support the design and delivery of services for children with disabilities and delays and their families (Paul et al., 2006).

The transdisciplinary approach requires the team members to share roles and systematically cross discipline boundaries. The purpose of the approach is to combine and integrate the expertise of team members so that more efficient and comprehensive assessment and intervention services are offered. Communication among team members involves continuous give and take between all members on a consistent basis. Evaluation and assessment, as well as intervention services, are typically conducted jointly by designated members of the team assigned to the child and family; one team member will then serve as the primary service provider and will deliver direct services that relate to all of the developmental disciplines for the child and family (Paul et al., 2006; Paul & Roth, 2010).

Evidence-Based Interprofessional Collaborative Practices

The most current and collaborative approach in EI, and a combination of the layers of teamwork presented thus far, is interprofessional education (IPE) and interprofessional collaborative practice (IPP). Consistent with the WHO definitions, ASHA (2021) defines IPE as "an activity that occurs when two or more professions learn about, from, and with each other to enable effective collaboration and improve outcomes for the individuals and families we serve." ASHA (2021) defines IPP as services that occur "when multiple service providers from different professional backgrounds contribute comprehensive health care or educational services by working with individuals and their families, caregivers, and communities to deliver the highest quality of care across settings."

EI is an interdisciplinary field with a history of collaborative teamwork that has consistently contributed to and benefits from IPP. We need to engage with other service providers and family members within the EI system through interprofessional collaboration to ensure effective and meaningful service delivery. As members of interprofessional teams, our contributions may vary depending on the knowledge and skills we possess as well as those represented by other service providers and professionals on the team. The Interprofessional Education Collaborative (IPEC, 2016) presents guiding principles and core competencies that intersect with the collaborative team approach required within EI services to give the highest quality of services. The IPEC core competencies define the goals and outcomes for both preprofessional preparation and professional practice across disciplines. To provide effective services in EI, we must embrace and demonstrate services defined and delivered by the framework of these competencies. Table 2–1 presents the IPEC competencies and their intersection with the EI core principles and our own roles and responsibilities.

Table 2–1. Intersection Between IPEC Core Competencies, Early Intervention (EI) Core Principles, and Speech-Language Pathologist (SLP) Roles and Responsibilities

Interprofessional Education Collaborative Core Competencies	Relationship to EI Core Principles and SLP Roles and Responsibilities
Competency 1: Values/Ethics for Interprofessional Practice Work with individuals of other professions to maintain a climate of mutual respect and shared values.	Each member of an EI team embraces collaboration and works together through a comprehensive approach that is inclusive, sensitive, responsive, and embedded in natural contexts. The team maintains a climate of mutual respect and shared values. The SLP needs to be sensitive to unique cultural and linguistic differences among families and also contributes to their team members' understanding of how these differences and priorities affect all aspects of service delivery.
Competency 2: Roles/Responsibilities: Use the knowledge of one's own role and those of other professions to appropriately assess and address the health care needs of patients and to promote and advance the health of the population.	Competency 2 relates directly to the eight specific responsibilities that are defined within the ASHA Scope of Practice for SLP (ASHA, 2016). Students preparing for entry into the profession must demonstrate foundational knowledge and skills related to psychological, physical, social, cultural, linguistic, cognitive, and biological human functions. While this role is common to all professions, SLPs are successful

	within a team when they are able to bring their unique knowledge of human communication together with that of their team members' professions. SLPs must use knowledge of our own role and those of other professionals to address the needs of the populations we serve.
Competency 3: Interprofessional Communication Communicate with patients, families, communities, and professionals in health and other fields in a responsive and responsible manner that supports a team approach to the promotion and maintenance of health and the prevention and treatment of disease.	The development of an effective team requires dynamic, open communication among all members. Teams must work together to become more effective. The early intervention SLP must communicate with the team in a manner that is free of jargon and relevant to each child and family. The SLP must be able to effectively explain how evidence from research relates to the family and child of concern. This requires disclosure and transparency among team members to build trust in our ability and that of others to fulfill our professional role.
Competency 4: Teams and Teamwork Apply relationship-building values and the principles of team dynamics to perform effectively in different team roles to plan, deliver, and evaluate patient- and population-centered care and population health programs and policies that are safe, timely, efficient, effective, and equitable.	The fourth core competency requires collaborative planning and problem solving that is systematic, ongoing, and frequently evaluated. When caregivers are active members of the team, they become more proficient in their ability to contribute to decision making, and are more engaged in fulfilling their role as primary interventionists for their child. SLP students need to develop their skills through clinical immersion in interprofessional learning contexts to develop the underlying foundations and applied skills necessary to function as effective members of an interprofessional team.

Note. Adapted from "Interprofessional collaborative practice in EI," by K. L. Coufal and J .J.

Woods, 2018; "Core competencies for interprofessional collaborative practice: 2016 update," by the Interprofessional Education Collaborative, 2016.

Services Based on the Highest Quality Internal and External Evidence

As SLPs, we strive to provide the most effective services to the infants, toddlers, and families with whom we work. To ensure this is the case, we now know we must use methods that have been demonstrated to be effective through scientific evidence, clinical experience, and client needs. The foundation of support for our practice includes both internal and external evidence. Internal evidence is based on policy, informed clinical opinion, values and perspectives of professionals and consumers, and professional consensus; external evidence is drawn from empirical research published in peer-reviewed journals. All of these considerations are evaluated in the delivery of EI services to realize positive outcomes for infants, toddlers, and their families (DEC, 2014). The combination of these variables gives us the evidence on which we base our practices.

As introduced in Chapter 1, as well as in the preceding narrative, services that are family-based, provided in the natural environment, culturally and linguistically responsive, and focused on the interprofessional, collaborative team are currently used in EI. These practices are based on the integration of the highest quality and most recent research, informed professional judgment and expertise, and family preferences and values (ASHA, 2023; DEC, 2014). The empirical research currently supporting these practices and approaches in EI is thoroughly discussed in Chapter 3.

Summary

EI is a federally mandated system that operates under the IDEA. The system, which has been restructured multiple times since its inception in 1997, authorizes services to meet the needs of infants and toddlers and their families, from birth to age 3 who have been or could be at risk for developmental delays or disabilities. In 2008, ASHA presented five guiding principles that continue to reflect best practices for those of us who are providing EI services to young children and their families; these principles were updated more recently to reflect current evidence-based practices in the field. This chapter discussed how each of those five guiding principles can be effectively implemented within the EI system. Cultural responsiveness, including the definitions and the considerations that influence the provision of effective and appropriate services, was addressed. This chapter defined family-centered practices, based on the family systems model, and presented the rationale for incorporating natural environments, routines, and everyday activities into the provision of EI services. Each step of the EI process, including final regulations and considerations regarding eligibility and the creation of the IFSP, was introduced. The chapter outlined interprofessional collaborative practice and the team approach to EI and different team formats. We were also reminded of the importance of research to serve as the foundation for the pathways and processes we incorporate into our practices.

Critical Thinking Questions

1. While all principles are of equal value, what would you say are the two guiding principles of evidence-based EI services in which you are most interested or intrigued by, as a future clinician? Why?

2. What are some examples of supports and resources for families in EI? Why is it so important we focus our attention on family-centered services?

3. What does it mean to be a culturally and linguistically responsive service provider?

4. What are the comprehensive and coordinated steps of service delivery in EI?

5. What does it mean for an infant or toddler to qualify for EI services based on a developmental delay? What does it mean for an infant or toddler to be considered "at-risk"? How are these distinctions different?

6. What are the required components of the IFSP? When is transition considered during this process? Why is transitioning out of EI services considered an integral component of the IFSP process?

7. Describe what a natural environment is, to a parent or caregiver who is new to the EI process. Why are services in the natural environment considered a foundation of effective practice?

8. What are the pros and cons of the different team approaches? Which is the one that IDEA recommends? Why?

References

American Speech-Language-Hearing Association. (2007). *ASHA SLP health care survey 2007: Caseload characteristics.* https://www.asha.org/uploadedFiles/research/memberdata/HC07CaseloadRprt.pdf

American Speech-Language-Hearing Association. (2008a). *Core knowledge and skills in early intervention speech-language pathology practice.* https://doi.org/10.1044/policy.KS2008-00292

American Speech-Language-Hearing Association. (2008b). *Roles and responsibilities of SLPs in early intervention: Guidelines.* https://doi.org/10.1044/policy.GL2008-00293

American Speech-Language-Hearing Association. (2016). *Scope of practice in speech-language pathology.* https://www.asha.org/policy/sp2016-00343/

American Speech-Language-Hearing Association. (2021). *Demographic profile of ASHA members providing bilingual services, year-end 2020.* https://www.asha.org/siteassets/surveys/demographic-profile-bilingual-spanish-service-members.pdf

American Speech-Language-Hearing Association. (2023). *Early intervention* [Practice portal]. https://www.asha.org/practice-portal/professional-issues/early-intervention/

Balthrop, C., & Coleman, W. (2003, March). *Why is Suzy so weird? Understanding cultural differences in the classroom* [Paper presentation]. Virginia Association for Early Childhood meeting, Richmond, VA.

Boyer, V. E., & Thompson, S. D. (2014). Transdisciplinary model and EI: Building collaborative relationships. *Young Exceptional Children, 17,* 19–32.

Caesar, L. G. (2013). Providing EI services to diverse populations: Are speech-language pathologists prepared? *Infants and Young Children, 26*(2), 126–146. https://doi.org/10.1097/IYC.0b013e3182848340

Coufal, K. L., & Woods, J. J. (2018). Interprofessional collaborative practice in EI. *Pediatric Clinics, 65,* 143–155. https://doi.org/10.1016/j.pcl.2017.08.027

Crawford, M. J., & Weber, B. (2014). *EI every day! Embedding activities in daily routines for young children and their families.* Brookes.

Division for Early Childhood. (2014). *DEC recommended practices in EI/early childhood special education 2014.* http://www.dec-sped.org/recommendedpractices

Dunst, C. J. (2002). Family-centered practices: Birth through high school. *Journal of Special Education, 36*(3), 139–147. https://doi.org/10.1177/00224669020360030401

Dunst, C. J. (2017). Family systems early childhood intervention. In H. Sukkar, J. Kirby, & C. J. Dunst (Eds.). *Early childhood intervention: Working with families of young children with special needs* (pp. 36–58). Routledge.

Dunst, C. J., Bruder, M. B., Trivette, C. M., Hamby, D., Raab, M., & McLean, M. (2001). Characteristics and consequences of everyday natural learning opportunities. *Topics in Early Childhood Special Education, 21*(2), 68–91. https://doi.org/10.1177/027112140102100202

Dunst, C. J., & Espe-Sherwindt, M. (2016). *Family-centered practices in early childhood intervention.* In B. Reichow, B. A. Boyd, E. E. Barton, & S. L. Odom (Eds.), *Handbook of early childhood special education* (pp. 37–55). Springer International.

Dunst, C. J., & Trivette, C. M. (2009). Capacity-building family-systems intervention practices. *Journal of Family Social Work, 12,* 119–143. https://doi.org/10.1080/10522150802713322

Early Childhood Personnel Center. (2017). *Cross-disciplinary personnel competencies alignment.* https://ecpcta.org/cross-disciplinary-competencies/

Hanft, B. E., Rush, D. D., & Shelden, M. L. (2004). *Coaching families and colleagues in early childhood.* Brookes.

Hanson, M. J., & Lynch, E. W. (1990). Honoring the cultural diversity of families when gathering data. *Topics in Early Childhood Special Education, 10*(1), 112–132. https://doi.org/10.1177/027112149001000109

Hebbeler, K., Spiker, D., Bailey, D., Scarborough, A., Mallik, S., Simeonsoon, R., … Nelson, L. (2007). *Early intervention for infants & toddlers with disabilities and their families: Participants, services, and outcomes. Final report of the National EI Longitudinal Study (NEILS).* https://www.sri.com/wp-content/uploads/2021/12/neils_finalreport_200702.pdf

Individuals With Disabilities Education Improvement Act of 2004, Pub. L. No. 108-446, § 632, 118 Stat. 2744 (2004). http://idea.ed.gov/

Individuals With Disabilities Education Improvement Act. (2011). Part C Final Regulations. 34 C.F.R. §§ 303 (2011). https://www.gpo.gov/fdsys/pkg/FR-2011-09-28/pdf/2011-22783.pdf

Infant & Toddler Connection of Virginia. (2003). *Individualized Part C EI supports and services in everyday routines, activities and places.* http://www.infantva.org/documents/wkg-ITF09302003IndividualizedSupportsandServices.pdf

Interprofessional Education Collaborative. (2016). *Core competencies for interprofessional collaborative practice: 2016 update.* https://ipec.memberclicks.net/assets/2016-Update.pdf

Jung, L. A., & Grisham-Brown, J. (2006). Moving from assessment information to IFSPs: Guidelines for a family-centered process. *Young Exceptional Children, 9*(2), 2–11. https://doi.org/10.1177/109625060600900201

Kashinath, S., Woods, J., & Goldstein, H. (2006). Enhancing generalized teaching strategy use in daily routines by parents of children with autism. *Journal of Speech, Language, and Hearing Research, 49*, 466–485. https://doi.org/10.1044/1092-4388(2006/036)

McWilliam, R. A. (2004). EI where it counts: Natural environments. *All Together Now!, 10*(3), 3–6.

McWilliam, R. A. (2010a). Assessing families' needs with the routines-based interview. In R. A. McWilliam (Ed.), *Working with families of young children with special needs* (pp. 27–60). Guilford.

Paul, D., Blosser, J., & Jakubowitz, M. (2006). Principles and challenges for forming successful literacy partnerships. *Topics in Language Disorders, 26*(1), 5–23.

Paul, D., & Roth, F. (2010). Guiding principles and clinical applications for speech-language pathology practice in early intervention. *Language, Speech, and Hearing Services in Schools, 42*(3), 320–330. https://doi.10.1044/0161-1461(2010/09-0079)

Paul-Brown, D., & Caperton, C. J. (2001). Inclusive practices for preschool-aged children with specific language impairment. In M. J. Guralnick (Ed.), *Early childhood inclusion: Focus on change* (pp. 433–463). Brookes.

Peña, E., & Fiestas, C. (2009). Talking across cultures in EI: Finding common ground to meet children's communication needs. *Perspectives on Communication Disorders and Sciences in Culturally and Linguistically Diverse Populations, 16*, 79–85. https://doi.org/10.1044/cds16.3.79

Peredo, T. N. (2016). Supporting culturally and linguistically diverse families in EI. *Perspectives of the ASHA Special Interest Groups, 1*(1), 154–167. https://doi.org/10.1044/persp1.SIG1.154

Puig, V. I. (2012). Cultural and linguistic alchemy: Mining the resources of Spanish-speaking children and families receiving EI services. *Journal of Research in Childhood Education, 26*(3), 325–345. https://doi.org/10.1080/02568543.2012.684421

Raspa, M., Bailey, D. B., Olmsted, M. G., Nelson, R., Robinson, N., Simpson, M. E., Houts, R. (2010). Measuring family outcomes in EI: Findings from a large-scale assessment. *Exceptional Children, 76*(4), 496–510. https://doi.org/10.1177/001440291007600407

Raver, S. A., & Childress, D. C. (2015). *Family-centered EI: Supporting infants and toddlers in natural environments.* Brookes.

Roberts, M. Y., Hensle, T., & Brooks, M. K. (2016). More than "Try this at home"— Including parents in EI. *Perspectives of the ASHA Special Interest Groups, 1*(1), 130–143. https://doi.org/10.1044/persp1.SIG1.130

Ross, K. D. (2018). *Speech-language pathologists in early childhood intervention: Working with infants, toddlers, families, and other care providers.* Plural Publishing.

Rush, D. D., & Shelden, M. L. (2011). *The early childhood coaching handbook.* Brookes.

Searcy, K. L. (2018). Funding and documentation for early intervention (0 to 3 years). In N. Swigert (Ed.), *Documentation and reimbursement for speech-language pathologists: Principles and practice* (pp. 251–291). Slack Incorporated.

Segal, R., & Beyer, C. (2006). Integration and application of a home treatment program: A study of parents and occupational therapists. *American Journal of Occupational Therapy, 60*, 500–510. https://doi.org/10.5014/ajot.60.5.500

SpecialQuest Multimedia Training Library. (2007). *Creating bright futures: Building relationships with families* [Facilitator's guide]. https://eclkc.ohs.acf.hhs.gov/children-disabilities/inclusion-children-disabilities-training-guide/creating-bright-futures-building-relationships-families

Turnbull, A. P., Summers, J. A., Turnbull, R., Brotherson, M. J., Winton, P., Roberts, R., & Stroup-Rentier, V. (2009). Family supports and services in EI: A bold vision. *Journal of EI, 29*(3), 187–206. https://doi.org/10.1177/105381510702900301

Wayman, K., & Lynch, E. W. (1991). Home-based early childhood services: Cultural sensitivity in a family systems approach. *Topics in Early Childhood Special Education, 10*(4), 56–76. https://doi.org/10.1177/027112149101000406

Woods, J., Kashinath, S., & Goldstein, H. (2004). Effects of embedding caregiver-implemented teaching strategies in daily routines on children's communication outcomes. *Journal of EI, 26*(3), 175–193. https://doi.org/10.1177/105381510402600302

Workgroup on Recommended Knowledge and Skills for Service Coordinators (RKSSC), National Service Coordination Leadership Institute Group. (2020). *Knowledge and Skills for Service Coordinators.* https://tinyurl.com/KSSC-8-12-20Final

Chapter 3

Evidence-Based Approaches and Practices in Early Intervention

Learning Outcomes

When we have completed this chapter, we will be able to:

- Discuss research that confirms the period from birth to age 3 years as a critical time in a child's development and the rationale for serving children as early as possible.

- Present current evidence to support family-centered and relationship-based practices, particularly those services offered in the natural environment and based on strengths, routines, and coaching.

- Describe the evidence that supports the importance of collaboration among the EI team and the consideration of a primary provider approach.

- Present current evidence that supports the provision of EI services in the natural environment.

- Share the research that supports how and why family-centered and relationship-based practices are accepted as best practice in EI.

- Recount the empirical data that children learn and develop best within everyday routines, activities, and play as part of their family and community life.

- Provide evidence to support the use of a strengths-based approach to promote the development of new competencies for both young children and families.

- Report the data that support the use of practice-based coaching to teach families and caregivers support strategies that facilitate and expand their children's receptive and expressive language skills.

- Describe the evidence that supports collaboration among the team and consideration of a primary provider approach in EI.

What Will We Learn and How Can We Apply It?

EI services based on evidence-based practices include those that consider the integration of the highest quality research, informed professional judgment and expertise, and family preferences and values (ASHA, 2023; DEC, 2014). The foundation of support for our practice includes both internal and external evidence. Internal evidence is based on policy, informed clinical opinion, values, perspectives of professionals and consumers, as well as professional consensus. External evidence is drawn from empirical research published in peer-reviewed journals. All of these considerations are evaluated in the delivery of EI services to realize positive outcomes for infants, toddlers, and their families (DEC, 2014). Within this chapter, research is presented that supports the period from birth to age 3 as a critical time in a child's development and provides the rationale for serving children as early as possible. The most current evidence regarding family-centered and relationship-based practices, particularly those services offered in the natural environment and based on strengths, routines, and coaching, is shared. Finally, evidence that further supports the importance of collaboration among the EI team and the consideration of a primary provider approach is presented.

Why does the research matter? As SLPs, we want to use strategies and approaches that we know are going to work. We make decisions about our services based on scientific evidence, clinical experience, and the needs of the children and families we serve. Although the data is still emerging and always evolving, it is important we are aware of the available empirical evidence as we consider our options, make our decisions, and provide our services to ensure the children and families in EI are receiving the best evidence-based practices possible. The research matters because it lays the foundation for us to succeed in our role as SLPs in the EI world.

The Importance of Engaging Early

Decades of research yields evidence that a child's earliest experiences play a critical role in brain development. Neural circuits, which create the foundation for learning, behavior, and health, are most flexible during the first 3 years of life. Over time, these circuits become increasingly difficult to change. The neural plasticity, or types and number of neural connections in the brain and the way a child's genes are expressed, can be altered either negatively or positively between birth and 3 years of age (Medina, 2011; National Scientific Council on the Developing Child, 2010). The brain is strengthened by positive early experiences, particularly those that include strong relationships with caring and responsive adults, safe and supportive environments, and appropriate nutrition. Persistent negative stress, such as extreme poverty, abuse and neglect, or lack of connection with caring adults, on the other hand, can damage the developing brain, leading to lifelong problems in learning, behavior, and physical and mental health. Early social and emotional development and physical health serve as the foundation on which cognitive and language skills develop (Medina, 2011; National Scientific Council on the Developing Child, 2010).

There is no doubt EI effectively addresses the development of infants and toddlers who are at risk of delay or who have established disabilities (CDCHU, 2008, 2010; Guralnick, 2019). High-quality EI services can change the trajectory of a child's development and improve outcomes for children, families, and communities. The foundation for all learning over the course of a child's life is established during the first 5 years of life (CDCHU, 2008, 2010; Ramey & Ramey, 2004). As a child ages, this foundation shifts. The best time to begin providing support to children with exceptional needs or to those who are at risk for development difficulties, therefore, is during infancy. A child's brain is highly responsive to early experiences, as these experiences have a direct effect on the neural connections and functions of the brain. EI is important because, although the services cannot eliminate most disabilities, they can have a positive impact on the development of young children and, in fact, lessen the effects of a disability or delay on the child's interactions and participation in everyday life. Services to young children who have or are at risk for developmental delays have been shown to positively affect outcomes across developmental domains, including health (CDCHU, 2010), language and communication (ASHA, 2008b; Joint Committee on Infant Hearing, 2007; McLean & Cripe, 1997; Ward, 1999), cognitive development (Hebbeler, 2009; Hebbeler et al., 2007), and social and emotional development (Hebbeler, 2009; Hebbeler et al., 2007; Landa et al., 2011). Early experiences can have a significant long-term impact on the developmental outcomes of young children regardless of the breadth or depth of their delay or disability (Ramey & Ramey, 2004).

The engagement of family has also been recognized and determined to be of vital importance as children develop (Bailey et al., 2012; Guralnick, 2011; Innocenti et al., 2013). When infants and toddlers who are at risk or have a diagnosed disability and their families are supplied with knowledge, skills, and the support necessary to build a strong developmental foundation, the outcomes are clear. The groundwork is established to develop the communication, language, and social-emotional skills every child needs to enjoy learning, growing, and developing through everyday activities and routines with the people who are most important to them, and to succeed academically. The research is clear: Families who receive EI services are better able to meet their children's special needs from an early age and throughout their lives (Hebbeler, 2009; Hebbeler et al., 2007; Landa et al., 2011).

Some children with established disabilities have delays in one developmental domain (e.g., physical or sensory), whereas others will have delays across multiple domains. Although it is difficult to determine exactly how much children with complex issues benefit from EI, there is strong evidence that the declines in functioning that occur in the absence of EI can be significantly reduced by providing services to a child and their family during the early years (Guralnick, 1997, 1998, 2005; Pungello et al., 2006). The evidence also shows that the stressors and challenges associated with families and children with delays or disabilities are mitigated by EI services (Barnett, 2000; Trohanis, 2008). Intervention is also likely to be more effective and less expensive when offered earlier rather than later in life. As a whole, society benefits economically when EI services are accessible to all families via a decreased need for special education and academic success in the school years (Hebbeler, 2009). The research consistently underscores the importance of EI and supports the positive impact of IDEA Part C services on children, families, and society as a whole (Dawson et al., 2010; Guralnick, 2005, 2011; Hebbeler, 2009; Howlin et al., 2009; Landry et al., 2008; Love et al., 2005; Ludwig & Phillips, 2008; Thomaidis et al., 2000).

Services in the Natural Environment

As presented in Chapter 1, IDEA (2004) states that services for infants and toddlers are to be provided "to the maximum extent possible, in the natural environments including home and community settings in which children without disabilities participate." The philosophy supporting EI within natural environments envisions the parent or caregiver and child interacting and learning as they participate in the typical activities and routines of the family. The natural environment of a young child can include any location where young children, with or without disabilities or developmental delays, spend their time. For most families, natural environments include the family home and child-care setting; they might also include a family member's house, a park, the library, a grocery store, a restaurant, or even a favorite place in the backyard. The evidence-based literature demonstrates that natural environments offer the best opportunities for EI activities and promote inclusion in both family and community activities. Most infants and toddlers learn and develop through caregiving activities embedded within family routines and play in the home and other locations in which they engage, play, and learn. These spaces ensure a safe base for the child to explore and learn.

The provision of EI in natural environments is a legal requirement, but it is also understood as more than a place; engaging with a child and family in a natural environment means more than visiting a home with a bag of toys or treatment materials. Instead, the practice involves engaging in intervention in a location familiar and comfortable for the child, including everyday routines, activities, and events, and involving the family members and caregivers as our partners. Our goal, as EI SLPs, is to help families support their children's development within their natural environments and through their everyday routines and activities. Young children learn best when they are in familiar places, with familiar people, and engage in familiar activities. In 2007, the OSEP TA Community of Practice on Part C Settings: Services in Natural Environments convened a national workgroup and produced several consensus documents on principles and practices that had been validated through research, evidence-based practice, and outreach projects. To support our clarification and engagement of EI services in natural environments, the workgroup determined a set of evidence-based Key Principles and Practices for Providing Early Intervention Services in Natural Environments (Workgroup on Principles and Practices in Natural Environments, 2008). Table 3–1 presents these principles and practices for our consideration.

Table 3–1. Key Principles and Practices for Providing Early Intervention Services in Natural Environments

Infants and toddlers learn best through everyday experiences and interactions with familiar people in familiar contexts.
All families, with the necessary supports and resources, can enhance their children's learning and development.
The primary role of a service provider in early intervention is to work with as well as support family members and caregivers in children's lives.
The early intervention process, from initial contacts through transition, must be dynamic and individualized to reflect the child's and family members' preferences, learning styles, and cultural beliefs.
Individualized Family Service Plan outcomes must be functional and based on children's and families' needs and family-identified priorities.

The family's priorities, needs, and interests are addressed most appropriately by a primary provider who represents and receives team and community support.
Interventions with young children and family members must be based on explicit principles, validated practices, the best available research, and relevant laws and regulations.

Note. Adapted from "Agreed Upon Mission and Key Principles for Providing Early Intervention Services in Natural Environments," by Workgroup on Principles and Practices in Natural Environments, OSEP TA Community of Practice: Part C Settings, 2008. Printed with permission.

Empirical evidence of the efficacy of engaging in EI in natural environments, with a focus on family-centered and routines-based approaches and practices, consistently supports these principles and practices today, and is explored further in the following sections. We then dive deeper into special considerations related to engaging and providing intervention, as well as what it means to implement best practices, in natural environments in Chapter 4 and Chapter 9.

Family-Centered Practices

To ensure EI services are furnished in the natural environment, we must focus on the family's priorities and needs, as well as their capacity and ability to engage effectively with their own child(ren). To be effective SLPs, we must, therefore, engage in family-centered practice. Family-centered practice refers to a way of working with families across service systems to build their capacity to care for and optimize their child's development outcomes. The approach focuses on the important influence of the family on the child's development. Family-centered practice is based on the belief that the best way to meet children's needs is within their families and to engage in services that involve, strengthen, and support families. When family-centered practices are used in EI, we build on the strengths of the family, meet the family's changing needs, collaborate with the family, and support the family's ability to build partnerships with other people and organizations. In turn, the child benefits tremendously from the strong connection and sense of belonging through intentional engagement with their family.

The family-centered approach, which views families as having the capacity to make informed decisions and act on them, differs from models in which professionals make decisions alone or with only the assistance of the family (NRCFCP, 2023). According to the National Resource Center for Family Centered Practice (NRCFCP, 2023), key components of family-centered practice include:

- Spending time with the family to ensure we have comprehensive understanding of their lives, goals, strengths, and challenges and developing a relationship between family and practitioner.

- Engaging with the family to set goals, strengthen capacity, and make decisions.

- Providing individualized, culturally responsive, and evidence-based interventions for each family.

Significant evidence in the literature supports the family-centered model as an effective approach to EI (Cole et al., 2019; Heidlage et al., 2019; McWilliam, 2010a, 2010b; Roberts & Kaiser, 2011, 2015; Rush & Shelden, 2011, 2020; Stredler-Brown, 2017). First, this approach acknowledges and focuses on the important role parents and caregivers play in their child's development. Within the context of EI, both child and parent are the focus of intervention, as addressing the behavior of the family member inherently changes the behavior of the child. Multiple studies have demonstrated the impact of family-centered services on child outcomes. Parents and caregivers can be taught to use both general and specific play, turn-taking, and language support strategies with children with developmental delays, expressive language delays, and autism; outcomes indicate positive and significant effects on social communication, play, and language development in young children with varying degrees of language and cognitive impairment (Heidlage et al., 2019; Killmeyer et al., 2018; Roberts & Kaiser, 2011, 2015). A meta-analysis of 76 studies focused on the use of parent-implemented interventions found that children whose parents and caregivers were taught to use language facilitation strategies made more progress than children whose parents and caregivers were not taught these strategies (Roberts & Kaiser, 2011, 2015).

Using the family-centered approach in our EI practice also has a positive impact on parent empowerment, confidence, and self-efficacy. Research indicates that professionals' use of family-centered practices is positively related to both self-efficacy beliefs and the parents' sense of competence and confidence (Dunst et al., 2007). When working with families within their daily routines, it is important we engage family members as equals when discussing and making decisions. We need to be aware of and address the family's priorities and work on skills within activities and routines both familiar and comfortable to the parents and caregivers (Crawford & Weber, 2014). When we employ these practices, we tend to treat families with dignity and respect; share information to ensure parents can make informed decisions; acknowledge and build on family member strengths; actively engage family members in obtaining resources and support; and are responsive to each family's changing life circumstances (Dunst, 2002; Dunst & Espe-Sherwindt, 2016). The results of several other studies support these findings and report positive relationships between family-centered practices and parent self-efficacy beliefs and parents' psychological well-being (Dempsey & Dunst, 2004; Mas et al., 2018). Strengthening the self-efficacy and well-being of parents and caregivers is important in EI, as these positive outcomes lead to informed family choices and decision making, active involvement by families in achieving desired goals and outcomes, and our own ability to effectively teach developmental strategies and coach parents and caregivers.

Routines-Based Intervention

According to McWilliam (2010b), *daily routines* are defined as "naturally occurring activities happening with some regularity, including caregiving events and simply hanging-out times" (p. 69). RBI is an approach that supports EI within natural environments by embedding instruction within the context of these naturally occurring activities and routines to build the capacity of the family to address the child's strengths and needs (McWilliam, 2010b). Rather than bring toys, books, and other materials into the natural environment, RBI emphasizes family-focused and family-implemented intervention using toys and objects from the family's own home or other natural environments.

We incorporate RBI into our EI practice to establish techniques, such as naturalistic language facilitation or swallowing strategies, to ensure that families can use them to maximize the child's development and learning within their everyday routines and activities (Dunst et al., 2012). These techniques are based on collaboration with the parents, family, caregivers, and other providers to identify typical learning opportunities in the child's home and community; determine the child's interests, strengths, and motivation within their daily routines; and create communication and participation goals during learning opportunities (Dunst et al., 2012). When we practice RBI and collaborate with family members, caregivers, other providers, and educators, we develop child-specific strategies practiced within the family's natural environment (McWilliam, 2010a, 2010b, 2016; Raver & Childress, 2015). Embedding skills and language facilitation strategies within daily routines is an effective way to support parents and caregivers in determining and providing the help their child needs to develop. Because every family activity ultimately bears an opportunity for children to learn, it is important that we work with them to determine and address their priorities, and to teach and target skills within activities and routines familiar to the parent or caregiver. Implementation of this approach encourages practice by the child and their family on a consistent basis and facilitates generalization of the strategies used within treatment sessions between sessions (Crawford & Weber, 2014; Friedman et al., 2012; Woods et al., 2004).

As we have learned, the first guiding principle that supports current best practices in EI focuses on the delivery of family-centered services (ASHA, 2008a). This practice involves working collaboratively with families in all aspects of EI and recognizes the importance of our awareness and inclusion of the beliefs, values, principles, and practices that strengthen the family's capacity to enhance their child's development and learning (IDEA, 2004). RBI builds the capacity of the family to address the child's strengths and needs by embedding instruction within the context of their everyday activities and routines (McWilliam, 2010b). According to Bernheimer and Weisner (2007), "no intervention, no matter how well designed or implemented, will have an impact if it cannot find a slot in the daily routines of an organization, family, or individual" (p. 199). When working with families within their daily routines, it is therefore important that we engage the family members as equals when discussing and making decisions. We need to be aware of and address the family's priorities and work on skills within activities and routines both familiar and comfortable to the parents and caregivers (Crawford & Weber, 2014). It is important that we, as SLPs, work collaboratively with families and engage them in conversations about their values, principles, priorities, and practices. We need to discuss their daily routines, consider their everyday activities, and use these as the context for our intervention visits with the families (Rush & Shelden, 2020). Best practice involves choosing activities and settings that occur often and are considered "high frequency" to make the most of the opportunities for family members to practice and learn when we are not present. It is also important that we check in with the parents or caregivers to determine when or if they have any concerns related to the routines and activities in which we are engaging with their child; because not every skill or strategy might fit into a set time or activity within the day, discussing the outliers to routines could lead to conversations about other important events or issues that might be effectively addressed as well (McWilliam, 2010b; Rush & Shelden, 2020).

The research is clear that children learn and develop best when participating in natural learning opportunities that occur in everyday routines and activities as part of their family and community life; providing intervention within daily routines has been found within multiple studies to be an effective model of intervention delivery (Bernheimer & Weisner, 2007; Crawford & Weber, 2014; McWilliam, 2010b; Rush & Shelden, 2020). Zimmerman et al. (2019) demonstrated that caregivers used more utterances, and lexical diversity in particular during feeding routines than they did in play situations; not only do children engage in eating and feeding multiple times each day, these activities also offer opportunities to address cognitive, language, communication, and social-emotional skills in a functional context without specific or additional expectations on the child.

Empirical evidence supports the approach of embedding skills and strategies within everyday activities and daily routines as an effective way to help parents and caregivers give their children the support to encourage development, increase children's participation in activities with their families, and facilitate carryover of skills when we are not there (Crawford & Weber, 2014).

Learning is what happens between intervention visits, through child-initiated play during everyday routines and activities, with multiple repetitions, and lots of practice; children are more likely to master functional skills that occur through high-frequency activities embedded in their own routines (Dunst et al., 2012).

What About Play?

When we think about family-centered practices and RBI, we need to consider and address the role of play within our services. For those families for whom play is a regular part of their day, a child's natural ability and interest in play can be used when we observe, assess, and engage in EI.

As we work with our families to determine their priorities and goals, we might consider play-based strategies to assess and serve those children for whom play is an everyday activity. Guided interactive play, either modeled by us or through which the parents and caregivers are coached to use supportive strategies, can lead to improved socioemotional, physical, cognitive, and language development (What Works Clearinghouse, 2012). When coaching parents and caregivers, play is an important component of our work. Research supports the use of play, in addition to daily routines, as an effective activity to address parent–child turn-taking, caregiver responsiveness, and language development (Roberts & Kaiser, 2011). Coaching parents and caregivers to imitate their child's actions, gestures, and words in play has also been shown to have a positive impact on both parents' use of imitation strategies and child's use of social eye gaze (Killmeyer et al., 2018).

Play can and should also be considered when we determine goals and outcomes in EI. According to Barton and colleagues (2020), "Play is a critical intervention goal and should be intentionally taught using evidence-based practices" (p. 15). The research concluded that directly addressing play and play skills with toddlers who have developmental deficits and disabilities is effective. Furthermore, strong evidence supports the use of parent, caregiver, and provider modeling of play skills and language with young children with disabilities. Recommendations from this research include the inclusion of a variety of play behaviors, or types of play, the use of a variety of common toys to address play skills, and the incorporation of verbal models about the child's play, as they engage in play, to facilitate their actions and activities (Barton et al., 2020). Again, before targeting play as a foundation for assessment or intervention, we must determine whether it is a part of a family's everyday activities or is already embedded into their routines. Once we have made this determination, play becomes a powerful strategy, in and of itself, to motivate and engage the children with whom we work. Strategies we can use to incorporate play and facilitate the development of play skills with the children and families we serve are further explored in Chapter 9.

Strengths-Based Practice

One of the defining characteristics of family-centered practices is acknowledging and building on the strengths of the parents, family members, and caregivers. Not only is every family unique, but we know that young children respond, develop, and learn in different ways as well. With this knowledge, we need to include opportunities for infants and toddlers to show us what they know and to offer opportunities for children and their families to engage in meaningful and varied learning experiences. Rather than focusing on the child's delays or deficits, the *strengths-based approach* to EI focuses on identifying what works for the infant or toddler and their parents or caregivers.

The evidence supports the consideration and use of the strengths of both children and families as building blocks for promoting the development of new competencies (Campbell et al., 2001; Fenton et al., 2015; Swanson et al., 2011; Trute et al., 2010). McCashen (2005) was one of the earliest architects of the strengths approach, which is based on principles of respect, self-determination, empowerment, social justice and the sharing of power; within the arena of EI, this approach focuses on facilitating and maintaining positive attitudes about the child's and family's dignity, capacities, rights, uniqueness, and commonalities (McCashen, 2005, 2017). The strengths approach emphasizes the capacity of families to take ownership of their priorities, needs, and preferences and to identify, value, and mobilize their strengths, capacities, and resources. Rather than focusing on their deficits and their child's delays or disorder, the approach guides us, as EI providers, to work with families to identify their social, personal, cultural, and structural constraints and empower them to take control of their goals (McCashen, 2005).

The nature of the strengths-based approach to practice in EI also acknowledges and supports the family's language(s) and culture(s) as positive contributors to a child's development (McCashen, 2017). Particularly because of our unique role in regard to a child's communication and language development, this practice also encourages us to view multilingualism as an asset and to support children in maintaining their first language while learning English as a second or additional language (Fenton et al., 2015). We thoroughly examine best practices for providing inclusive services in Chapter 8.

This approach requires that we also engage in a more reflective practice, examine our own values and professional practice, and determine how these could affect each child's learning and development. By developing a reflective stance toward our practice, we are better positioned to develop the skills, knowledge, and approaches necessary for achieving the outcomes that will be most successful and most appropriate for each child and family (McCashen, 2017). We will learn more about how difficult the process of reflection can be for us, as well as for the families with whom we work, as we move into the next discussion regarding practice-based coaching.

Practice-Based Coaching

As SLPs, we might often find it easier to simply "do it ourselves." Empirical data support the empowerment of families by EI providers when we coach caregivers to support their children in their natural environments (Hanft et al., 2004; Roberts et al., 2014; Rush & Shelden, 2020). With the shift to family-centered services under IDEA Part C in 2004, there has also been a shift away from direct one-to-one intervention with the child and toward implementation of an early childhood *practice-based coaching model*. Coaching models focus on family-implemented interventions and collaborative consultation between the service providers and the family members. Coaching in EI is an adult learning strategy that intends to build the family's capacity to enhance their child's development using everyday interactions and activities. EI providers support families during visits by joining the family in their routines and activities and coaching caregivers as they practice using intervention strategies with their children (Roberts et al., 2019; Roberts et al., 2014; Rush & Shelden, 2020). During the initiation of the coaching process, the door is opened to engage in a conversation regarding this approach. We develop a plan together with the parents, which includes the purpose and specific outcomes of the coaching. As noted previously, the purpose within EI is typically to support the child's participation and development in ordinary family and community life. Following the initial discussion, we might choose to observe the parents as they use an existing strategy, try out a new skill, or demonstrate a skill that has been used between visits. We could also observe the parent engaging in an activity with the child. When we have an opportunity to see the parent and child interact, it allows us to (a) see what the parent or family member is doing well, and (b) offer additional suggestions or modifications. Such active guidance serves as an opportunity to build partnerships with families. These partnerships enhance the family members' effectiveness as they engage in everyday learning opportunities with their children (Shelden & Rush, 2001, 2011, 2020).

Although there are various definitions and frameworks of coaching in EI, the most commonly accepted and adopted version is authored by Rush and Shelden (2001, 2011, 2020). They defined coaching as "an adult learning strategy in which the coach promotes the learner's (coachee's) ability to reflect on his or her actions as a means to determine the effectiveness of an action or practice and develop a plan for refinement and use of the action in immediate and future situations" (Rush & Shelden, 2020, p. 8) and presented five evidence-based strategies that lead to the intended and desired outcomes of coaching in EI. Rush and Shelden (2020) recognized that understanding the characteristics of the coaching practice is important to ensure we, as providers, know what steps to take to achieve the desired outcomes. The foundation of these coaching strategies for our work in EI, therefore, is based on evidence that examined the characteristics of coaching that were related to variations in the use of newly learned practices or improvement of existing skills (Rush & Shelden, 2020). Although the literature presents varying steps in the coaching process (Doyle, 1999; Flaherty, 1999; Hanft et al., 2004; Kinlaw, 1999), the research suggests that coaching that leads to intended outcomes includes five characteristics: joint planning, observation, action/practice, reflection, and feedback. Practice-based coaching in EI highlights these characteristics and focuses on the ways in which they are used within natural environments to improve existing abilities, develop new skills, and deepen the understanding of the evidence-based practices by the parents or caregivers being coached (Rush & Shelden, 2020).

Inbar-Furst et al. (2020) identified the plan, act, and reflect (PAR) strategy for coaching parents and caregivers in the natural environment. In the first step of PAR, plan, we collaborate with caregivers to identify goals for the child and family and develop a plan to achieve these goals. During the second step of this approach, in which we act, we observe the parents or caregivers as they interact with the child and demonstrate the identified strategy. As we engage in the third step, reflect, we encourage the parents or caregivers to reflect on their knowledge and skills regarding the strategy they are modeling; we then provide supportive feedback and reflect with them about what went well and how they might engage more effectively with their child (Inbar-Furst et al., 2020). Researchers explored the PAR strategy and found that EI providers report that although they feel comfortable implementing the plan and act components of the strategy, they often struggle to engage family members in the reflection component and often have difficulty providing feedback to caregivers (Inbar-Furst et al., 2020).

Even as service providers in the study highlighted their difficulty with reflection, they also noted the benefits of engaging in this strategy with and for the family. Reflection is an important and empowering tool for families and caregivers and the evidence suggests that those of us who engage in reflection with the families we serve demonstrate better outcomes and more independence in implementation of strategies with their children between sessions (Lorio et al., 2020).

The teach–model–coach–review (TMCR) approach (Roberts et al., 2019; Roberts & Kaiser, 2014) is of particular interest to us, as SLPs, as one that incorporates the practice-based coaching practice to teach families and caregivers support strategies, particularly within the context of play, to facilitate and expand their children's receptive and expressive language skills, and to teach them how to use enhanced milieu teaching (Roberts et al., 2019; Roberts & Kaiser, 2015). This approach is also supported by empirical data, is rooted in adult learning principles, and incorporates the five key strategies of the coaching model presented in Table 3–1 (Dunst & Trivette, 2009; Rush & Shelden, 2020).

Teamwork and Collaborative Practice

Best practice in EI includes coordinated intervention through collaborative practice among and between the service providers. To effectively support the family within the child's natural environment and to support the child's relationship with the family, teamwork is essential. The most current and collaborative approach in EI, and a combination of the layers of teamwork as previously presented, is IPE and IPP. Consistent with the WHO definitions, ASHA (2023) defines IPE as an "activity that occurs when two or more professions learn about, from, and with each other to enable effective collaboration and improve outcomes for individuals and families we serve." ASHA (2023) defines IPP as a service that occurs "when multiple providers from different professional backgrounds furnish comprehensive health care or educational services by working with individuals and their families, caregivers, and communities to deliver the highest quality of care across settings." EI is an interdisciplinary field with a history of collaborative teamwork that has consistently contributed to and benefits from IPP. We need to engage with other service providers and family members within the EI system through interprofessional collaboration to ensure effective and meaningful service delivery. As a member of an interprofessional team, your contributions could vary depending on the knowledge and skills you possess as well as those represented by other service providers and professionals on the team. The Interprofessional Education Collaborative (IPEC, 2016) presented guiding principles and core competencies that intersect with the collaborative team approach required within EI services to ensure the highest quality of services. The IPEC core competencies define the goals and outcomes for both preprofessional preparation and professional practice across disciplines. To deliver effective services in EI, we must embrace and demonstrate services defined and delivered by the framework of these competencies. Table 2–4 presented the IPEC competencies and their intersection with the EI core principles and our own roles and responsibilities.

Potential EI team members include the family, other health care providers, social workers, infant mental health specialists, physicians, caregivers, and preschool teachers. In addition to our role, an EI service team often also consists of an occupational therapist (OT) and physical therapist (PT). OTs work in the development of occupations such as play, social participation, and activities of daily living. Physical therapy offers services to address the physical aspects of the child's development, including gross motor development and mobility. We, of course, focus on verbal and nonverbal communication. We often collaborate with OTs to facilitate feeding and play development, and OTs and PTs often collaborate to encourage the development of motor skills and positioning for play.

Primary Service Provider Approach

IDEA (2004) requires that eligible children and their families have access to a team of professionals from a variety of disciplines. As presented in Chapter 2, the three common models identified in the teaming literature are multidisciplinary, interdisciplinary, and transdisciplinary. These models vary based on levels of team interaction, parent involvement, and approaches to assessment and intervention. We know IDEA Part C requires that services are offered in the child's natural environment because young children learn in the context of everyday activities with the important people in their lives. We also know a child's learning is not restricted to the window of time during which we, or other EI providers, are present. Our role, therefore, is to ensure that parents and caregivers have the knowledge and tools to promote their child's participation and development during everyday natural learning opportunities. The transdisciplinary team model is one in which a group of professionals work collaboratively to share the responsibilities of evaluating, planning for, and implementing EI services for infants and toddlers; this model is widely accepted as best practice in EI (ASHA, 2008a). Typically, one provider is chosen to serve as the primary provider in the transdisciplinary approach. The Mission and Key Principles for Providing Early Intervention guides us to set up our teams to ensure that families are supported by a primary provider, who then receives team and community support to address family priorities (Workgroup on Principles and Practices in Natural Environments, 2008).

The *primary service provider approach* is one way a team is operationalized in accordance with the EI mission and key principles. This evidence-based approach is defined as a process for supporting families of young children engaged in EI services, in which one provider, often the SLP, is identified as the primary service provider for each family. The primary service provider is selected by the team based on the match between their expertise, availability, and the family's needs, preferences, and priorities. The primary service provider then serves as the family's main contact; the close and frequent interaction in this model offers the opportunity for families to establish strong working relationships with one provider (Boyer & Thompson, 2014). The primary service provider then receives support from other team members through consultation and coaching of strategies to specifically include during dynamic assessment and intervention with the child to promote and address a range of child and family priorities (Shelden & Rush, 2022). In the role of primary service provider, one provider dispenses consistent support to the family, backed up by a team of other EI providers who typically engage in services with the child and family through joint home visits with the primary service provider. The intensity of joint home visits depends on child, family, and primary service provider needs. This approach is designed to address some of the problems with the multidisciplinary approach, in which different providers work directly with the child and family, but communication across providers is limited. The primary service provider focuses on EI services that emphasize how children really learn, determines a plan unified around the family's functional needs, capitalizes on the opportunity for families to form close relationships with the primary service provider, and uses the time of the specialist providers as efficiently as possible (Shelden & Rush, 2022).

According to Shelden and Rush (2022), the primary service provider is a member of a larger team and is identified by the team to be the family's main source of support and interaction on behalf of the team. Depending on the needs and priorities of the family, the primary service provider might need minimal consultative support from the team, or they might collaborate more directly with other team members. This approach to teaming is characterized by the use of coaching practices by all service providers to build the capacity of parents, family, friends, or anyone who is a part of the child's support network to promote child learning, growth, and development. This approach also includes building the capacity of other members of the team using a coaching interaction style. The purpose of the teaming interactions is to improve existing abilities, develop new skills, and gain a deeper understanding of how to promote child learning and development within the context of interest- and routine-based, everyday learning opportunities (Shelden & Rush, 2022).

When a team is using a primary service provider approach, each family is a member of the team and has access to the expertise of other providers on the team through the primary service provider. The primary service provider works alongside and collaborates with parents and caregivers to implement the plan developed by the team; they use strategies and information that other providers on the team have shared through collaboration during team meetings or while on joint visits (Workgroup on Principles and Practices in Natural Environments, 2008). This does not mean that families do not interact with more than one team member; instead, all interactions include the primary service provider and serve to support the working relationship between the primary service provider and the caregivers (Shelden & Rush, 2022).

All service providers on each team meet on a consistent basis to ensure the primary service provider is aware when new referrals might be needed (Bell et al., 2010), to coordinate services, and to engage in colleague-to-colleague coaching (Shelden & Rush, 2022). Team meetings also offer facilitated time for ongoing interactions among team members, enabling them to pool and exchange information, build their knowledge and skills, and work together cooperatively (King et al., 2009). Joint visits could occur when primary service providers need support beyond what is gained in team meetings through information sharing and peer coaching. Joint visits in this approach are planned in advance of the sessions and both providers engage in debriefs with the family and each other after the session (Hong & Reynolds-Keefer, 2013; Rush & Shelden, 2008).

The literature supports evidence-based outcomes of the primary service provider approach for both providers and the families who receive EI services. When the primary service provider approach is implemented with these evidence-based guidelines, the impact increases the capacity of both providers and caregivers. This approach has been determined to promote increased caregiver participation and a sense of ownership over the EI process. Additionally, the research indicates each member of the professional team, including primary service providers and supporting providers, experience increases in their own competence and confidence in supporting caregivers, and parents and caregivers experience increased confidence and competence in supporting their children during daily routines and activities (Bell et al., 2010; Moore et al., 2012; Rausch et al., 2021; Shelden & Rush, 2022; Sloper et al., 2006; Yang et al., 2013).

Summary

This chapter provided us with the evidence-based foundations for family-centered practices, practice-based coaching, and strengths-based practices, as well as the rationale for incorporating natural environments, routines, and everyday activities into the provision of EI services. We now have a clear definition of family-centered practices, based on the family systems model, and the foundation of a structure within which to collaborate interprofessionally with colleagues, caregivers, and family members.

We have learned about the evidence that supports a primary service provider approach, as well as how this approach benefits the children and families, and why this is considered best practice within EI. , Our goal is to ensure we engage in exceptional services that come from the heart. With the knowledge covered in this chapter, we can feel confident that the services we are providing are based on a solid foundation of evidence-based practices from which we make our decisions, engage in discussions, and implement intervention with the families with whom we work.

Critical Thinking Questions

1. Why is the period from birth to age three years considered a critical time in a child's development?

2. Present the current research that supports EI practices that are family-centered and provided in the natural environment.

3. What do the family's strengths and routines have to do with the services we provide in EI?

4. Describe the steps involved, and our role within each, when engaged in practice-based coaching with a family.

5. Why is it important we engage in collaboration among our EI team? What is the evidence to support the inclusion of a primary provider approach?

6. How do we know that children learn and develop best within everyday routines, activities, and play as part of their family and community life? How can we apply the evidence to best practice in EI?

7. Provide evidence that supports the use of a strengths-based approach to promote the development of new competencies for both young children and their families.

8. Explain, as if to a family member, why and how the use of practice-based coaching will help them support strategies that facilitate and expand their children's receptive and expressive language skills.

References

American Speech-Language-Hearing Association. (2008a). *Core knowledge and skills in early intervention speech-language pathology practice.* https://doi.org/10.1044/policy.KS2008-00292

American Speech-Language-Hearing Association. (2008b). *Roles and responsibilities of speech-language pathologists in early intervention: Technical report.* https://doi.org/10.1044/policy.TR2008-00290

American Speech-Language-Hearing Association. (2023). *Early intervention* [Practice portal]. https://www.asha.org/practice-portal/professional-issues/early-intervention/

Bailey, D. B., Raspa, M., & Fox, L. C. (2012). What is the future of family outcomes and family-centered services? *Topics in Early Childhood Special Education, 31*(4), 216–223.

Barnett, W. S. (2000). Economics of early childhood intervention. In S. I. Meisels (Ed.), *Handbook of early childhood intervention* (2nd ed., pp. 589–610). Cambridge University Press.

Barton, E. E., Murray, R., O'Flaherty, C., Sweeney, E. M., & Gossett, S. (2020). Teaching object play to young children with disabilities: A systemic review of methods and rigor. *American Journal on Intellectual and Developmental Disabilities, 125*(1), 14–36. https://doi.org/10.1352/1944-7558-125.1.14

Bell, A., Corfield, M., Davies, J., & Richardson, N. (2010). Collaborative transdisciplinary intervention in early years—Putting theory into practice. *Child: Care, Health and Development, 36*(1), 142–148. https://doi.org/10.1111/j.1365-2214.2009.01027.x

Bernheimer, L. B., & Weisner, T. S. (2007). "Let me just tell you what I do all day" … The family story at the center of intervention research and practice. *Infants and Young Children, 20*(3), 192–201.

Boyer, V. E., & Thompson, S. D. (2014). Transdisciplinary model and EI: Building collaborative relationships. *Young Exceptional Children, 17*, 19–32.

Campbell, P. H., Milbourne, S. A., & Silverman, C. (2001). Strengths-based child portfolios: A professional development activity to alter perspectives of children with special needs. *Topics in Early Childhood Special Education, 21*, 152–161. https://doi.org/10.1177/027112140102100303

Center on the Developing Child at Harvard University. (2008). *In brief: The science of early childhood development.* https://harvardcenter.wpenginepowered.com/wp-content/uploads/2007/03/InBrief-The-Science-of-Early-Childhood-Development2.pdf

Center on the Developing Child at Harvard University. (2010). *The foundations of lifelong health are built in early childhood.* https://developingchild.harvard.edu/wp-content/uploads/2010/05/Foundations-of-Lifelong-Health.pdf

Cole, B., Pickard, K., & Stredler-Brown, A. (2019). Report on the use of telehealth in early intervention in Colorado: Strengths and challenges with telehealth as a service delivery method. *International Journal of Telerehabilitation, 11*(1), 33–40. https://doi.org/10.5195/ijt.2019.6273

Crawford, M. J., & Weber, B. (2014). *Early intervention every day! Embedding activities in daily routines for young children and their families.* Brookes.

Dawson, G., Rogers, S., Munson, J., Smith, M., Winter, J., Greenson, J., & Varley J. (2010). Randomized, controlled trial of an intervention for toddlers with autism: The Early Start Denver model. *Pediatrics, 125*, 17–23.

Dempsey, I., & Dunst, C. J. (2004). Help giving styles and parent empowerment in families with a young child with a disability. *Journal of Intellectual & Developmental Disability, 29*, 40–51. https://doi.org/10.1080/13668250410001662874.

Division for Early Childhood. (2014). *DEC recommended practices in EI/early childhood special education 2014.* http://www.dec-sped.org/recommendedpractices

Doyle, J. S. (1999). *The business coach: A game plan for the new work environment.* Wiley.

Dunst, C. J. (2002). Family-centered practices: Birth through high school. *Journal of Special Education, 36*(3), 139–147. https://doi.org/10.1177/00224669020360030401

Dunst, C. J., & Espe-Sherwindt, M. (2016). *Family-centered practices in early childhood intervention.* In B. Reichow, B. A. Boyd, E. E. Barton, & S. L. Odom (Eds.),

Handbook of early childhood special education (pp. 37–55). Springer International.

Dunst, C. J., Raab, M., & Trivette, C. M. (2012). Characteristics of naturalistic language intervention strategies. *Journal of Speech-Language Pathology & Applied Behavior Analysis, 5*, 8–16. https://www.thefreelibrary.com/Characteristics+of+naturalistic+language+intervention+strategies.-a0299887454

Dunst, C. J., & Trivette, C.M. (2009). Capacity-building family-systems intervention practices. *Journal of Family Social Work, 12*, 119–143. https://doi.org/10.1080/10522150802713322

Dunst, C. J., Trivette, C. M., & Hamby, D. W. (2007). Meta-analysis of family-centered help giving practices research. *Mental Retardation and Developmental Disabilities Research Reviews, 13*, 370–378. https://doi.org/10.1002/mrdd.20176.

Fenton, A., Walsh, K., Wong, S., & Cumming, T. (2015). Using strengths-based approaches in early years practice and research. *International Journal of Early Childhood, 47*(1), 27–52.

Flaherty, J. (1999). *Coaching: Evoking excellence in others.* Butterworth-Heinemann.

Friedman, M., Woods, J. & Salisbury, C. (2012). Caregiver coaching strategies for EI providers: Moving toward operational definitions. *Infants & Young Children, 25*(1), 62–82. https://doi.org/10.1097/IYC.0b013e31823d8f12

Guralnick, M. J. (1997). *The effectiveness of early intervention.* Brookes.

Guralnick, M. J. (1998). Effectiveness of early intervention for vulnerable children: A developmental perspective. *American Journal on Mental Retardation, 102*, 319–

345. https://doi.org/10.1352/0895-8017

Guralnick, M. J. (2005). Early intervention for children with intellectual disabilities: Current knowledge and future prospects. *Journal of Applied Research in Intellectual Disabilities, 18*, 313–324. https://doi.org/10.1111/j.1468-3148.2005.00270.x

Guralnick, M. J. (2011). Why early intervention works: A systems perspective. *Infants & Young Children, 24*, 6–28. https://doi.org/10.1097/IYC.0b013e3182002cfe.

Guralnick, M. J. (2019). *Effective early intervention: The developmental systems approach.* Brookes.

Hanft, B. E., Rush, D. D., & Shelden, M. L. (2004). *Coaching families and colleagues in early childhood.* Brookes.

Hebbeler, K. (2009, June 11). *First five years fund briefing; Education that works: The impact of early childhood intervention on reducing the need for special education services* [Paper presentation]. 2019 Congressional Briefing, Washington, D.C., United States. https://files.eric.ed.gov/fulltext/ED522123.pdf

Hebbeler, K., Spiker, D., Bailey, D., Scarborough, A., Mallik, S., Simeonsoon, R., … Nelson, L. (2007). *Early intervention for infants & toddlers with disabilities and their families: Participants, services, and outcomes. Final report of the National EI Longitudinal Study (NEILS).* https://www.sri.com/wp-content/uploads/2021/12/neils_finalreport_200702.pdf

Heidlage, J. K., Cunningham, J. E., Kaiser, A. P., Trivette, C. M., Barton, E. E., Frey, J. R., & Roberts, M. Y. (2019). The effects of parent-implemented language interventions on child linguistic outcomes: A meta-analysis. *Early Childhood Research Quarterly, 50*, 6–23. https://doi.org/10.1016/j.ecresq.2018.12.006

Hong, B. S., & Reynolds-Keefer, L. (2013). Transdisciplinary team building: Strategies in creating early childhood educator and health care teams. *International Journal of Early Childhood Special Education, 5*(1), 30–44.

Howlin, P., Magiati, I., & Charman, T. (2009). Systematic review of early intensive behavioral interventions for children with autism. *American Journal on Intellectual and Developmental Disabilities, 114*, 23–41.

Inbar-Furst, H., Douglas, S. N., & Meadan, H. (2020). Promoting caregiver coaching practices within early intervention: Reflection and feedback. *Early Childhood Education Journal, 48*(1), 21–27.

Individuals With Disabilities Education Improvement Act of 2004, Pub. L. No. 108-446, § 632, 118 Stat. 2744 (2004). http://idea.ed.gov/

Individuals With Disabilities Education Improvement Act. (2011). Part C Final Regulations. 34 C.F.R. §§ 303 (2011). https://www.gpo.gov/fdsys/pkg/FR-2011-09-28/pdf/2011-22783.pdf

Innocenti, M. S., Roggman, L. A., & Cook, G. A. (2013). Using the PICCOLO with parents of children with a disability. *Infant Mental Health Journal, 34*, 307–318. https://doi.org/10.1002/imhj.21394

Interprofessional Education Collaborative. (2016). *Core competencies for interprofessional collaborative practice: 2016 update.* https://ipec.memberclicks.net/assets/2016-Update.pdf

Joint Committee on Infant Hearing. (2007). Year 2007 position statement: Principles and guidelines for early hearing detection and intervention programs. *Pediatrics, 120*(4), 898–921. https://pediatrics.aappublications.org/content/120/4/898

Killmeyer, S., Kaczmarek, L., Kostewicz, D., & Yelich, A. (2018). Contingent imitation and young children at-risk for autism spectrum disorder. *Journal of Early Intervention, 41*(2), 141–158. https://doi.org/10.1177/1053815118819230

King, G., Strachan, D., Tucker, M., Duwyn, B., Desserud, S., & Shillington, M. (2009). The application of a transdisciplinary model for early intervention services. *Infants & Young Children, 22*(3), 211–223. https://doi.org/10.1097/ IYC.0b013e3181abe1c3

Kinlaw, D. C. (1999). *Coaching for commitment: Interpersonal strategies for obtaining superior performance from individuals and teams.* Jossey-Bass.

Landa, R., Holman, K., O'Neill, A., & Stuart, E. (2011). Intervention targeting development of socially synchronous engagement in toddlers with autism spectrum disorder: A randomized controlled trial. *Journal of Child Psychology and Psychiatry, 52*(1), 13–21. https://doi.org/10.1111/j.1469-7610.2010.02288.x

Landry, S. H., Smith, K. E., Swank, P. R., & Guttentag, C. A. (2008). Responsive parenting intervention: The optimal timing across early childhood for impacting maternal behaviors and child outcomes. *Developmental Psychology, 44*, 1335–1353.

Lorio, C. M., & Woods, J. J. (2020). Multi-component professional development for educators in an Early Head Start: Explicit vocabulary instruction during interactive shared book reading. *Early Childhood Research Quarterly, 50*, 86–100.

Love, J. M., Kisker, E. E., Ross, C., Raikes, H., Constantine, J., Boller, K., & Vogel, C. (2005). The effectiveness of Early Head Start for 3-year-old children and their parents: Lessons for policy and programs. *Developmental Psychology, 41*, 885–901.

Ludwig, J., & Phillips, D. A. (2008). Long-term effects of Head Start on low-income children. *Annals of the New York Academy of Science, 1136*, 257–268.

Mas, J. M., Cañadas, M., Balcells, A., Giné, C., Serrano, A., & Dunst, C. J. (2018). Psychometric properties of the Spanish version of the Family-Centered Practices scale for use with families of young children receiving early childhood intervention. *Journal of Applied Research in Intellectual Disabilities, 31*(5), 851–861. https://doi.org/10.1111/jar.12442

McCashen, W. (2005). *The strengths approach*. St. Luke's Innovative Resources.

McCashen, W. (2017). *The strengths approach: Sharing power, building hope, creating change* (2nd ed.). Innovative Resources.

McLean, L. K., & Cripe, J. W. (1997). The effectiveness of early intervention for children with communication disorders. In M. J. Guralnick (Ed.), *The effectiveness of early intervention* (pp. 349–428). Brookes.

McWilliam, R. A. (2010b). *Routines-based EI: Supporting young children and their families*. Brookes.

McWilliam, R. A. (2016). The routines-based model for supporting speech and language. *Revista de Logopedia, Foniatría y Audiología, 36*, 178–184.

Medina, J. (2011). *Brain rules for baby: How to raise a smart, happy child from zero to five*. Pear Press.

Moore, L., Koger, D., Blomberg, S., Legg, L., McConahy, R., Wit, S., & Gatmaitan, M. (2012). Making best practice our practice: Reflections on our journey into natural environments. *Infants & Young Children, 25*(1), 95–105. https://doi.org/10.1097/IYC.0b013e31823d0592

National Resource Center for Family Centered Practice. (2023). *What is family centered practice?* https://nrcfcp.uiowa.edu/what-is-family-centered-practice

National Scientific Council on the Developing Child. (2010). *Early experiences can alter gene expression and affect long-term development*. http://developingchild.harvard.edu/index.php/download_file/-/view/666/

Pungello, E. P., Campbell, F. A., & Barnett, W. S. (2006). *Poverty and early childhood educational intervention*. http://www.law.unc.edu/documents/poverty/publications/pungelloandcampbellpolicybrief.pdf

Ramey, C. T., & Ramey, S. L. (2004). Early learning and school teadiness: Can early intervention make a difference? *Merrill-Palmer Quarterly, 50*(4), 471 491. https://doi:10.1353/mpq.2004.0034

Rausch, A., Bold, E., & Strain, P. (2021). The more the merrier: Using collaborative transdisciplinary services to maximize inclusion and child outcomes. *Young Exceptional Children, 24*(2), 59–69. https://doi.org/10.1177%2F1096250620922206

Raver, S. A., & Childress, D. C. (2015). *Family-centered EI: Supporting infants and toddlers in natural environments*. Brookes.

Roberts, M. Y., Curtis, P. R., Sone, B. J., & Hampton, L. H. (2019). Association of parent training with child language development: A systematic review and meta-analysis.

Journal of the American Medical Association Pediatrics, 173(7), 671–680. https://doi.org/10.1001/jamapediatrics.2019.1197

Roberts, M. Y., & Kaiser, A. P. (2011). The effectiveness of parent-implemented language interventions: A meta-analysis. *American Journal of Speech-Language Pathology, 20*, 180–199.

Roberts, M. Y., & Kaiser, A. P. (2015). Early intervention for toddlers with language delays: A randomized controlled trial. *Pediatrics, 135*(4), 686–693. https://doi.org/10.1542/peds.2014-2134

Roberts, M. Y., Kaiser, A. P., Wolfe, C., Bryant, J., & Spidalieri, A. (2014). The effects of the Teach-Model-Coach-Review instructional approach on caregiver use of language support strategies and children's expressive language skills. *Journal of Speech, Language, and Hearing Research, 57*, 1851–1869. https://doi:10.1044/2014_JSLHR-L-13-0113

Rush, D. D., & Shelden, M. L. (2008). Guidelines for team meetings when using a primary-coach approach to teaming practices. *CASE Tools, 4*(2). https://fipp.ncdhhs.gov/wp-content/uploads/casetools_vol4_no2.pdf

Rush, D. D., & Shelden, M. L. (2011). *The early childhood coaching handbook*. Brookes.

Rush, D. D., & Shelden, M. L. (2020). *The early childhood coaching handbook* (2nd ed.). Brookes.

Shelden, M. L., & Rush, D. D. (2001). The ten myths about providing EI services in natural environments. *Infants and Young Children, 14*(1), 1–13.

Shelden, M. L., & Rush, D. D. (2022). *The early intervention teaming handbook: The primary service provider approach* (2nd ed.). Brookes.

Sloper, P., Greco, V., Beecham, J., & Webb, R. (2006). Key worker services for disabled children: What characteristics of services lead to better outcomes for children and families? *Child: Care, Health & Development, 32*(2), 147–157. https://doi.org/10.1111/j.1365- 2214.2006.00592.x

Shelden, M. L., & Rush, D. D. (2001). The ten myths about providing early intervention services in natural environments. *Infants and Young Children, 14*(1), 1–13.

Swanson, J., Raab, M., & Dunst, C. J. (2011). Strengthening family capacity to provide young children everyday natural learning opportunities. *Journal of Early Childhood Research, 9*, 66–80. https://doi.org/10.1177/1476718X10368588

Thomaidis, L., Kaderoglou, E., Stefou, M., Damianou, S., & Bakoula. C. (2000). Does early intervention work? A controlled trial. *Infants and Young Children, 12*, 17–22.

Trohanis, P. L. (2008). Progress in providing services to young children with special needs and their families: An overview to and update on the implementation of the

Individuals with Disabilities Education Act (IDEA). *Journal of Early Intervention, 30*(2), 140–151. https://doi.org/10.1177/1053815107312050

Trute, B., Benzies, K. M., Worthington, C., Reddon, J. R., & Moore, M. (2010). Accentuate the positive to mitigate the negative: Mother psychological coping resources and family adjustment in childhood disability. *Journal of Intellectual and Developmental Disability, 35*, 36–43. https://doi.org/10.3109/13668250903496328

Ward, S. (1999). An investigation into the effectiveness of an early intervention method on delayed language development in young children. *International Journal of Language & Communication Disorders, 34*(3), 243–264.

What Works Clearinghouse. (2012). *Play-based interventions.* https://ies.ed.gov/ncee/wwc/FWW

Woods, J., Kashinath, S., & Goldstein, H. (2004). Effects of embedding caregiver-implemented teaching strategies in daily routines on children's communication outcomes. *Journal of EI, 26*(3), 175–193. https://doi.org/10.1177/105381510402600302

Workgroup on Principles and Practices in Natural Environments, OSEP TA Community of Practice: Part C Settings (2008, March). *Agreed upon mission and key principles for providing early intervention services in natural environments.* http://ectacenter.org/~pdfs/topics/families/Finalmissionandprinciples3_11_08.pdf

Yang, C. H., Hossain, S. Z., & Sithartham, G. (2013). Collaborative practice in early childhood intervention from the perspectives of service providers. *Infants & Young Children, 26*(1), 57–73. https://doi.org/10.1097/ IYC.0b013e3182736cbf

Zimmerman, E., Connaghan, K., Hoover, J., Alu, D., & Peters, J. (2019). Is feeding the new play? Examination of the maternal language and prosody used during infant-directed speech. *Infant Behavior and Development, 54*, 120–132.

Part II
Early Intervention in Practice

Chapter 4

Considerations for Early Intervention Services in the Natural Environment

Learning Outcomes

When we have completed this chapter, we will be able to:

- Present the primary principles of adult-based learning and how to integrate them into EI sessions.

- Describe three models of practice-based coaching commonly incorporated in EI, general and specific coaching strategies, and considerations for the implementation of effective coaching with families.

- Discuss the importance and ways in which to connect and collaborate with families to provide routines-based intervention that is meaningful and effective.

- Recount strategies to facilitate communication among EI team members, including child-care providers who foster support, development, and growth of all service providers.

- Explain the barriers and opportunities involved in connecting with parents and caregivers when engaged in family-centered practices.

- Provide information related to challenges, approaches, and best practices related to remote service delivery in EI.

- Describe general considerations, including those related to the environment and provide safety and health, which we must address when engaging in EI services.

What Will We Learn and How Can We Apply It?

As an SLP working in EI, engaging with children, families, and caregivers in natural environments should be simple, right? Beyond our current knowledge and skills as SLPs, as EI providers, we also need to teach adults, coach caregivers, collaborate with colleagues, and provide consultative services. These are unique sets of knowledge and skills that support us in our roles of consultant, family educator, and team member. These are in addition to, rather than replacements of, those skills we learn in a traditional speech-language pathology curriculum. Although our traditional training focuses on our abilities to assess and provide intervention with young children, we must also be able to connect with and teach adults, using effective and relationship-enhancing instruction in an environment specifically tailored to meet the needs, priorities, and goals of each individual family. We must be able to engage with our colleagues to engage in consultation in our areas of expertise, as they relate to those areas connected to speech, language, communication, and feeding.

Now, more than ever before, we also need to know how to connect with families via remote learning platforms and telehealth technology. In this chapter, we focus on the awareness, knowledge, and skill set an SLP must have to ensure effective services with young children and their families in natural environments; we also address the unique opportunities and challenges we face to maintain safety and hygiene practices for both ourselves and the families we serve as providers in EI.

The Natural Environment

We have now heard several times that services for infants and toddlers must be offered "to the maximum extent possible, in the natural environments including home and community settings in which children without disabilities participate" (IDEA, 2004, 2011). We have discussed ASHA's five guiding principles of evidence-based best practice in EI as well; the principle that focuses on services that are developmentally supportive and promote children's participation in their natural environments also leads us to the ways in which we implement our services (ASHA, 2008a).

As SLPs, we engage in these services by engaging in authentic experiences, active exploration, and interactions consistent with a child's age, cognitive and communication skills, strengths, and interests to address the family's routines, concerns, and priorities (DEC, 2014). We have also learned that natural environments are not just places where children and their families spend a typical day. They also include those locations where all young children, with or without disabilities or developmental delays, spend their time. For most families, natural environments include the family home and day care, but they might also include a family member's house, a park, the library, a grocery store, a restaurant, or even a favorite place in the backyard. Table 4–1 provides variables, including settings, materials, people, and activities to consider when discussing natural environments with our families in EI.

Table 4–1. Variables Related to Natural Environments

• **Settings** The home and yard, as well as other locations, where the child and family live, learn, and play; settings might include, but are not limited to, a child-care site, relative's home, family member's place of work, park, grocery store, or library.
• **Materials** Any object that is available in the child's physical environment; these materials might include, but are not limited to, toys, rocks, books, swings, grass, spoons, a highchair, or any favorite comfort item.
• **People**

> Anyone with whom the child might interact in their environment on a consistent or regular basis, including (but not limited to) parents, siblings, relatives, friends, neighbors, and teachers.

- **Activities**

> Any activity in which the child and family consistently engages; these activities often involve daily activities and routines (e.g., eating, bathing, and dressing); recreation (e.g., playing, reading, walking, camping, swimming, going to the playground); and community participation (e.g., family and holiday celebrations, cultural practices, faith traditions, shopping, as well as different forms of transportation).

Note. Adapted from "DEC recommended practices in early intervention/early childhood special education 2014," by the Division for Early Childhood, 2014 (http://www.dec-sped.org/recommendedpractices); "Natural Environments Support Early Intervention Services," by the Pacer Group, 2020 (https://www.pacer.org/parent/php/PHP-c178.pdf); "Part C Final Regulations," by the Individuals with Disabilities Education Improvement Act, 2011 (https://www.gpo.gov/fdsys/pkg/FR-2011-09-28/pdf/2011-22783.pdf).

The evidence-based literature demonstrates that natural environments offer the best opportunities for EI activities and promote inclusion in both family and community activities—and these environments do not include a clinical setting. Our goal, therefore, is to help families support their children's development within their natural environments and through their everyday routines and activities. The research indicates that young children learn best, and tend to generalize the skills they acquire, when they are engaged in everyday, natural learning opportunities in familiar places and with familiar people (Chiarello, 2017; Dunst et al., 2001; Hwang et al., 2013; Rush & Shelden, 2020; Trivette et al., 2004). We explore these opportunities and the ways in which to deliver them throughout this chapter.

Adult-Based Learning

Focusing on the adult learner during the visit is something we do not tend to consider often in our SLP training in the EI arena. Integrating *adult-based learning* into our EI visits, however, has the potential to have a big impact on our interactions with the parents or caregivers and the positive outcomes for the child and family. Adult learning strategies are based on several theories and their accompanying principles that support the ways in which we build learning experiences for adults (Dunst & Trivette, 2009b, 2012; Knowles et al., 2005; Trivette et al., 2009). There are multiple ways in which the following adult learning principles can and should be incorporated into our EI services.

Adults Need to Relate New Information to What They Already Know

Adults need to know how new information they are learning relates to what they already know. We need to ask good questions before jumping into intervention. We should find out what, from the parent or caregiver, they have already tried with their child—and build from there. This type of reflection also helps parents learn to connect any new information that we might be presenting with the knowledge and experience they might already have. This type of reflection and discussion will also support the family members in drawing from their own experiences in the future to solve problems when we are not present to offer support.

Adults Need Learning to Be Relevant and Immediately Useful

Adults are motivated when they learn to use new strategies that are relevant, when they recognize their purpose and connection to their current and past experiences and can see how they will be immediately useful to their life and in working with their children. This is the principle on which building intervention on family priorities is based. When we focus on the family's priorities and immediate needs, the parents and caregivers tend to be more involved during decision-making and coaching processes.

Adults Learn Through Active Hands-On Experiences

As adults, we learn much more efficiently and effectively by "doing" than by listening and observing. When we focus on joining the parents or caregivers when they interact with their child during routines or everyday activities, and coach them while they engage with their child, they learn to use the strategies we present much more easily than if they passively observe us with their child. We need to work as a triad, where the child and parent interact, and we support that interaction.

Adults Learn Through Practice and Feedback

Adults need to practice what they are learning and receive feedback to ensure they are on the right track. As SLP students, this is the most effective way in which we learn! When working with families in EI, we need to reflect on how the interaction went between the parent and child with the family by inviting the parent to be an active participant in the reflection process. We can problem-solve together to overcome any challenges and create a plan to ensure the parent will use strategies during other routines, in our absence. The literature supports joint problem-solving as one of the biggest benefits of EI from the perspective of parents and caregivers (Barton et al., 2013; Ingersoll & Dvortcsak, 2006; Wlodkowski & Ginsberg, 2017). When we work together to develop strategies and plan for their use, rather than prescribing activities for the parent and child to do, the result is most often positive outcomes for both family and child.

The Practice of Coaching

We have now learned that evidence-based best practice in EI involves the utilization of adult learning strategies to ensure positive outcomes. Coaching in EI is a collaborative process through which we use a variety of adult learning strategies to support parents and caregivers in developing the skills that will lead to the developmental and learning outcomes of their children (Rush & Shelden, 2011; Shelden & Rush, 2020). Practice-based coaching with the parents, caregivers, and family members, rather than "doing therapy" ourselves, is rooted in adult learning principles (Dunst & Trivette, 2009b, 2012; Trivette et al., 2009). This means we need to meet families where they are; share the knowledge, skills, and strategies we have learned; and build their capacity to support, engage, and teach their children every day and within their own activities and routines. To be effective in our role as SLPs in EI, we cannot keep our strategies to ourselves; we need to teach families how to help their children. This is where coaching becomes an empowering tool to support our services to families. Through effective coaching, parents and caregivers can learn and implement new strategies with their children. They become empowered and feel more prepared to support their children and their needs, and they can carry out EI goals when we are not present or available (Douglas et al., 2017, 2018; Mahoney & MacDonald, 2007; Meadan et al., 2013, 2016; Rush & Shelden, 2011, 2020). To effectively support family-centered practices through coaching, there are different components we need to learn and implement. Three models, in particular, include these components, are frequently encouraged in the literature, and are currently supported by the evidence. All three of these coaching models include activities related to planning, action, and reflection and are based on proven adult learning strategies (Dunst et al., 2010; Trivette et al., 2009).

The first of the three coaching models included in this chapter, the PAR strategy for coaching parents and caregivers in the natural environment, was identified by Inbar-Furst et al. (2020).

- In the first step of PAR, plan, we collaborate with caregivers to identify goals for the child and family and develop a plan to achieve these goals.

- During the second step of this approach, in which we act, we observe the parents or caregivers as they interact with the child and demonstrate the identified strategy.

- As we engage in the third step, reflect, we encourage the parents or caregivers to reflect on their knowledge and skills regarding the strategy they are modeling; we then provide supportive feedback and reflect with the parents or caregivers about what went well and how they might engage more effectively with their child (Inbar-Furst et al., 2020).

The second model, the TMCR approach (Roberts et al., 2014), is of particular interest to us as SLPs, as it incorporates the practice-based coaching practice to teach families and caregivers to support strategies, particularly within the context of play, to facilitate and expand their children's receptive and expressive language skills, and to teach them how to use enhanced milieu teaching (Roberts et al., 2014; Roberts & Kaiser, 2015). Table 4–2 presents the four steps involved in implementation of the TMCR approach and supports our use of this practice in EI.

Table 4–2. Steps to the Teach–Model–Coach–Review Approach

Step 1: Teach	At the beginning of the visit, define and provide a rationale for the strategy that will be used. Describe and explain how and when to use the strategy with the child. Provide examples by engaging in role-play with the parent

	or caregiver or relating the strategy to a previous example. Clarify the parent's understanding and offer an opportunity for questions. If available, provide a handout that reaffirms the information we have provided.
Step 2: Model	Model the strategy with the child. As we demonstrate the strategy, explain to the parent or caregiver when and why we used it. Relate the strategy back to the child's language, behavior, or both. Be sure to include a discussion about when and why we also choose not to use the strategy (i.e., when and how it is effectively used).
Step 3: Coach	Provide the parent or caregiver an opportunity to practice the strategy with their child. Coach the parent to use the strategy effectively by providing feedback, including clearly defined praise, reinforcement, and constructive correction. When we provide constructive feedback, be sure to clarify how the parent might improve or change how they implement the strategy.
Step 4: Review	Discuss how the parent or caregiver felt about the session and, specifically, the use of the strategy. Provide an opportunity for the parent to ask questions. Reinforce how the parent used the strategy and the outcomes of the child's behavior, language, or communication skill. Address any challenging moments or situations that occurred during the session, or that could occur when the parent uses the strategy in the future. Create a plan for the parent to incorporate the strategy into the child's everyday activities or routines.

Note. Adapted from "Effects of the Teach-Model-Coach-Review Instructional Approach on Caregiver Use of Language Support Strategies and Children's Expressive Language Skills," by M. Y. Roberts, A. P. Kaiser, C. E. Wolfe, J. D. Bryant, & A. M. Spidalieri, 2014; "More than 'Try this at home'—Including parents in early intervention," by M. Y. Roberts, T. Hensle, & M. K. Brooks, 2016.

As presented in Chapter 3, the most commonly adopted model of coaching is that which has been consistently studied and supported by Rush and Shelden (2011, 2020). This practice-based coaching tool includes five evidence-based strategies that lead to our implementation of and desired outcomes of coaching in EI (Rush & Shelden, 2020). These strategies include joint planning, observation, action/practice, reflection, and feedback. Table 4–3 illustrates these strategies and presents a description of each for us to include when working with the children and families we serve.

Table 4–3. Characteristics and the Role of the Provider When Coaching in Early Intervention

Joint planning	• At the beginning of the visit, discuss the plan and goals from the last visit with the family members. • Encourage the family to share what they have tried with their child as well as what did and did not work. • Ask the parent or caregiver what they would like to work on this session.
Observation	• Watch the family member(s) play, interact, and engage in their everyday routines and activities with the child. • Ask the parent or caregiver what new strategies they have tried with their child since the last visit. • Show them a strategy to use and encourage them to try the strategy with the child while we observe.
Action	• After observing and learning what they have already tried, choose and model one or more strategies that they might try with the child. • Give the parent or caregiver the opportunity to practice the strategy we modeled for them. • Support the family in their practice of new ways to help their child meet their goals within the context of their everyday routines and activities. • Encourage the family to consider ways in which they can put into action the strategies we consider together.
Reflection	• Ask open-ended questions about what the family members have already tried with their child and what is typical for their family. • Ask questions to help the family reflect on their use of past and new strategies. Inquire about differences they have noted between previous and current practice. • Listen to the family and discuss what has and has not worked, and why their efforts have or have not been successful. Ask the parent or caregiver how they feel as they implement strategies.
Feedback	• In response to the family's reflections, share information, including thoughts, ideas, and

		feedback that might facilitate the determination of additional strategies to best support the family as they work with their child to meet their goals. • Provide the parent or caregiver with verbal coaching as or in response to their use of strategies. Be sure to provide informative feedback that affirms the family's strengths and capacity to support their child's learning and development.
	Joint planning	• At the end of the visit, return to joint planning. • Work with the family to develop a specific plan to address the child's goals between now and the next visit. Schedule our next visit.

Note. Adapted from "The early childhood coaching handbook, 2nd edition," by D. D. Rush & M. L. Sheldon, 2020; "The early intervention teaming handbook: The primary service provider approach," by M. L. Sheldon & D. D. Rush, 2013; "The early childhood coaching handbook," by D. D. Rush & M. L. Sheldon, 2011.

Coaching Strategies

We use both general and specific coaching strategies in EI to ensure services are family-centered and implemented within everyday activities and routines. Although these strategies overlap with those presented by Shelden and Rush (see Table 4–3), they offer our coaching practice an additional layer of support. General strategies include information sharing and observation; specific strategies include direct teaching, demonstration with narration, guided practice, caregiver practice, general and specific feedback, problem solving, reflection, and review (Friedman et al., 2012; Woods et al., 2011). Let's take a closer look at each of these.

General Coaching Strategies

Information sharing: As simple as it sounds, sharing information in each session with the families is an important component of effective coaching. When engaged in this strategy, we exchange information with the parent or caregiver related to the child's and family's IFSP and outcomes. We participate in the exchange by asking and answering questions, sharing comments, and supporting one another. Information sharing is used to gather updates about the family status, child and family outcomes, developmental information resources, and intervention.

Observation: This coaching strategy should occur during routines or family-based activities. The primary role of the parent or caregiver is to interact with the child within a routine or activity, while the role of the SLP is to observe, gather information, and share feedback. We are not a part of the activity itself, although we should be in close proximity.

We should not comment or give specific feedback or suggestions to the family while we are engaged in observation.

Specific Coaching Strategies

Direct teaching: When engaged in direct teaching, we furnish the family with information about a specific strategy, routine, or developmental milestone; the intent of our information sharing is to add to the parents' or caregivers' knowledge and ability to support their child in new ways. This is often an opportunity to share and discuss a handout or view a video clip with the family.

Demonstration with narration: During a coaching session, we will typically take the lead and demonstrate a strategy with the child while the parent or caregiver observes. We want to set up the demonstration by informing the caregiver what we will be doing and why we are choosing to do so. Both during and after the demonstration, we should narrate our actions and intentions with the purpose of modeling for the caregiver how to use the strategy. Demonstration can be repeated as needed or requested by the family, although our goal is to evolve into guided practice by the parent or caregiver.

Guided practice: In guided practice, we support the caregiver when they are practicing intervention strategies in the context of a routine. We guide the interaction by providing specific suggestions about how to use a strategy. The caregiver takes a turn (or multiple turns) to practice using the strategy with the child as we make suggestions during the interaction, or following the routine or activity.

Caregiver practice: The parent or caregiver now takes the lead in their interaction with the child while we observe and support the interaction, as needed. We offer support by giving the parent or caregiver feedback specific to their behavior or the behavior of the child. Our support might include encouragement, verbal prompts, or asking a reflective question following the activity. We are less actively involved when engaged in this strategy than in either guided practice or joint interaction.

General and specific feedback: This strategy is as simple or as complex as the label suggests. We need to give the family feedback regarding their child's behavior or responses or about their own use of strategies with the child. Our feedback might be specific (sharing something we observed) or it could be more general in nature, including encouragement or reinforcement of their efforts and the child's participation. Feedback can be issued both during and after the routine, and we can direct it to either the child or the parent or caregiver. Feedback should occur after observation, guided practice, and caregiver practice.

Problem solving: When we problem solve with the family, we should consider and discuss strategies to improve routines and activities, outcomes, and strategies. Everyone should be offered the opportunity to contribute, define, or clarify solutions to a problem, situation, or concern, and we should work together to develop an action plan for when or how the strategy will be used in the routine.

Reflection: As noted before, reflection is an extremely powerful, evidence-based strategy for us to include in our coaching approach. When engaged in the process of reflection, we communicate with the parent or caregiver to reflect on a particular routine, home visit, strategy, or behavior by the child. We might ask questions or make comments to encourage the family to reflect. We could share our own reflections and impressions and build or expand on the parent's or caregiver's comments to encourage continued reflection. We might also use videos or other tools to create opportunities for reflection.

Considerations for Effective Coaching

One of the most challenging parts of coaching can be finding effective ways to invite parents and caregivers to participate and join in interactions with their children. When families first enter EI services, they are often unfamiliar with family-centered intervention, coaching, or their own role in the process of serving their children. It is important that we explain to families the policies and evidence-based support for parent and caregiver collaboration within EI. Once families understand what is involved in effective collaboration through coaching, they will be empowered to make informed decisions, consider opportunities for the implementation of interventions within their routines and activities, and embrace the practices now inherent in effective EI. What are some of the variables we might consider to support a family's understanding of, and engagement in collaborative coaching?

Consider Proximity and Location

As SLPs, it is natural for us to think first about the relationship between ourselves and the children we serve. When we are working within EI and approaching our services through coaching, however, our role is to teach and collaborate with the family. When we look at our services through this lens, our relationship with the parent or caregiver, and the parent's relationship with the child, suddenly becomes much more important. As coaches, we know the interactions that parents have with their child are primary. One strategy we can use to keep those interactions at the forefront is to either physically place ourselves behind the child rather than in front of them, or to create a triangle between ourselves, the parent, and the child when engaged in an activity. This format breaks up the traditional child–provider dyad and supplies the parents with a physical location from which to engage directly with their child and at their level. Locations that can make this spacing and proximity easier include the couch, a highchair, a table, the floor, or wherever the parent and child typically spend time together.

Begin with Routines

Even after we have described and discussed the use of coaching in our sessions with families, many parents and caregivers will continue to expect traditional therapy when we arrive for our initial visits. Rather than starting with an activity that we initiate, it is often helpful to observe the family engaged in their own natural routines first. We can set the stage for parents and caregivers to get involved by asking what they would be doing if we were not there. This prompt can lead naturally into a mutual discussion about ways to increase interaction and language in everyday activities. If it is snack time and the child heads for the refrigerator or brings us their cup, we can take the opportunity to introduce a word or sign for "eat" or "drink," model and practice prompts for choices to build language, or encourage and accept intentional eye gaze as an initial request. Snack time, diaper changes, and dressing are activities in which families typically engage. Parents are more likely to take the lead, based on their own expectations and activities; this then provides us with the opportunity to naturally support and encourage their interaction.

Model through Play

Often in the early stages of EI with a family, there may be times when we need to engage in traditional therapy or play activities during our visits. If we observe a parent or caregiver who seems less inclined to join the activity or to take the lead, indicates that their child normally plays by themselves while they do other things, or is otherwise hesitant, we might need to be cautious about pushing them too far into a coaching situation. We need to be careful about taking the lead ourselves, however, because we are more likely to lose family interaction when we do not keep it at the forefront of the session. We might need to work intentionally on keeping the parent–child interaction at the forefront. If we are looking at a book and working on pointing out pictures, we might stand or sit behind the child and put the parent or caregiver in front of us or next to the child on the couch. We can then gently coach the parent to ask those "Where's the … ?" questions and help the child point out the pictures. This form of interaction tends to feel much more natural and might be less intimidating for the family. It also increases the chance that the next time the child brings a book to their parent, the parent will point out a few pictures, rather than reading complicated text, because we have practiced this strategy together. If we are engaged in a reciprocal activity (e.g., rolling a ball back and forth), we might have the parent or caregiver join the game more naturally (e.g., rolling the ball to the parent). Most parents and caregivers want to participate with us; we might, however, need to invite them in to play.

Build on Trust

Coaching begins to become effective once we have created positive physical spacing, observed and focused on routines, and successfully engaged the family in interactions with their child. Once we have the parents or caregivers involved, our job is to get out of the way. This might involve gauging your own awareness of your physical presence during the visit and ensuring that the parent–child dyad is in place, even when all you really want to do is jump in between them. We should bring forth suggestions to coach the parent or caregiver and to ensure the child is learning within the activity but should be aware of doing so only as necessary. We want to encourage and reinforce the family's capacity to make the difference and engage in intervention with their child as much as possible by showing them that we trust their abilities.

Wait It Out

When we are building trust and reinforcing the capacity of the families with whom we work, we often need to nod our encouragement and simply wait as they are learning how to engage intentionally together. Once the parents are engaged, we want to avoid pulling them out of an activity and putting attention on ourselves, even if we see an opportunity to model and teach. Once the child initiates a shift in activities, however, we might take the opportunity to open a discussion with the parent or caregiver. Following an initial statement of reinforcement (e.g., "Wow, you were able to get their attention quickly when you blew that bubble"), we might reflect together on the strengths and challenges of the interaction. We can then engage in brainstorming strategies. When parents reflect first, we give them an opportunity to think about how an activity went before we add to their thoughts. This reflection encourages them to seek out and focus on opportunities for even greater interaction during the time when we are not with them.

Although it can be challenging to encourage parents to join in on interactions during visits, paying attention to our words and actions can help us to create space for parents and caregivers to actively participate, rather than watching us play or engage with their child.

Coaching is a tool for us to use when we interact with families and caregivers, to help them think purposefully about what they are doing and how they are engaging with their child. When we successfully incorporate coaching into our EI practice, we discover that our visits become more about what the parent or caregiver is learning than about which questions we ask or which skill the child needs to learn. Coaching is a powerful tool to ensure families are empowered and recognize their capacities to make the difference for and with their young children—and for the rest of their lives.

Routines-Based Intervention

As is now evident, each of the approaches, models, and tools we have been discussing overlap intentionally within EI. We have learned that RBI supports EI within natural environments by embedding instruction, often within the context of coaching, through activities and routines that occur as a daily part of each family's life; this approach builds the capacity of the family and supports their abilities to address their child's strengths and needs (McWilliam, 2010b; Woods et al., 2011). Rather than bringing toys, books, and other materials into the natural environment, RBI means that we focus on the family and the intervention by using toys and objects from the family's own home or other natural environments.

When working with families within their daily routines, it is important that we engage with them as equal members of our team, particularly when discussing plans for intervention and making decisions. We must be aware of and address the family's priorities, needs, and choices to focus on skills within activities and routines both familiar and comfortable to the parents and caregivers (Crawford & Weber, 2014; McWilliam, 2010b). It is important that we work collaboratively with families and engage them in conversations about their values, principles, priorities, and practices (DEC, 2014). To base intervention on routines, we must determine, with the families, what their everyday routines and activities are; we can then use these as the context for our intervention visits with the families (McWilliam, 2010b; Rush & Shelden, 2020). Best practice involves choosing activities and settings that occur often and are considered high-frequency activities to make the most of the opportunities for family members to practice and learn when we are not present.

It is also important that we check in with the parents or caregivers to determine when or if they have any concerns related to the routines and activities in which we are engaging with their child; because not every skill or strategy might fit into a set time or activity within the day, discussing the outliers to routines could lead to conversations about other important events or issues that might be effectively addressed as well (McWilliam, 2010b; Rush & Shelden, 2020). RBI is regarded as best practice in EI because we know that embedding strategies in everyday routines results in increased opportunities for the child to learn. When we consider and discuss family routines, we can think about either general or specific activities. If we think more generally, we might consider that all families eat meals, have snack times, give their children baths, and change their child's diaper or use the bathroom throughout the day. Although this is generally true, how any given routine works for each family will be unique. To really understand how each routine or activity works within the dynamics of each unique family, we need to ask parents and caregivers specific questions to find out what makes them work. When we consider that our role is to help the family think through how to support their child, and we are not expected to, nor should we provide all the answers, we discover that intervention strategies become more individualized because we work together to brainstorm, and problem solve. We can engage in RBI with the family on a meaningful level. With this goal in mind, Table 4–4 presents a series of questions we may ask families that support the focus of our practice on routines and everyday activities.

Table 4–4. Questions to Support the Focus of Families on Routines and Everyday Activities

Choose a routine (e.g., bath time, bedtime, snack time) or individualized activity in which the family and child already engage every day. What are the questions we can ask the family to focus on intervention?	**How does this question support and empower the family to take ownership of and focus on intervention with their child?**
How does [routine] work for you and your child? Tell me about what happens before, during, and after [routine].	Present this question to explore the specifics of the routine. Ideally, we want to observe the routine as we ask these questions. If this is not possible, these questions provide us with the opportunity to brainstorm and problem-solve with the family for the next time they are engaged in the activity. We want to think and talk broadly and beyond the routine; be sure to explore what happens before and after, especially when a routine is difficult for the family.
Which parts of [routine] do you think go well? Which parts are challenging and/or tricky for you, your child, or both? Why?	Help the family reflect on their thoughts about the routine and avoid making any assumptions.

	This question helps parents and caregivers learn to think through how to solve problems and use strategies during routines on their own.
What do you do during [routine]? What does your child do? Why?	We want to determine what the child and each family member does (or does not do) during the routine. This information can provide great insight into both interactions and expectations. It also provides opportunities to brainstorm shifts in roles and responsibilities within routines.
Which parts of this routine does your child like to do? What parts does he not enjoy doing?	When we learn what the child likes to do, family members and we are better equipped to build interventions around the child's interests and what is naturally motivating to them. This question also helps us figure out where the problems might be and what might be causing them.
If you could change one part of [routine], what would it be? Why?	Asking this question provides us with another layer to coach the parent or caregiver and to build on their ability to problem-solve and plan for using strategies independently.
How do you think your child could learn to _____ during [routine]?	We want to help the family think through how a strategy might work, how their child might engage differently, and what their child might learn within a routine or everyday activity. We will often be impressed by the amazing ideas families have, once provided with the opportunity to think through an activity with their child. This question also supports the sense of confidence and competence by parents and caregivers as they realize how well they know their own child.

What strategy would you like to try during [routine] this week?	It is always important to be intentional with a plan to ensure the family knows how to use strategies between visits. We should encourage the parent or caregiver to identify which strategies they want to try and plan together for how the strategy will be implemented. Remember to check back in about how everything went during the next visit.

Note. Adapted from "7 specific questions to ask when exploring family routines," by D. Childress, 2012 (https://www.veipd.org/earlyintervention/2012/12/12/6-specific-questions-to-ask-when-exploring-family-routines/)

To ensure focused and effective routines-based services, we must embed the practice within each step of the EI process. The processes involved in a routines-based approach will be integrated into our professional development throughout this textbook, as we learn more about best practices for evaluation and assessment in Chapter 6, how to determine and write functional outcomes in Chapter 7, the integral elements to inclusive practice in Chapter 8, and treatment in Chapter 9.

Collaboration and Teamwork

The coordination and collaboration of the team is critical to ensuring EI outcomes are successful. EI teams include providers from different disciplines working together to present the most effective services for children and their families. Every member of the EI team, including each family member with whom we work, brings unique knowledge, skills, abilities, and experiences. When team members collaborate and communicate well with one another, all participants reap the benefits from the comprehensive services. Access to all necessary supports and services, the provision of skills and resources from multiple agencies, and the sharing of information and opinions across areas of expertise are just a few of the benefits of teams collaborating within the system. Collaboration among team members gives us all the opportunity to develop and coordinate services that complement one another. When we communicate well, and collaborate with our colleagues across disciplines, as well as with family members, we also benefit from joint professional development and consultation that results in enhanced knowledge and skills (Boyer & Thompson, 2014; Coufal & Woods, 2018). There are numerous ways in which we might assist our team members, and for our team members to assist us that result in expanding our knowledge, learning new practices and implementing novel strategies with each family with whom we engage.

Connecting With Other Service Providers

Just as there are strategies involved in coaching and communicating with families, strategies to facilitate communication and collaboration among team members to help one another learn and grow as providers exist as well. These all lead back to the practice of mutual support among and between the providers on the EI team. How do we effectively engage and practice support of one another?

- It is important to take the time to become acquainted with our team members' professional interests, skills, and areas of expertise. Getting to know one another furnishes us with the knowledge and ability to identify who on the team might need specific or unique assistance.

- Engaging in authentic learning experiences with our team members ensures everyone has opportunities to explore novel concepts, ideas, and theories; and to learn new strategies, tools, and approaches. Through these experiences we also learn to trust one another and to recognize how and when we can lean on each other as needed.

- We need to maintain an open mind and a willingness to both share and receive information and expertise with our team members. By establishing an environment in which honesty, respect, and supportive feedback are typical among its members, our team will consistently develop and learn new knowledge and skills to share with children and families.

- We can and should receive and offer support and guidance to our team members in a nonjudgmental manner. Knowing that we can receive constructive support from our team members and being able to offer advice or assistance without a team member having to ask, are effective practices for a successful collaborative and interprofessional team.

- It is important to offer sufficient time for each team member, ourselves included, to expand knowledge and skills through practice and reflection. Using a coaching practice similar to one we might use with our families, we can mentor (and be mentored by) other team members to learn new strategies, methods, and models of working with young children and their families in EI.

Connecting With Families

In keeping with the legal requirements and spirit of IDEA (2004), we know families are expected and encouraged to play a central role in the EI process. Family-centered practices include both relationship building and participation by and with the parents and caregivers. Involving parents and caregivers seems like a logical and even natural thing to do, but engaging parents as equal and inclusive members of the EI team is not always an easy or simple process. In EI, developing a relationship between ourselves and the families we serve is essential. Developing a collaborative relationship, however, might not always be easy. There are three potential barriers to creating and ensuring collaboration. First, we are typically taught to engage in services through the traditional "expert" model. We work within their disciplinary area to evaluate, make recommendations, and treat individual children. It is difficult for some

SLPs to consider, and even more so to shift, from a discipline-specific to a transdisciplinary model. The transdisciplinary model requires us to serve in different roles and to share our knowledge openly with others. This approach requires effective communication with other providers and families. Most important, the goal of the transdisciplinary model is to serve families, rather than just the child. Second, parents often expect to engage in a more passive role when involved in EI services; they expect that their children will be the recipients of our services. Based on what we now know is best practice and will result in the most positive outcomes, parents are expected to play an active role in their child's evaluation and intervention services. To this end, parents need to have a stronger knowledge of the available services and the system. They also need to have effective communication skills, and in general, be a contributing member of the team. Most parents have not been prepared in any way to fulfill these expectations. It might be difficult, therefore, for some family members to participate as active members of our EI team. Third, the engagement by parents and caregivers on our EI teams requires a collaborative relationship. The evidence supports effective collaboration as a method to provide better services for young children and their families. What belief systems and qualities, however, need to be in place for us, as providers, and parents or caregivers to engage in truly collaborative relationships? According to Edmondson (n.d.), the personal qualities necessary for effective relationships include mutual respect, honesty, trust, openness, listening skills, sensitivity, communication skills, and empathy.

How might we connect with the families and build on the personal qualities that serve to ensure we are building a strong relationship and encouraging the family to be active and involved members of the EI team? We need to remember that building a relationship takes time. Developing mutual trust and respect only comes when we work together with parents and caregivers to listen, demonstrate respect for all perspectives and experiences, and contribute to the achievement of the family's desired goals and outcomes.

Maintaining Professional Boundaries

Establishing and maintaining a collaborative relationship with families while upholding *professional boundaries* adds an additional challenge to our role and can be tricky for any provider in EI. It is therefore important to build rapport while also maintaining boundaries. To build rapport, sharing some personal information can be helpful when getting to know the family. Knowing what is appropriate to share, how much, and how to handle situations when families want more information about us is an important consideration when working closely with families. Another aspect of maintaining professional boundaries involves knowing how deeply to become involved in a family member's personal life. Parents often share a great deal about their lives with us, particularly when presented with challenging circumstances. It is ultimately our responsibility to know when we are becoming too involved. When professional boundaries are crossed, it becomes difficult to serve the family objectively in a manner that makes them feel empowered to help themselves. Maintaining professional boundaries is an ongoing and important process for every EI provider. Because we work so closely with families, the boundaries can become blurred. This can happen for both provider and parent or caregiver; ultimately, it is our responsibility to maintain the boundary. EI providers often meet families at emotionally charged times and continue to support them over an average of 18 months or longer. Working together, week after week, it is natural that close relationships will develop. It is also likely that interventionists will offer different kinds of support, depending on the needs of the family. Providing informational and emotional support is a very real part of this work and can be done in a professional manner. Table 4–5 examines several strategies we might consider using to maintain professional boundaries while supporting the children and families with whom we work.

Table 4–5. Strategies to Establish and Maintain Professional Boundaries

Be mindful of how much and what type of personal information we share	Before we share personal information and experiences with a family, we need to consider how it will benefit or possibly harm the relationship we are building or have already built. We should be cautious about sharing information about our own families. Visits are a time for us to focus on what is happening in the child's and family's life—not in ours.
Be thoughtful about our role as a supporter and partner	Part of building rapport and trust with families is developing a friendly relationship around the services we provide. Being friendly, however, is not the same as being friends. Developing friendships with parents and caregivers is often discouraged; there is a risk that once a professional boundary is crossed, it can compromise our ability as service providers to remain objective. A personal friendship can also compromise the parent's ownership of and ability to ask for changes to the Individualized Family Service Plan, if and as needed.
Redirect requests for personal information or advice	Parents and caregivers will occasionally ask for information or advice as part of casual conversation. When we work closely with families, this is not unexpected. If we are asked for information that crosses a professional boundary, however, we should try to redirect the conversation back to the intervention activity. If necessary, it is appropriate to respond more directly as well; we might tell the parent or caregiver we are not allowed to disclose certain personal information (e.g., home phone number).
Offer to link families with others to	Many programs have parent groups or ways in

provide them with an effective support structure	which parents can connect with families with similar interests or whose children have similar needs; these groups provide a support structure in which they can learn from and lean on one another. When a parent is in need of social support, we should take the initiative to connect them with others who can fill that need.

Connecting With Child-Care Providers

A natural environment in which we often engage in EI services is a child-care or home day-care center. Many children spend their entire day, up to 5 days a week, in a center with their peers while growing, learning, and developing under the supervision of their child-care providers. We will often implement EI services in these centers, but this environment might present its own unique challenges. Keeping in mind that the child-care providers in these centers serve as primary caregivers to the children we serve, a challenge worth considering is creating a connection and effectively collaborating with child-care providers.

Strategies for Working in Child-Care Centers and With Child-Care Providers

Child-care settings are ideal for EI services. Because many children spend up to 10 hours per day and 5 days per week in their child-care center, this environment is certainly considered a natural setting for us to engage with the children. These centers typically have consistent schedules, embedded routines, child-centered and play-based activities, and consistent opportunities for peer interaction. Child-care providers and teachers who serve as primary caregivers in these settings are considered viable EI team members; effective collaboration with child-care providers facilitates intervention, including generalization of services when we are not present, support for child outcomes, and the opportunity for us to share EI information with families through the providers. Additionally, there is evidence to support that inviting child-care providers to join the EI team and coordinate our services with intention can improve child and family outcomes (Weglarz-Ward et al., 2020).

The research indicates that child-care providers have a strong interest and willingness to participate in the EI process (Mohay & Reid, 2006; Weglarz-Ward et al., 2019). Yet, providers in both childcare and EI struggle to effectively communicate and collaborate with each other (DeVore & Hanley-Maxwell, 2000; Mohay & Reid, 2006; Wong & Cumming, 2010). When working in a child-care setting, however, it is not unusual for the expectation of the child-care provider to be that we will remove the child from the classroom to engage in our services. Child-care providers are often not aware of or knowledgeable about best practices in EI and might expect that we will take the child to another room to engage in traditional therapy. When we do remain in the classroom, we can be surrounded by a cadre of children and struggle to address the needs of the child we are visiting. What are the strategies for addressing the child-care provider's expectations and effectively shifting our services to implement best practices in the natural environment of the child's classroom?

If a family requests that we engage with their child in their child-care setting, it is important to first establish a respectful and collaborative relationship with the child-care provider(s). We should take time to learn about the child-care center and its programs, including their philosophy, approach, schedule, routines, and provider responsibilities and expectations. In turn, we can share information about the EI process, our own role, our expectations, and what the child-care provider can expect during an EI visit. With the family's permission, we should share and discuss the child's IFSP, including the child's and family's priorities, needs, challenges, and goals. We should communicate and clarify the child-care provider's role in EI as well. Table 4–6 offers strategies and points for discussion when working with child-care providers as SLPs in EI.

Table 4–6. Strategies for Collaborating Effectively With Child-Care Providers

Be respectful of child-care providers and their authority in their own classroom. Recognize the multiple responsibilities of the child-care providers, including oversight of an entire group of children, and be flexible within visits.
Verbalize to child-care providers how important they are as members of the EI team. Clearly provide information about the EI process, our own role and expectations, and what the child-care provider can expect during a visit.
Take the time to observe the center and the specific classroom in which we are providing services. Learn the schedule, routines, and expectations of the child-care providers working with the child. We want to ensure we are making suggestions for strategies that are relevant, functional, and meaningful within this environment.
Model techniques for child-care providers and discuss how these support the child's outcomes. Help the providers brainstorm their own strategies, try them out, and problem solve to ensure that they feel confident using them when we are not present.
Embed intervention techniques and strategies within the center's daily routines, materials, activities, and peer interactions.
Use the coaching tools and embed time with child-care providers to discuss and reflect on what has been working with the child and where the challenges lie. Be sure to let the child-care providers know we will spend a lot of time talking with them, modeling for them, and coaching them through various strategies during their activities in the classroom.

Once we have explored the possibilities for coaching and intervention with the child-care provider and have helped them understand what our purpose and approach is in serving the child in EI at their center, we should have the stage set for effective engagement and collaboration. Mutual respect, clear communication, and teamwork will keep us in the classroom and support our EI services in this natural setting.

Remote Service Delivery

Multiple terms are currently used to describe the methodology in which services are implemented with young children and families through video or audio technology to connect service providers and educators with parents and other caregivers in ways that support their child's development throughout everyday activities and routines. These terms include *remote service delivery, remote learning, distance learning, telehealth, teletherapy, telepractice, virtual home visits,* and *virtual learning* (Poole et al., 2022). The term *telehealth* is the most common when specifically addressing reimbursement of live video conferencing under Medicaid and private health insurance plans. Therefore, the term *remote service delivery* is used to discuss the range of services available via technology, and the term *telehealth* is used to discuss the use of video conferencing to proffer services in EI (Poole et al., 2022).

Just a few years ago, providing EI via remote service delivery or telehealth was already possible through the use of advanced tools; several remote training programs for families, caregivers, and service providers; and protocols for direct clinical services (Buzhardt & Meadan, 2022). At that point in time, these protocols and processes were viewed as an option through which to expand access to evidence-based practices, regardless of location. Remote services in EI were typically used in special circumstances and with specific populations, including families who lived in remote areas or those who were restricted in participating in home visits. In the spring of 2020, however, the landscape shifted when the COVID-19 pandemic forced EI programs to stop, or severely limit, face-to-face interactions between children, families, caregivers, and providers. Suddenly, we had an immediate need to engage in both remote and telehealth services, including screening and diagnostics, direct intervention services, clinical consultation, professional development and training, assessment administration, and support for services in natural environments (Buzhardt & Meadan, 2022). Over the past 4 years, the demand for remote services and telehealth in EI has resulted in swift, widespread changes in how infants, toddlers, and their families receive services. These changes have included the way in which technology is used to afford access across diverse populations, practical considerations for providers, and the evidence that has emerged to support the approaches through which we should engage and connect with children, parents, and caregivers when providing remote services in EI.

When technology is used to engage in remote EI services, it is imperative that it is used effectively for all participants. Although telehealth has been the most common service to support remote EI services, this requires broadband internet access for all participants. Because not all families, caregivers, or service providers have adequate resources to support remote engagement, we need to consider other approaches as well (Poole et al., 2022). These remote approaches could include web-based training modules, email or text communications between telehealth sessions, telephone consultations, and the creation of videos by parents and caregivers for our review and later coaching and feedback. Many families might also find these remote alternatives to telehealth to be as or more effective, as either an alternative or supplement to video conferencing, and some even prefer the option to participate in EI via remote services. Both the DEC (2020) and the Early Childhood Technical Assistance Center (ECTA, 2020) have published recommendations related to features of video conferencing platforms to consider for use in EI (Edelman, 2020).

In addition to using approaches that are accessible and effective for everyone involved, there are several practical considerations when providing remote services in EI. These include updates that have been made regarding the sources of funding that support services. The ECTA (2023) has also compiled resources to support the navigation of billing for telehealth services through Medicaid and private insurance. According to the U.S. Department of Health and Human Services (DHHS, 2023), the Centers for Medicare and Medicaid Services have also expanded the types of telehealth services now reimbursable, including EI services. An additional practical consideration involves the secure delivery of remote services. It is important to protect the personal information of the families when engaging in telehealth, but they might have limited home resources that do not adhere to strict Health Insurance and Portability and Accountability Act (HIPAA) security requirements. Within the past 2 years, in response to the overwhelming need for telehealth services during the COVID-19 pandemic, the U.S. Department of Health and Human Services (DHHS, 2023) stated that providers "may use popular applications that allow for video chats, including Apple FaceTime, Facebook Messenger video chat, Google Hangouts video, Zoom, or Skype, to provide telehealth without risk [of] penalty for noncompliance with the HIPAA rules delivering services securely."

In regard to best practices in EI when engaging in remote service delivery, recent research supports our use of telehealth as an effective alternative or supplement to face-to-face methods to offer diagnostic and assessment services (Ferguson et al., 2019; Greenwood et al., 2022; Wallisch et al., 2019). According to the literature, we primarily and effectively use coaching when providing remote services to parents, caregivers, and even siblings by embedding strategies into their everyday routines and activities that promote the child's engagement, development, and learning. Current evidence indicates that our use of coaching and direct intervention in the EI arena is effective (Akemoglu et al., 2022; McCarthy et al., 2019; Poole et al., 2022).

Despite the current evidence that supports our use of telehealth and remote service delivery in EI, the practice is often easier discussed than implemented and comes with its own challenges. In Chapter 9, we explore challenges and opportunities we could face when engaging in remote service delivery in EI.

General Considerations

When working in the natural environment and engaging with families, we need to be ready for anything. We will often need to problem solve when confronted with safety, health, and hygiene (or lack thereof) situations. We might be faced with and need to handle difficult situations that involve when and how to report suspected child abuse and neglect. We must be flexible in our approaches to these challenges and see them as opportunities to connect, as each family requires a unique approach to benefit from EI services.

Safety and Health Considerations

Providing best practices and quality services in EI are our greatest priorities. Because these best practices mean providing services primarily in settings considered natural to the family, we consider our own personal safety and other issues unique to providing services outside of clinic or center-based settings. Visiting families in natural environments means we are often on our own in unfamiliar locations. It is important that we share our schedule with others, including the dates and times during which we will be at specific locations. It is also a good idea to keep a cell phone with us, for safety purposes, when engaged in visits; we should keep the ringer turned off out of respect for the family we are visiting. Visiting families with another staff person is also considered appropriate, particularly when we feel uncomfortable in an environment on our own. Maintaining our own safety ensures that we will have the opportunity to effectively share our knowledge and skills with families. Additional suggestions for ensuring our safety during EI visits in natural environments include the following (Partnership for People with Disabilities, 2010):

- Always have our cell phone on our body.

- Car keys should be kept in our pocket or on our body; do not leave them on a table or place them on the floor.

- Be aware of our clothing; dress in comfortable clothing and wear only simple jewelry.

- Do not take a wallet or purse into a family's home. Any personal belongings should be kept in the trunk of the car prior to arriving at our destination.

- Clearly document visits, particularly if there is anything that feels uncomfortable or causes concern. These concerns should be discussed with a supervisor as soon as possible.

- Visit families who live in areas where safety may be a concern with a colleague.

- Engage in visits during daylight hours.

- Survey the area thoroughly before leaving the car or the home; be aware of any signs of danger.

- When possible, park on the street instead of in the driveway. Ensure the car will not be blocked in by other vehicles.

- When walking to the car, always have keys available.

- Make eye contact and be friendly with people in the area while walking to and from a family's home.

- Be aware of limits and ask for help when needed. We need to learn to trust our instincts; if we feel uncomfortable in a home or in a situation, do not hesitate to politely leave.

As SLPs, we should also take precautions to ensure we are considering the health and wellness of all participants when engaging in EI visits. There are a number of ways in which we can protect ourselves as well as the children, and their family members. These include washing hands before and after the EI session, wearing a mask during the visit, particularly if anyone is not feeling well or has recently recovered from an illness, and practicing social distancing between ourselves and family members. When possible, the EI visit might be held outside to limit close contact between individuals in an indoor environment; effective outdoor natural environments in which to connect with children and families could include a backyard, playground, or open space in the neighborhood.

Managing an Unclean Environment

Each environment in which we engage in services might present a different level of cleanliness. The challenge that faces us is maintaining the balance between respect for the family and comfort for ourselves while providing services in these environments. The Partnership for People with Disabilities (2010) offers several suggestions to increase our comfort while providing family-centered services:

- Wear clothing that can be easily laundered; keep a change of clothing in the car.

- Keep hand sanitizer in the car and approved disinfecting wipes in the trunk to clean any materials used during the visit.

- Bring a large book or small blanket to spread out on the floor on which everyone can sit and play.

- Keep in mind that we are in someone's home and, although it may not be as clean as our own standards, it may suit the family's needs and expectations.

- Recognize that, if the unclean environment is truly a health hazard to the child (e.g., roaches in the child's bedroom, spoiled formula in the infant's bottle, an unsafe heating element), we need to communicate with the family about the issue and offer to assist in finding a solution. If the family is unable or unwilling to act to correct the health hazard, we may need to speak with our supervisor and file a report with Child Protective Services (CPS).

In addition to our own comfort, we also want to be sure we are connected to and recognize the needs of the child and family. This means we need to keep an open mind and avoid sharing our own judgments about the living situation. Unless we have health or safety concerns, we need to ignore the challenges in the environment as much as possible. If we do determine a need to address our concerns, we must do so in a respectful manner and be specific about how our concern relates to the child's health or safety. At the same time, we should not be expected to ignore our own discomfort. It is our responsibility to be flexible and meet families wherever they are, but we also have our own feelings to consider. If we are in an environment that makes us uncomfortable, we should talk to our supervisor for support and guidance.

Reporting Child Abuse and Neglect

EI personnel, including SLPs, are mandated reporters of suspected child abuse or neglect in all states. As mandated reporters, service providers are required to report suspected child abuse or neglect. The circumstances under which a mandatory reporter must make a report vary from state to state. Therefore, it is important we become familiar with how to make a report in our area, what information CPS needs, and any documentation required when making a report. We should also be aware of internal policies within our agency for making CPS reports.

According to the Child Welfare Information Gateway (2019), a report must be made if or when we, in our official capacity, suspect or have reason to believe that a child has been abused or neglected. Another frequently used standard is the requirement to report in situations in which we have knowledge of, or observe a child being subjected to, conditions that would reasonably result in harm to the child. As mandatory reporters, we are required to report the facts and circumstances that could lead us to suspect that a child has been abused or neglected. We do not have the burden of providing proof that abuse or neglect has occurred. Although it is an aspect of the job that we hope we will not have to think about often, reporting suspected child abuse or neglect is always difficult.

Summary

This chapter offered an evidence-based foundation and advice for providing best practices within natural environments, in addition to suggestions for establishing a positive and safe work environment. As providers working in EI, we often need to think and work beyond our traditional SLP knowledge and skill set. Although our traditional training focuses on our abilities to assess and engage in intervention with young children, we must also be able to connect with and teach adults, using effective and relationship-enhancing instruction in an environment specifically tailored to meet the needs, priorities, and goals of each individual family. We must be able to offer consultation to both families and colleagues in our areas of expertise, as they relate to those areas connected to speech, language, communication, and feeding. We need to know how to teach adults, coach caregivers, collaborate with colleagues, and furnish consultative services. More than ever before, we also need to know how to connect with families via remote learning platforms and telehealth technology. In this chapter, we discussed the tools, strategies, skills, and considerations needed to provide effective services to young children and their families in natural environments; we also considered the unique opportunities and challenges regarding safety and hygiene we might face when engaging in EI.

Critical Thinking Questions

1. Describe the primary principles of adult-based learning and how to integrate them into EI sessions.

2. What are the three models of practice-based coaching commonly incorporated in EI? Name at least 3 general and 3 specific coaching strategies. What do we need to consider in order to effectively implement effective coaching practices with the families we serve?

3. How can we connect and collaborate with families to provide routines-based intervention that is meaningful and effective?

4. Present at least 2 strategies we can incorporate to facilitate effective communication among our EI team members to foster support, development, and growth of all service providers. Are these the same strategies we might incorporate into our work with childcare providers? Why or why not?

5. What are the barriers and opportunities involved in connecting with parents and caregivers when engaged in family-centered practices?

6. What are the challenges we may face, approaches we may take, and best practices we can incorporate when working with families in EI via remote service delivery?

7. Describe general considerations, including those related to the environment and provider safety and health, we must address when engaging in EI services.

8. Present at least two do's and two don'ts for maintaining professional boundaries. What strategies can we use to establish and maintain professional boundaries?

9. What strategies can we use when visiting a home that would be considered an unclean environment? What advice can we give to a new EI provider faced with this situation?

References

Akemoglu, Y., Hinton, V., Laroue, D., & Jefferson, V. (2022). A parent-implemented shared reading intervention via telepractice. *Journal of Early Intervention, 44*(2), 190–210.

American Speech-Language-Hearing Association. (2007). *ASHA SLP health care survey 2007: Caseload characteristics.* https://www.asha.org/uploadedFiles/research/memberdata/HC07CaseloadRprt.pdf

American Speech-Language-Hearing Association. (2008b). *Roles and responsibilities of speech-language pathologists in early intervention: Guidelines.* https://doi.org/10.1044/policy.GL2008-00293

Barton, E. E., Pribble, L., & Chen, C. I. (2013). The use of e-mail to deliver performance-based feedback to early childhood practitioners. *Journal of Early Intervention, 35*(3), 270–297.

Boyer, V. E., & Thompson, S. D. (2014). Transdisciplinary model and early intervention: Building collaborative relationships. *Young Exceptional Children, 17*, 19–32.

Buzhardt, J., & Meadan, H. (2022). Introduction to the special issue: A new era for remote early intervention and assessment. *Journal of Early Intervention, 44*(2), 104–109.

Chiarello, L. (2017). Excellence in promoting participation: Striving for the 10 Cs—Client-centered care, consideration of complexity, collaboration, coaching, capacity building, contextualization, creativity, community, curricular changes, and curiosity. *Pediatric Physical Therapy, 29*, 16–22. https//doi.10.1097/PEP.0000000000000382

Child Welfare Information Gateway. (2019). *Mandatory reporters of child abuse and neglect.* Washington, DC: U.S. Department of Health and Human Services, Children's Bureau. https://www.childwelfare.gov/pubpdfs/manda.pdf

Childress, D. (2012). 7 specific questions to ask when exploring family routines. *Early Intervention Strategies for Success: Tips, Insight, and Support for EI Practitioners.* https://www.veipd.org/earlyintervention/2012/12/12/6-specific-questions-to-ask-when-exploring-family-routines/

Coufal, K. L., & Woods, J. J. (2018). Interprofessional collaborative practice in early intervention. *Pediatric Clinics, 65*, 143–155. https://doi.org/10.1016/j.pcl.2017.08.027

Crawford, M. J., & Weber, B. (2014). *Early intervention every day! Embedding activities in daily routines for young children and their families.* Brookes.

Department of Health and Human Services. (2023). *Telehealth for providers: What you need to know.* https://www.cms.gov/files/document/telehealth-toolkit-providers.pdf

DeVore, S., & Hanley-Maxwell, C. (2000). "I wanted to see if we could make it work": Perspectives on inclusive childcare. *Exceptional Children, 66*, 241–255.

Division for Early Childhood. (2014). *DEC recommended practices in early intervention/early childhood special education 2014.* http://www.dec-sped.org/recommendedpractices

Douglas, S. N., Kammes, R., & Nordquist, E. (2018). Interactive online communication training for parents of children with autism spectrum disorders. *Communication Disorders Quarterly, 39*(3), 415–425.

Douglas, S. N., Nordquist, E., Kammes, R., & Gerde, H. (2017). Online parent communication training for young children with complex communication needs. *Infants & Young Children, 30*(4), 288–303.

Dunst, C. J., Bruder, M. B., Trivette, C. M., Hamby, D., Raab, M., & McLean, M. (2001). Characteristics and consequences of everyday natural learning opportunities. *Topics in Early Childhood Special Education, 21*(2), 68–91. https://doi.org/10.1177/027112140102100202

Dunst, C. J., & Trivette, C. M. (2009b). Let's be PALS: An evidence-based approach to professional development. *Infants and Young Children, 22*(3), 164–176.

Dunst, C. J., & Trivette, C. M. (2012). Moderators of the effectiveness of adult learning method practices. *Journal of Social Sciences, 8*(2), 143–148.

Dunst, C. J., Trivette, C. M., & Hamby, D. W. (2010). Meta-analysis of the effectiveness of four adult learning methods and strategies. *International Journal of Continuing Education and Lifelong Learning, 3*(1), 91–112.

Early Childhood Technical Assistance Center. (2023). *Remote service delivery and distance learning.* https://ectacenter.org/~pdfs/topics/disaster/Planning_for_the_Use_of_Video_Conferencing_in_EI_during_COVID-19_Pandemic.pdf

Edelman, L. (2020). Planning for the use of video conferencing for early intervention home visits during the COVID-19 pandemic. Author. https://ectacenter.org/~pdfs/topics/disaster/Planning_for_the_Use_of_Video_Conferencing_in_EI_during_COVID-19_Pandemic.pdf

Ferguson, J., Craig, E. A., & Dounavi, K. (2019). Telehealth as a model for providing behaviour analytic interventions to individuals with autism spectrum disorder: A systematic review. *Journal of Autism and Developmental Disorders, 49*(2), 582–616. https://doi.org/10.1007/s10803-018-3724-5

Friedman, M., Woods, J., & Salisbury, C. (2012). Caregiver coaching strategies for early intervention providers: Moving toward operational definitions. *Infants & Young Children, 25*(1), 62–82. https://doi.org/10.1097/IYC.0b013e31823d8f12

Greenwood, C., Higgins, S., McKenna, M., Buzhardt, J., Walker, D., Ai, J., ... Grasley-Boy, N. (2022). Remote use of individual growth and development indicators (IGDIs) for infants and toddlers. *Journal of Early Intervention, 44*(2), 168–189.

Hwang, A. W., Chao, M. Y., & Liu, S. W. (2013). A randomized controlled trial of routines-based early intervention for children with or at risk for developmental delays. *Research in Developmental Disabilities, 34*(10), 3112–3123. https://doi.org/10.1016/j.ridd.2013.06.037

Inbar-Furst, H., Douglas, S. N., & Meadan, H. (2020). Promoting caregiver coaching practices within early intervention: Reflection and feedback. *Early Childhood Education Journal, 48*(1), 21–27.

Individuals With Disabilities Education Improvement Act of 2004, Pub. L. No. 108-446, § 632, 118 Stat. 2744 (2004). http://idea.ed.gov/

Individuals With Disabilities Education Improvement Act. (2011). Part C Final Regulations. 34 C.F.R. §§ 303 (2011). https://www.gpo.gov/fdsys/pkg/FR-2011-09-28/pdf/2011-22783.pdf

Ingersoll, B., & Dvortcsak, A. (2006). Including parent training in the early childhood special education curriculum for children with ASD spectrum disorders. *Journal of Positive Behavior Interventions, 8*(2), 79–87.

Knowles, M. S., Holton, E. F., & Swanson, R. A. (2005). *The adult learner: The definitive classic in adult education and human resource development* (6th ed.). Elsevier.

Mahoney G., & MacDonald J. (2007). *Autism and developmental delays in young children: The responsive teaching curriculum for parents and professionals.* PRO-ED.

McCarthy, M., Leigh, G., & Arthur-Kelly, M. (2019). Telepractice delivery of family-centered early intervention for children who are deaf or hard of hearing: A scoping review. *Journal of Telemedicine and Telecare, 25*(4), 249–260.

McWilliam, R. A. (2010b). *Routines-based early intervention: Supporting young children and their families.* Brookes.

Meadan, H., Ostrosky, M. M., Santos, R. M., & Snodgrass, M. R. (2013). How can I help? Prompting procedures to support children's learning. *Young Exceptional Children, 16*(4), 31–39. https://doi.org/10.1177/1096250613505099

Meadan, H., Snodgrass, M. R., Meyer, L. E., Fisher, K. W., Chung, M. Y., & Halle, J. W. (2016). Internet based parent-implemented intervention for young children with autism: A pilot study. *Journal of Early Intervention, 38*, 3–23.

Mohay, H., & Reid, E. (2006). The inclusion of children with a disability in child care: The influences of experience, training and attitudes of child care staff. *Australian Journal of Early Childhood, 31*, 35–42.

Partnership for People with Disabilities. (2010). *Kaleidoscope: New perspectives in service coordination* [Trainer's notebook]. Virginia Commonwealth University: Author.

Poole, M., Fettig, A., McKee, R., & Gauvreau, A. (2022). Inside the virtual visit: Using tele-intervention to support families in early intervention. *Young Exceptional Children, 25*(1), 3–14. https://doi.org/10.1177/109625620948061

Roberts, M. Y., Hensle, T., & Brooks, M. K. (2016). More than "Try this at home"—Including parents in early intervention. *Perspectives of the ASHA Special Interest Groups, 1*(1), 130–143. https://doi.org/10.1044/persp1.SIG1.130

Roberts, M. Y., & Kaiser, A. P. (2015). Early intervention for toddlers with language delays: A randomized controlled trial. *Pediatrics, 135*(4), 686–693. https://doi.org/10.1542/peds.2014-2134

Roberts, M. Y., Kaiser, A. P., Wolfe, C. E., Bryant, J. D., & Spidalieri, A. M. (2014). Effects of the teach-model-coach-review instructional approach on caregiver use of language support strategies and children's expressive language skills. *Journal of Speech-Language and Hearing Research, 57*(5), 1851–1869. https://doi.org/10.1044/2014_JSLHR-L-13-0113

Rush, D. D., & Shelden, M. L. (2011). *The early childhood coaching handbook.* Brookes.

Rush, D. D., & Shelden, M. L. (2020). *The early childhood coaching handbook* (2nd ed.). Brookes.

Shelden, M. L., & Rush, D. D. (2013). *The early intervention teaming handbook: The primary service provider approach*. Brookes.

Trivette, C. M., Dunst, C. J., & Hamby, D. (2004). Sources of variation in consequences of everyday activity settings on child and parenting functioning. *Perspectives in Education, 22*(2), 17–36. https://eric.ed.gov/?id=EJ687912

Trivette, C. M., Dunst, C. J., Hamby, D. W., & O'Herin, C. E. (2009). Characteristics and consequences of adult learning methods and strategies. *Research Brief, 3*(1), 1–33.

Wallisch, A., Little, L., Pope, E., & Dunn, W. (2019). Parent perspectives of an occupational therapy telehealth intervention. *International Journal of Telerehabilitation, 11*(1), 15–22.

Weglarz-Ward, J. M., Santos, R. M., & Hayslip, L. A. (2020). What early intervention looks like in child care settings: Stories from providers. *Journal of Early Intervention, 42*(3), 244–258. https://doi.org/10.1177/1053815119886110

Weglarz-Ward, J. M., Santos, R. M., & Timmer, J. (2019). Factors that impact inclusion in child care settings: Perspectives from child care and early intervention providers. *Early Childhood Education Journal, 47*(163), 163–173. https://doi.org/10.1007/s10643-018-0900-3

Wlodkowski, R. J., & Ginsberg, M. B. (2017). *Enhancing adult motivation to learn: A comprehensive guide for teaching all adults*. Wiley.

Wong, S., & Cumming, T. (2010). Family day care is for normal kids: Facilitators and barriers to the inclusion of children with disabilities in family day care. *Australian Journal of Early Childhood, 35*, 4–12.

Woods, J. J., Wilcox, M. J., Friedman, M., & Murch, T. (2011). Collaborative consultation in natural environments: Strategies to enhance family-centered supports and services. *Language, Speech, and Hearing Services in Schools, 42*(3), 379–392.

Chapter 5
Current Levels of Functioning

Learning Outcomes

When we have completed this chapter, we will be able to:

- Explain why it is important for SLPs in EI to have a solid foundation of knowledge regarding all early development domains.

- Present detailed expectations and milestones related to early communication development, including those associated with prelinguistic communication and use of gestures, receptive and expressive language development, and speech sound development.

- Define domains and concepts related to cognitive development and executive functioning, the development of play, social-emotional development, adaptive development, and physical development including motor, oral motor, and sensory development.

- Share expectations and developmental milestones between birth and 3 years in the areas of cognition and executive functioning, play, social-emotional, adaptive, and physical development, including those related to motor, oral motor, vision, and hearing.

- Discuss how all developmental domains intersect and affect one another as a child learns and grows, and why SLPs need to consider all areas of development over time.

- Recount the influence of cultural and linguistic diversity, as well as many other factors, on a young child's acquisition of knowledge and skills across all developmental domains.

What Will We Learn and How Can We Apply It?

As SLPs at this point in our education and practice, we have a solid foundation of knowledge regarding communication, speech, and language development. If we are committed to providing effective services to children and families through EI, we must also be confident in our grasp of all early developmental domains. From birth, the minds of children are active and inquisitive and many of the foundations of learning are established in their earliest years of life. To implement best practices for infants and toddlers who have or could be at risk for developmental delays or disabilities (and their families), therefore, we need to have a broad and deep view of early development and expected milestones in all areas.

Our awareness must be focused on a child's holistic development. In addition to speech, language, and communication, it is our responsibility to be able to define terms, concepts, and development expectations related to the following domains: Cognition and executive functioning; play; adaptive, self-help, and feeding skills; social connections and emotions; and physical skills, including gross and fine motor, vision, and hearing.

This chapter presents developmental milestones across each of these domains and provides us with information about how each relates and is connected to speech, language, and communication development. We need to understand how these domains intersect and affect one another as a child learns and grows and consider all areas of development to ensure every child's communication, speech, and language skills will continue to develop over time. As we review the milestones presented throughout this chapter, it is important to recognize the influence of cultural and linguistic diversity, as well as many other factors, on a child's acquisition of knowledge and skills across all developmental domains. We consider these variables in this chapter, and we discuss those factors involved in providing inclusive services in detail in Chapter 8.

Communication, Language, and Speech Development

When serving children and families in EI, we can only be effective providers if we have a clear understanding of the holistic development of a child and how the development of one domain, or lack thereof, contributes to and affects the others. At the same time, as SLPs, our expertise lies in our knowledge regarding communication, speech, and language development. We will, therefore, begin with a review of these developmental skills and expectations of the young children we serve.

Communication Development

Communication is the active process of exchanging information and ideas (ASHA, n.d.). The process includes the use of both nonverbal behavior (i.e., eye gaze, facial expression, and gestures) and verbal behavior (i.e., speech or spoken language) to tell others what we want, express our feelings, share ideas, and solve problems. Becoming a successful communicator means a child can send clear messages to others as well as tune into, understand, and respond to other people's messages. When children communicate effectively, they express their needs, wants, feelings, and preferences. Even before children begin developing speech sounds and formal language, however, they learn to communicate with their parents and caregivers through gestures and nonverbal means. Infants and toddlers also learn to share experiences, thoughts, and emotions through social communication strategies. It is important we understand prelinguistic and social communication expectations to encourage and support.

Prelinguistic Communication and the Use of Gestures

Prelinguistic communication describes behaviors children display, both intentional and unintentional, to communicate their wants and needs (ASHA, n.d.). Some behaviors are natural reactions, whereas others are more purposeful to access and refuse items, participate in a social interaction, and give and receive more information. The prelinguistic stage is considered the period between birth and when a child begins to use words and signs to interact with others. During this time, young children begin to use eye gaze, attend to sounds and words, and use facial expressions and affective vocalizations to communicate. Their use of gestures and other nonverbal means begins to emerge. The development of prelinguistic communication builds the foundation for later developing skills, including the use of words (or signs) and the ability to combine these into sentences to communicate. As children engage in intentional attempts to receive and send messages, they begin to demonstrate an understanding and emerging appreciation of the details related to successful communication (Crais & Ogletree, 2016).

When we consider our interactions with young children, their earliest communication is through use of their hands rather than their mouths (Goldin-Meadow, 2015). Infants begin to use gestures as early as 8 or 9 months of age. Within the window of 8 to 18 months, infants and toddlers demonstrate several important milestones in gesture development. Table 5–1 presents these milestones and the ages at which they are expected to emerge.

Table 5–1. Gesture Development of Infants and Toddlers

What type of gesture?	When should we expect this gesture to emerge?	What does the use of this form of gesturing look like?
Deictic gestures	10 months (prior to the onset of spoken language)	• Pointing to or drawing attention to an object or event in the child's immediate environment. • The child first holds up an object to show someone; they then give an object to someone; they eventually point toward a specific object, location, or event.
Ritualized requests	9–13 months	• Requesting gestures include reaching with an open-and-closed grasping motion, putting an adult's hand on an object, and pulling an adult's hand toward a desired item or action.
Play schemes	12 months	• Actions carried out on an object to demonstrate the object's function (e.g., drinking out of a toy cup). • Through their use of play schemes, children demonstrate

		a capacity for symbolic representation and provide insight into their semantic knowledge.
Iconic gestures	Before a child has acquired 25 words	• Also known as representational or symbolic gestures. • A child uses these gestures to illustrate an aspect of the item or action they represent (e.g., blowing to indicate bubbles; flapping their arms to represent a bird). • Some iconic gestures are culturally defined, such as waving as a form of greeting
Gestures or spoken words	12–18 months	• Children use either a gesture or a word; they do not yet combine them.
Gesture + speech combinations	18 months	• Children first use complementary gestures (e.g., points to a dog and says "dog"). • Quickly begin to produce supplementary gestures (e.g., points to a dog and says "big").

Note. Adapted from "Gesture development: A review for clinical and research practices," by N. Capone & K. McGregor, 2004; "Gesture as a window onto communicative abilities: Implications for diagnosis and intervention," by S. Goldin-Meadow, 2015; "Gestural communication in children with autism spectrum disorders during mother-child interaction," by M. Mastrogiuseppe, O. Capirci, S. Cuva, & P. Venuti, 2015.

Recognizing and supporting the development of gestures with the young children we serve is important. The milestones related to infant and toddler gestural development provide us with an index of developing cognitive abilities and help us predict when certain language milestones might emerge. The use of specific gestures also precedes the onset of spoken language. This is exciting because it means we can use a young child's gestures as a gauge to anticipate and encourage the development of language (Goldin-Meadow, 2015). Based on research by Goldin-Meadow (2015) and Capone Singleton and Saks (2015), empirical data support the following connections between the use of gestures and emerging language skills in early childhood:

- Children who produce more gestures early develop larger expressive vocabularies.

- When parents and caregivers are coached in EI and model gesture–word pairs within routines and everyday interactions with their infants, the children begin to use symbols earlier.

- An infant or toddler who points intentionally at objects is likely to learn the words for those objects within 3 months.

- Children produce gesture + word combinations before word + word combinations.

- Those children who frequently use gestures to supplement or support their communication attempts are likely to use relatively complex sentences several years later.

- Children who convey a wide variety of different meanings via gestures early are likely to have larger expressive vocabularies than those children who use limited gestures.

- The age at which a young child first produces a complementary gesture about a noun (e.g., points to a ball and verbalizes "ball") precedes and predicts the onset of their use of determiner + noun combinations in speech (e.g., "the ball").

We discuss how to assess gestures and ways in which we might incorporate the use of gestures with our families to support their child's speech and language development in later chapters.

Social Communication

By the age of 5 years, children are expected to have the skills needed to engage in conversation with others (ASHA, n.d.). To become successful communicators, we must be aware of and understand the unspoken rules of conversation. Acquiring these skills, however, is a process that begins at birth and develops as infants and toddlers acquire a specific set of skills; it is important that we, as SLPs serving families in EI, know what these milestones are to support the children's development of social communication.

In the first few months of life, children are fascinated with faces, especially their mother's or primary caregiver's face. Being interested in their mother is the first step an infant takes toward socializing with others. Toward the end of the first year of life, an infant becomes even more sociable, indicating interest in the things their caregivers point to, and sometimes even saying their first words. Even when a child is not talking as they enter toddlerhood, they are expected to be sending clear messages through their attention toward others and their use of gestures. They begin by giving or holding objects with the intention of getting their parents' attention and then progress to simple gestures (Sussman, 2016). By the end of the second year, children are socializing with others by using words to communicate a variety of needs and wants or to simply engage with others. Table 5–2 presents the social communication milestones young children are expected to meet between birth and age 3.

Table 5–2. Social Communication Milestones from Birth to Age 3

Age Range Within Which Skill Is Expected	Milestone
Birth–12 months	• Prefers looking at the human face and listening to the human voice • Looks for the source of a voice • Differentiates between tones of voice (e.g., angry vs. friendly) • Smiles back at the parent or caregiver • Vocalizes to call others, and also when another person calls • Indicates a desire for a change in activities • Participates in speech routine games (e.g., peek-a-boo) • Performs for social attention
12–18 months	• Imitates other children • Initiates turn-taking routines • Points to, shows, or gives objects to others • Uses more words to engage in during turn-taking • Uses words to protest
18–24 months	• Uses words to interact with others • Takes one-two turns within a conversation • Able to maintain topic in adjacent pairs of utterances (e.g., responds to a question with a related answer) • Uses vocalizations and words when engaged in pretend play
24–36 months	• Take 4-5 turns within a conversation • Verbally introduces and changes topic • Expresses emotion • Relates own experiences • Begins to provide descriptive details to support the listener's comprehension • Use attention-getting words • Uses some politeness terms or markers • Understands and begins to follow rules • Incorporates familiar activities in play (e.g., haircut, grocery shopping)

Note. Adapted from "Components of Social Communication," by the American Speech-Language and Hearing Association, n.d. (https://www.asha.org/practice-portal/clinical-topics/social-communication-disorder/components-of-social-communication/); "The Rossetti Infant Toddler Language Scale," by L. Rossetti, 2005.

Language Development

Based on the presentation of milestones related to both prelinguistic and social communication, it is clear why we must consider the early development of these skills as an integral component of the development of language.

Receptive Language Development

Receptive language encompasses our ability to understand and comprehend spoken language. Typically, young children can understand language before they are capable of producing it. Within just the first month of a child's life, he or she begins to show awareness of a speaker by quieting to a familiar voice, moving in response to a voice, and even attending to the speaker's mouth. Early in their development, infants learn where information seems to come from and to focus their attention toward that specific direction. Newborns are also able to discriminate between angry and friendly voices, and react accordingly, by the end of their first month of life. Between birth and the first birthday, an infant is learning to comprehend the world. These little humans continue to show awareness of a speaker as they grow, and their receptive language skills continue to develop. By 1 year of age, children can recognize, stop, and look at person when their own name is called, look at familiar people when named, and maintain attention to the speaker. Infants are also able to follow simple directions embedded within routines or everyday activities. They learn to respond with gestures or vocalizations to adult verbalizations. Even though they do not yet have the expressive language skills to verbalize, they are beginning to understand when an adult or older child talks to them, they are expected to respond. Ultimately, before a child is 1 year old, he or she is already learning to understand the rules of conversation. By the time toddlers are 18 months old, they should understand an entire arsenal of vocabulary and are learning approximately six new words a day. These words will typically relate, again, to the child's everyday activities and routines. They learn through repetition of the words and the objects, actions, or pictures that go along with the words. At this stage, a young child will only learn words and concepts that have a concrete symbol that goes along with them (Levey, 2014; Owens, 2019).

By the time children are between 2 and 3 years of age, their receptive language skills are becoming more refined and more complex. They are beginning to understand more abstract concepts, and vocabulary does not have to be quite as concrete as it once was for older toddlers to process the meaning. With this in mind, 2-year-olds can answer more questions, follow more complex directions, and process information beyond the "whole" to understand and identify features and parts of objects and people (Levey, 2014; Owens, 2019).

Receptive language is closely linked to an infant's cognitive skills. Until a child is 3 years or older, it is often difficult to separate receptive language and cognition. Although it is true that some children might demonstrate cognitive strengths, such as a good memory or exceptional visual skills, we often discover that poor language comprehension skills are linked to underlying cognitive deficits. We review additional details about early cognitive development and the skills about which we need to be aware in this domain later in this chapter.

Expressive Language Development

Whereas receptive language is considered the input of language, *expressive language* is often thought of as the output. Expressive language is the ability to express our wants and needs through verbal or nonverbal communication. Infants learn to communicate as soon as they are born; they express themselves when they are hungry, uncomfortable, or tired by crying or via facial expressions. They learn to laugh when they are engaged in an enjoyable interaction with a parent or caregiver and smile in response to joy. Infants learn to use differentiated cries and begin to coo. By 6 months of age, infants are engaging in vocal play when they are occupying themselves or are being entertained by familiar adults. They begin babbling at this age as well, and often sound like they are talking. Their use of both vowels and consonants continues to expand throughout infancy and they will use speech or other sounds to gain and keep their parents' attention. First words typically emerge right around a child's first birthday. Over the next 2 years, expressive language explodes. Toddlers learn and use new words every day and the types of words they use vary with their experiences. They begin using two-word utterances to make requests, commands, and statements, and to ask questions. These young children tend to listen to and imitate everything; their vocabulary continues to grow quickly. By 2 years of age, a child could have more than 250 words. By 3 years old, their lexicon could be comprised of more than 1,000 words and their use of language is much more complex and intentional. Sentences are often comprised of one, two, or three (if not longer) words and they are more easily understood by family members. They are often able to talk about things that have happened both at home and in other environments; they are also interested in talking about current activities and events that have happened in the recent past (Levey, 2014; Owens, 2019).

As SLPs, we are already knowledgeable about the milestones for infants and toddlers in the areas of expressive and receptive language. Table 5–3 presents a list of the key developmental expectations of infants and toddlers and the ages at which we expect acquisition of each skill; please note this table is not exhaustive. We should refer to the arsenal of available evidence-based tools and materials to ensure we are using comprehensive resources regarding receptive and expressive language expectations and outcomes within our EI practice.

Table 5–3. Receptive and Expressive Language Milestones from Birth to 3 Years

Age Range Within Which Skill Is Expected	Language Milestones
Birth–3 months	• Vocalizes to gain attention • Plays with a rattle or noise-inducing toy
3–6 months	• Smiles at familiar people • Looks at an adult; engages in eye gaze • Engages in vocal turn-taking with an adult

	• Responds to their name • Produces reduplicated babbling • Laughs
6–9 months	• Responds to request "Come here" • Responds to "Want up?" • Wants to be with people • Responds to "no" most of the time • Waves "bye" • Uses a few gestures (give five, reach up, wave "bye") • Participate in games with adults by using gestures • Plays with toys without mouthing/banging them • Attends to pictures • Participates in song with adults by vocalizing • Produces early variegated babbling
9–12 months	• Perform or repeats actions for attention • Points to objects • Resists the removal of a toy • Plays with toys with purpose (e.g., pushes a car, stirs a spoon in a bowl) • Beginning to understand questions (e.g., responds to "Where's mom?" by looking for her) • Beginning to understand directions (e.g., "Give me [object]") • Points to at least two body parts • Verbalizes "mama" or "dada." • Imitates sounds (e.g., moo, beep-beep) • Produces expanded variegated babbling
12–15 months	• Demonstrates the use of objects (e.g., brushes teeth, feeds others) • Shakes head "no" • Follows one-step directions when provided with both gestures and words during play • Points to at least two action words in pictures • Points to ask for something or to get help • Understands early prepositions (e.g., in, on) • Vocalizes at least three animal sounds • Verbalizes at least two words, in addition to "mama" and "dada," spontaneously
15–18 months	• Plays independently • Hands a toy to an adult for help

	- Follows directions for two objects (e.g., "Give me [object] and [object]") - Identifies object by category (e.g., food, animal, clothes) - Verbalizes at least five words meaningfully - Adds new words to their vocabulary every day - Asks "What's that?" - Responds to "What's this?" accurately for five to seven familiar objects
18–21 months	- Uses two turns during conversation - Leads parent or caregiver to desired object - Plays with a group of toys (e.g., farm animals) - Identifies four body parts on self - Uses single words frequently - Repeats a few phrases (e.g., "I love you," "What's that?")
21–24 months	- Chooses one object from a group of five - Puts toys away upon request - Follows a two-step related direction - Combines two words together to create early sentences (e.g., "More ball")
24–27 months	- Points to four action words in pictures - Recognizes family members' names - Understands the concept of "one" - Understands size concepts - Repeats two numbers or words - Uses a variety of gestures to get needs and wants met - Uses two- to three-word phrases frequently - Uses action words
27–30 months	- Identify four objects by function - Uses early pronouns consistently (including me, mine, my, I, you) - Uses negation in phrases (including no, not) - Answers simple *wh-* questions - Verbalizes at least 50 words - Uses action words within two-word sentences (e.g., "Doggie go")

30–33 months	• Sequences actions during play (e.g., eat, go to bed) • Understands five common action words • Understands quantity concepts (including one, all) • Uses plural -*s* • Verbalizes early prepositions (in, out, off, on, up, down, here, there) • Answers "yes" and "no" questions
33–36 months	• Identifies parts of an object (e.g., wheel, tail) • Follows three-step directions • Follows directions with two familiar descriptions (e.g., big red ball) • States first name • Talks to an adult in conversation using at least two back-and-forth exchanges • Asks *wh-* questions • Uses verb forms (including -*ing*, -*ed*, and -*s*) • Expresses physical state (tired, hungry) • Verbalizes three- to five-word sentences

Note. Adapted from "Developmental Milestones," by the Centers for Disease Control and Prevention, 2022; "The Rossetti Infant Toddler Language Scale," by L. Rossetti, 2005.

Speech Sound Development

Speech sound disorders refer to any difficulty or combination of difficulties a child might have with perception, motor production, or phonological representation of speech sounds, speech segments, or both. Speech sound disorders can be organic and result from an underlying motor, neurological, structural, or sensory/perceptual cause. These disorders can also be functional and have no known cause. In the past, we have referred to functional speech sound disorders as either articulation disorders or phonological disorders. Articulation disorders focus on errors made in the production of individual speech sounds. Phonological disorders focus on predictable, rule-based errors that affect more than one sound. As SLPs, we know it is often difficult to clearly differentiate between articulation and phonological disorders, especially in the early years; therefore, in more recent years, we have turned to the broader term speech sound disorder when referring to speech errors of unknown cause (ASHA, 2023).

Table 5–4 presents the expected ages of acquisition of speech sounds for our review of developmental expectations. We review these expectations and take a closer look at speech sound development, including articulation, phonology, and intelligibility, as well as milestones for infants and toddlers within each of these areas in Chapter 10. We also dissect our role in monitoring, assessing, and providing intervention related to speech development in EI. In Chapter 8, we address considerations and differences regarding the speech sound development of monolingual and multilingual children and the variables that guide us to differentiate between speech disorders and differences.

Table 5–4. Age of Acquisition of English Consonants

Average Age of Acquisition	English Consonants
2 years	p, b, d, m, n, h, w
3 years	t, k, g, ng, f, y
4 years	v, s, z, sh, ch, j, l
5 years	th (voiced), zh, r
6 years	th (voiceless)

Note. Adapted from "Children's English Consonant Acquisition in the United States: A Review," by K. Crowe & S. McLeod, 2020.

Cognitive Development and Executive Functioning

Cognitive and executive functioning skills begin developing at birth and are affected by a young child's environment and everyday interactions with those around them. *Cognitive development* describes how a child acquires knowledge, thinks, and learns about their environment. *Executive functioning* refers to how children regulate their behavior, attention, persistence, problem-solving, memory, organization, and planning skills. Infants and toddlers draw on social-emotional, language, motor, and perceptual experiences and abilities to support cognitive development. They are attuned to relationships between features of objects, actions, and the physical environment; infants are particularly attuned to people. Parents, family members, friends, and caregivers play a vital role in supporting the cognitive development of infants and toddlers by providing the healthy interpersonal or social-emotional context in which cognitive development unfolds. Responsive adults create the foundation from which infants fully engage in behaviors and interactions that promote learning. The healthy development of skills associated with cognition and executive functioning is considered by many developmental experts to be the most important for a child's success later in life (National Research Council and Institute of Medicine, 2000). Cognition and executive functioning are closely linked to the other developmental domains, including communication, speech, and language. The primary skills within this domain we need to recognize, and which we must support and encourage in our EI practices, are presented next.

Object Permanence

The concept of *object permanence* involves the recognition by a young child that an object still exists even though they can no longer see, hear, or smell it. Examples of object permanence that we can look for when visiting a child and their family include observing an infant's demonstration of interest in a toy even though they can no longer see it; continued interest by the infant in their dog after it has been called to another room; or a demonstration by the infant of separation anxiety when their primary caregiver is no longer in their line of sight. Object permanence is a key milestone in an infant's development and demonstrates early signs of memory formation. Research indicates that most infants will develop object permanence prior to the age of 6 months (Bremner et al., 2015; Bogartz et al., 2000).

Memory

The capacity to remember allows infants and toddlers to differentiate between familiar and unfamiliar people and objects, anticipate and participate in personal care routines, learn language, and recognize the rules of social interaction. As infants get older, they are able to retain information for longer periods of time (Bauer, 2004). In fact, infants demonstrate their ability to recall past events well before they are able to articulate their past experiences verbally (Bauer, 2002b). The emergence of memory is related to the development of a neural network with various components (Bauer, 2002b). According to Bauer (2002a), memory is made up of different systems or processes, each of which serves a distinct function, characterized by fundamentally different rules of operation. Empirical data provide evidence that infants are capable of storing information over the long term and their early experiences are held in their memories and affect later behaviors.

Cause and Effect

The concept of cause and effect is the understanding that one event brings about another event. Everyday experiences provide opportunities for infants to learn about cause and effect. This knowledge helps infants better understand the properties of objects, the patterns of human behavior, and the relationship between events and consequences. By developing an understanding of cause and effect, infants form a foundation from which to solve problems, make predictions, and understand the impact their behaviors could have on others (National Research Council and Institute of Medicine, 2000).

Problem-Solving

Infants and toddlers present a strong level of interest in solving problems. Even very young infants will work to solve a problem and might work hard to find their fingers to suck on them (National Research Council and Institute of Medicine, 2000). Older infants might demonstrate even more complex problem-solving by working hard to obtain an interesting toy out of their reach; they might attempt to roll toward the toy or gesture to an adult for help.

Infants and toddlers solve problems through a variety of methods, including physically acting on or toward objects, using learning schemes they have developed, imitating solutions they have observed in others, using objects or other people as tools, and using trial and error.

Imitation

As SLPs, we know how powerful imitation can be when we are attempting to learn a new skill. Almost immediately, newborns imitate their parents and caregivers, including their facial expressions, head movements, and tongue protrusions (Meltzoff & Moore 1983, 1989). Imitation by infants involves both perception and motor processes, and they engage in both immediate and delayed imitation (Meltzoff & Moore, 1999). Immediate imitation occurs when infants observe others and attempt to copy their behaviors almost immediately (e.g., an infant's parent sticks out their tongue and the infant sticks out their tongue in response). As infants develop, they can engage in delayed imitation, which involves repeating the behavior they have observed at a later time (e.g., a child reenacts a caregiver's earlier cleaning routine by pretending to dust their bed with a blanket at bedtime).

Number Sense

Number sense refers to the development of the concept of numbers and the relationships among numbers. Infants as young as 5 months of age are sensitive to numbers and are able to discriminate among small sets of up to three objects (Starkey & Cooper 1980; Starkey et al., 1990). Infants also demonstrate the ability to quickly and accurately recognize a quantity within a small set of objects without counting (Mix et al., 2002). Although it is unclear whether this skill is solely perceptual, or also numerical, it sets the foundation for the later development of a child's understanding of number and quantity. Between 18 and 24 months of age, children use relational words to indicate "more" or the "same." At this time, they also begin to use numbers to make requests and to describe what they see. They begin to count, although they might omit some numbers, including small collections of objects; accuracy is not a priority for children at this age.

Classification

Classification refers to the infant's developing ability to group, sort, categorize, and connect objects and people according to their attributes. By 3 months old, infants demonstrate their awareness that people act differently than objects and discriminate between smiling and frowning expressions (Barrera & Maurer, 1981). Infants present both perceptual and conceptual categorization skills (Mareschal & French, 2000). Perceptual categorization is related to the similarities or differences sensed by an infant (e.g., regarding visual appearance). Conceptual categorization is focused on grouping objects based on what their purpose is or how they act. Classification is an important cognitive skill, as it serves as a foundation for the development of both problem-solving and symbolic play.

Spatial Relationships

Infants learn about spatial relationships in a variety of ways, including the exploration of objects with their mouths, tracking of objects and people visually, squeezing into tight spaces, fitting objects into openings, and looking at things from different perspectives (Mangione et al., 1992). They spend a lot of time exploring the physical and spatial aspects of the environment, including the characteristics of and interrelationships between people, objects, and physical space around them (Clements, 2004). The development of an understanding of spatial relationships by young children is important because it is related to their emerging knowledge about the properties of objects and how things move and fit in and beyond their own environment.

Joint Attention

Joint attention occurs when two people share a common interest in an object or event and there is an understanding between them that they are both interested in the same object or event. Joint attention should emerge around 9 months of age and be very well-established by 18 months of age. It is a form of early social and communicative behavior and requires a young child to gain, maintain, and shift attention. Joint attention (also sometimes called shared attention) might include the use of eye contact, gestures, vocalizations, or verbalizations. Early joint attention skills could be as simple as an infant reaching out to be picked up by an adult or a toddler looking at the same page of a book with another person. Subsequent skills could include requesting a favorite item or joint attention on a game. By the age of 3, children have developed the ability to consistently gain and maintain joint attention from and with adults and peers. The development of joint attention provides a critical foundation for social, cognitive, and language development (Levey, 2014).

As young children become more aware of the world around them, their brains will grow and change. They gain more complex thinking, reasoning, and problem-solving skills and their expanding cognitive skills are closely linked to all other developmental domains. To support this holistic development, we must be aware of and recognize both development and delay within the cognitive domain. To support us in our EI practices, Table 5–5 presents the major cognitive milestones between the ages of birth and 3 years, and the ages at which we should expect them to emerge. Use of these skills by young children demonstrates an understanding of their development of the concepts just presented.

Table 5–5. Cognitive Milestones from Birth to 3 Years

Age at Which Skills Are Expected (90% of Children)	Milestone
Birth	<ul><li>Sees objects that are 8–12 inches from their face</li><li>Is sensitive to sounds in close proximity</li><li>Startles to loud noises by arching back, kicking legs, and flailing arms</li></ul>
1 month	<ul><li>Watches faces and objects briefly and follows moving objects with their eyes</li></ul>

	• Continues to startle to loud noises by arching back, kicking legs, and flailing arms
2 months	• Follows moving objects with eyes • Recognizes familiar people at a distance • Cries or fusses when bored • Startles to loud noises
3 months	• Recognizes the bottle or breast • Follows movements by turning head • Startles to loud noises
4 months	• Watches moving objects by moving eyes from side to side • Communicates when happy or sad • Watches faces and looks at parent's or caregiver's face while eating • Reaches for toys and brings toys to their mouth
6 months	• Uses hands and mouth to explore their surroundings • Transfers objects from one hand to the other hand • Tries to obtain objects that are out of reach • Look around at people and objects
9 months	• Watches objects as they fall • Looks for objects that they see a person hide • Transfers things easily from hand to hand • Uses thumb and index finger to pick up small objects • Turns pages in books • Puts everything into their mouth • Plays peekaboo

12 months	• Puts objects in and takes objects out of containers • Looks at the correct picture in a book when it is named • Bangs objects together • Begins to use common objects correctly (e.g., drinks from a cup) • Follows simple directions (e.g., "Pick up the ball") • Explores objects by banging, shaking, or throwing them
18 months	• Demonstrates knowledge of common objects and how to use them • Points to get the attention of others • Shows interest in stuffed animals or dolls and engages in pretend play • Enjoys books, stories, and songs • Turns the pages of a book
24 months (2 years)	• Builds a tower of four or more blocks • Finds things that are hidden under two or more covers • Explores how things work by touching them and trying them out • Begins to sort shapes and colors • Plays simple pretend and make-believe games • Completes sentences and rhymes in familiar books

36 months (3 years)	• Completes puzzles with three or four pieces • Draws or copies a circle with a crayon or pencil • Identifies several colors accurately • Matches and sorts objects by shape and color • Engages in play with mechanical toys (e.g., manipulates buttons, levers, and moving parts) • Plays make-believe with dolls, animals, and people • Uses imagination to create stories or to engage in play • Turns pages one at a time

Note. Adapted from "Developmental milestones," by Centers for Disease Control and Prevention, 2022; "Mary Sheridan's from birth to five years 4th edition," by A. Sharma & H. Cockerill, 2014.

The Development of Play

Play is important work for young children and their families. Engaging in and developing play skills supports the foundation from which children learn and prepares them to interact with the world around them. Children learn important developmental skills through different stages of play (Milteer et al., 2012). According to Milteer and colleagues (2012), play is essential to the social, emotional, cognitive, and physical well-being of children beginning in early childhood. It is a natural tool through which young children develop resiliency as they learn to cooperate, overcome challenges, and negotiate with others. Play also allows children to be creative. How do we define play? Gray (2013) presents several variables that characterize play in early childhood.

- Play is self-directed. Young children engage through play when they choose and direct their own activities. It is much more intriguing for an infant or toddler to participate in activities related to their own needs and interests and in which they are engaged.

- Play is about the process, not the product. An activity is considered play when a child is engaged in the moment and is not concerned about the outcome. Although play might include goals, the anticipated outcomes are generally focused on the creation of something, instead of the end product itself.

- Play is individually constructed. The structure of a play-based activity is directed by the child and intended to meet their needs and desires. Play is also self-governing, in the sense that children create boundaries for themselves.

- Play involves imagination. The structure of play can be imaginative when the activity is governed by rules that do not necessarily fit in the real world.

- Play is active. Play activities often take place when children are alert and active. Children think through their actions to engage in play; they actively think about what they are doing and how they are doing it.

Symbolic Play

Symbolic play is also called "pretend play, make-believe play, fantasy play, or imaginative play" (Gowen, 1995, p. 75). The development of symbolic play is crucial in early development; research suggests evidence to support a causal relationship between symbolic play and the emergence and development of skills across several other domains, including those related to communication, language, social-emotional, and cognitive development (Jarrold et al., 1993; Ungerer & Sigman, 1981).

Symbolic play occurs when a child uses objects or actions to represent other objects or actions. Representational thinking is a core component of symbolic play (Youngblade & Dunn, 1995). At or around 8 months of age, infants have learned the functions of common objects (e.g., holding a play telephone to "hear" Grandma's voice). By the time children are approximately 18 months of age, they use one object to stand for, or represent, another (e.g., an 18-month-old might pretend a long block is a telephone). At or around 36 months, children engage in make-believe play in which they represent an object without having that object, or a concrete substitute, available (e.g., they might make a "phone call" by holding their hand up to their ear). As children approach 36 months of age, they more frequently engage in pretend play in which they reenact familiar events. Make-believe play allows older infants to try to better understand social roles, engage in communication with others, and revisit and make sense of past experiences. The research suggests that engaging in pretend play could also be related to the early development of empathy, based on the understanding of other people's feelings and beliefs (Youngblade & Dunn, 1995).

Social Play

Social play is a type of play that provides children with an important learning environment in which to develop social-emotional, communication, language, and physical skills. This type of play also helps young children engage with the world around them, promotes resilience and builds confidence, facilitates problem-solving skills, and supports the emerging concepts of sharing and conflict resolution (Coplan et al., 2015; Milteer et al., 2012). Parten (1932) identified six stages of play through which each child progresses. Table 5–6 presents Parten's stages of play, descriptions of what we might observe within each stage, and examples of social play engagement by infants and toddlers during our EI visits.

Table 5–6. Six Stages of Social Play

Name of Stage	Age Range Observed	Characteristics and Expectations	Examples of Play
Unoccupied play	Birth – 3 months	• Children demonstrate a lack of social interaction, lack of sustained focus, and no clear storylines during play. • Language use is nonexistent or very limited. • During this stage, children practice manipulating materials, mastering self-control, and learning about how the world works.	• Picking up, shaking, and discarding objects within their reach • Hitting and giggling at a play mobile in their crib
Solitary play	3 months – 2.5 years	• Children demonstrate an increased focus and sustained attention on toys. • Emerging play narratives (e.g., symbolic play) are frequent. • Disinterest in other children or adults during play is observed. • Children engage in unstructured play and a lack of clear goals. • Children explore freely, master new motor or cognitive skills, and prepare themselves to play with others.	• Playing with another child with their own toys but never looking at or showing any interest in the other child • Developing the ability to sustain interest in any one toy for more than 60 seconds • Walking through the park and exploring their surroundings

Onlooker play	2.5 years - 3.5 years	• Children show interest in another child's play. • They often withhold from play due to fear, disinterest, or hesitation. • Children learn about the social rules of play and relationships by watching other children; they explore different ways of playing or using materials.	• Observing older children at play, but not getting involved • Watching peers play but keeping their distance

| Parallel play | 3.5 years – 4.0 years | • Children play in the same room and with the same resources, but not together.
• Evidence of independent exploration and discovery is observed.
• Children engage in observation and imitation of adults and peers.
• Children have separate goals and focus on different objectives during play.
• They engage in minimal communication with other children.
• Children work side by side on the same activity, practice skills, and learn new methods to engage together. | • Playing with the same Lego set with another child, but constructing different buildings
• Sharing brushes and paints, but painting on different paper or surfaces |

Associative play	4.0 years – 4.5 years	• Children negotiate the sharing of resources. • Emerging chatter and language skills are embedded in play. • Children ask each other questions about their play. • Children continue to play independently with different objectives and strategies. • Imitation and observation by the children continue to occur, but at a closer distance. • Children begin practicing what they have observed through onlooker and parallel play. They begin to use their new social skills to engage with other children and/or adults during an activity.	• Asking one another questions about their play, what they are doing, and how they are doing it. • Realizing there are limited resources in the play area and negotiating with one another to allocate and make choices.

Cooperative play	4.5 years +	• Children work together on a shared game. • Children share a common objective. • Children choose team roles or personas. • There can be an element of compromise and sacrifice for the common good of the game.	• Engaging in imaginative play during which the children take on the roles of their favorite movie characters to act out a scene or even create a new scene • Sharing board games with agreed-upon rules; the children take turns for the game to proceed • Playing organized sports

Note. Adapted from "Early childhood education: Becoming a professional," by K. Gordon Biddle, A. Garcia-Nevarez, W. Roundtree Henderson, & A. Valero-Kerrick, 2015; "Social participation among preschool children," by M. Parten, 1932.

As we consider these social stages of play, we must keep in mind that every child develops at their own pace, and children might vary in their engagement in the levels of play regardless of their chronological age (Bernard, 1970). Additionally, although these six stages of play are typically mastered in a linear fashion, a child could choose to return to any or all stages as they continue to learn and grow. It is also important for us to be aware that some children might present differences regarding which types of play they prefer and how they make choices when engaging in play. This leads us to consider and learn more about the importance of social-emotional development in early childhood.

Social-Emotional Development

Social-emotional development involves the way that children relate to their social world and their ability to understand and express emotions, both their own and those of other individuals, such as their parents, teachers, and other children (Joint Task Force on Social-Emotional Development, n.d.). Social development involves learning to form and value relationships with others, feelings about self, and social adjustment to a variety of interactions over time. Emotional development pertains to the child's feelings about themselves, the people in their lives, and the environment in which they live and play. It includes the child's ability to be aware of, express, and manage feelings, and to understand and respond to the feelings of others (Joint Task Force on Social-Emotional Development, n.d.). When we understand how critically important social and emotional development is for our youngest children, we can provide the most effective practices to the children and families we serve. As SLPs in EI, we recognize that supporting parents in understanding the importance of social-emotional development while sharing practical strategies to build social emotional skills will allow their child to regulate their emotional states appropriately, build relationships, learn to solve problems, gain confidence, and manage stress and anxiety. These skills are integral to the child's ability to communicate confidently and competently (Joint Task Force on Social-Emotional Development, n.d.). Keeping the importance of this developmental domain in mind as we provide EI services, Table 5–7 presents social-emotional milestones between birth and age 3.

Table 5–7. Social-Emotional Milestones from Birth to 3 Years

Age at Which Skill Is Expected (90% of Children)	Milestone
Birth–1 month	• Show their feelings by crying • Uses their face and body to show us how they are feeling • Shows interest in watching our faces • Quiets in respond to our touch
2 months	• Shows their feelings by crying and smiling • Begins to smile at their parents or caregivers • Follow their parents or caregivers with their eyes
3 months	• Quiets to a familiar voice or touch • Smiles at people • Enjoy being hugged and cuddled
4 months	• Smiles spontaneously, particularly at people • Shows excitement by waving their arms and legs • Becomes calm and stops crying when they are comforted • Enjoys playing with people; imitates facial expressions to play
6 months	• Knows familiar faces and demonstrates an understanding of "stranger danger" • Enjoys playing with others; engages in peekaboo • Like to look at themselves in the mirror • Responds to other people's emotions and often seems happy

	• Makes sounds to express emotions
9 months	• Shows feelings by smiling, crying, and pointing • Shows preference for certain toys • Clings to familiar adults • Cries when parents or caregivers leave; is shy around strangers • Responds to their own name
12 months	• Shows a preference for certain people and toys • Imitates sounds, gestures, and actions to get parent's or caregiver's attention • Cries when parent or caregiver leaves, and is shy around strangers • Puts arm or leg out to help with dressing • Enjoys engaging in social games (e.g., peekaboo; pat-a-cake)
18 months	• Shows interest in other children • Engages in pretend play (e.g., feeding a baby doll) • Imitates the behaviors of parents or caregivers • Tries new things when familiar adults are in close proximity • Hands things to others to engage in play • Shows feelings through actions (e.g., temper tantrums, fear of strangers, clinging behaviors in new situations, affection with familiar people)
24 months (2 years)	• Engages in parallel play for brief periods of time • Imitates the actions of adults and older children • Begins to play with peers (e.g., chasing each other) • Demonstrates increased independence and defiance through actions

36 months (3 years)	• Demonstrates spontaneous concern and affection for others • Imitates adults and peers • Takes turns in games • Separates easily from parents or caregivers • Presents a wide range of emotions • Enjoys routines; dislikes disruptions in routines

Note. Adapted from "Developmental milestones," by Centers for Disease Control and Prevention, 2022; "Mary Sheridan's from birth to five years 4th edition," by A. Sharma & H. Cockerill, 2014.

Important Concepts Related to Social-Emotional Development

Because it is so important that we have a solid grasp on the importance of this developmental domain, it is to our benefit to understand the following concepts.

Social Development

Social development refers to a young child's ability to create and sustain social relationships with both adults and other children. Infants begin developing and demonstrating social skills when they respond to a familiar voice, smell, or touch of the important people in their lives. When they receive positive reinforcement for their engagement, infants can move toward the next stage in social development. When they become toddlers with at least one secure relationship with a trusted adult, children will confidently explore novel objects and places. They are then able to learn to share, cooperate, take turns, compromise, and negotiate through these relationships (Michigan Department of Community Health, 2023). As children grow older, their relationships with peers take on greater importance. As they continue to grow and face new challenges, they also learn skills, including cooperation, negotiation, and appreciation for the needs and rights of others. This leads to the ability to sometimes put aside their own needs and desires to meet the needs of others.

Emotional Development

Emotional development is closely related to social development and refers to a young child's feelings about themselves, the people in their life, and the environments in which they play and live (Michigan Department of Community Health, 2023). Infants respond strongly to physical discomfort such as hunger and fatigue and their emotional behavioral repertoire is basic and shaped by temperament. They might respond by crying, screaming, or cooing to demonstrate how they are feeling at any given time. Toddlers are developing a range of emotions; as such, they might respond to external stimuli by having tantrums, acting out, or becoming easily frustrated. As children develop the ability to recognize, express, and manage feelings, and to understand and respond to the feelings of others, they are demonstrating their emotional development. Healthy emotional development allows a young child to respond to and engage in a full range of emotions in appropriate ways. Learning to manage their emotions and maintain focus and attention is a process that develops over time through reciprocal interactions with the adults in their lives. It is within our scope of practice as SLPs in EI to support this development and set the foundation for other areas of development.

Family Relationships

All relationships are integral to a young child's development, and they matter as early as the first few days of infancy. The evidence is clear: Best practice EI services are those delivered to children and parents through the family-centered approach, children need to be served within the context of strong relationships, parents and caregivers are coached to become their children's primary provider, and as needed, families receive supports and services along with their children (Joint Task Force on Social-Emotional Development, n.d.; ZERO TO THREE, 2009).

Attachment

Attachment refers to the emotional relationship that develops between an infant and the parent or primary caregiver during their first year of life. An infant's secure attachment to their parents is regarded as the primary source of a child's security, self-esteem, self-control, and social skills throughout their lifetime (Eliot, 1999). This relationship develops over time and is the result of many interactions and caregiving experiences; the most important of these interactions include those in which the parent or caregiver responds to the infant's needs and bids for attention, comfort, and protection (Michigan Department of Community Health, 2023). A child who has a secure attachment and engages in predictable and responsive relationships with primary caregivers has greater opportunities to learn and master the skills they need to be successful in both academics and throughout their lives (Children's Behavioral Health Initiative, 2015).

Trauma and Resilience

Trauma occurs when children experience an intense event that threatens or causes harm to their emotional and physical well-being. The cerebral cortex is responsible for many complex functions, including memory, attention, perceptual awareness, thinking, language, planning and organization. Early childhood trauma has been associated with reduced size of this part of the brain. These changes are related to intellectual ability and the ability to regulate emotions; a child who experiences early trauma, therefore, is more likely to become more fearful and might feel less safe or protected. In addition to experiencing one or more traumatic events, experiencing multiple adverse childhood experiences (e.g., poverty, domestic violence, parental substance abuse, homelessness) could also negatively affect a young child's development (National Child Traumatic Stress Network, n.d.).

The development of social-emotional learning serves as the foundation of a child's ability to approach life openly and to handle life's challenges effectively. The ability to relate to adults and other children and to learn from others influences the infant's development in all other domains. As children's interaction skills grow, they learn from others through imitation and communication. Language learning, problem-solving, imaginative play, and social games all depend on social-emotional development (ZERO TO THREE, 2009).

Adaptive Development

Adaptive development refers to the development of behaviors and self-help skills that assist children in coping with the natural and social demands of their environment, including sleeping, feeding, mobility, toileting, dressing, and higher-level social interactions. The development of adaptive skills, including those related to self-help and feeding, plays a significant role in a young child's daily life. Activities such as dressing, eating, and brushing teeth are often embedded in daily routines and present significant opportunities for young children to learn in natural environments. The developing abilities of infants and toddlers to anticipate, understand, and participate in these routines represent a significant aspect of their cognitive functioning, social-emotional engagement and the building of relationships with others, their abilities to take care of themselves along with their speech and language development. Young infants initially respond to an adult's actions during these routines. Over time, though, they begin to participate more actively and to initiate engagement through these activities. Understanding the steps involved in personal care routines and anticipating the next steps are skills related to the cognitive foundations of attention maintenance, imitation, memory, cause and effect, and problem-solving (O'Brien, 1997).

The cultural perspectives of parents and caregivers are often directly related to their expectations regarding degree of independence or initiation by their young children during personal care (i.e., self-help) routines and feeding activities. Depending on their cultural experiences, infants and toddlers could vary greatly in their understanding of and engagement in personal care routines. We address these considerations further in Chapter 8.

A young child who is experiencing delays in adaptive development has difficulty in learning and acquiring these behaviors and skills. Delays in adaptive development could be associated with delays or impairments in other areas of development, including fine and gross motor skills, cognitive development, communication development, and social-emotional development. Table 5–8 examines the adaptive milestones we should expect to observe and in which an infant or toddler should engage.

Table 5–8. Adaptive Milestones from Birth to 3 Years

Age Range Within Which Skill Is Expected	Milestone
0–6 months	<ul><li>Tracks objects with eyes</li><li>Communicates hunger, fear, or discomfort through crying</li><li>Coordinates suck, swallow, breath sequence</li><li>Sleeps for 4–10 hours at a time</li></ul>

6–12 months	- Tracks objects with eyes - Reaches for nearby objects - Tolerates a range of different textured foods - Holds a bottle or cup independently - Holds a cup with two hands and drinks with assistance - Uses tongue to move food around their mouth - Feeds themselves small crackers or other small pieces of food - Sleeps 10–12 hours overnight, waking up only once
12–24 months (1–2 years)	- Distinguishes between edible and inedible objects (by 18 months) - Understands common dangers such as hot objects, stairs, glass, and so on - Holds a cup with one hand and drinks unassisted - Chews food independently - Tolerates diaper changes - Attempts to brush their own teeth - Cooperates with dressing by extending an arm or leg - Removes their own shoes and socks - Unzips a large zipper - Settles themselves to sleep at night or during the day
24–36 months (2–3 years)	- Uses the toilet with assistance and has daytime control - Distinguishes between urination and bowel movements; names them correctly - Opens the door by turning the handle - Takes their socks and shoes off - Uses a spoon independently with little spilling - Washes and dries their hands with assistance - Puts on coat with assistance; takes off coat independently - Unbuttons large buttons - Tolerates a range of different textured foods - Uses a napkin to wipe their face and hands - Enjoys or at least tolerates messy play

Note. Adapted from "Self care development chart," by Kid Sense Child Development Corporation, 2022 (https://childdevelopment.com.au/resources/child-development-charts/self-care-developmental-chart/); "Early identification – Adaptive milestones," by National Joint Committee on Learning Disabilities, 2023 (https://www.ldonline.org/ld-topics/working-families/early-identification-adaptive-milestones).

Physical Development

Physical development, including hearing and vision, refers to physical changes throughout childhood. Aspects of physical development we address include gross and fine motor skills, the degree or quality of a child's motor and sensory development, health status, and physical skills. Physical development interacts with, and often affects, all the other development domains and developmental milestones of a young child. Physical development in early childhood is typically measured using growth charts and physical indicators (including measurements of height, weight, and head circumference); assessment of sensory functioning, including hearing and vision; and assessment of motor development. Physical therapists and occupational therapists are the service providers who typically provide assessment and treatment services in EI. As SLPs, it is important that we are also aware of the expectations related to a young child's physical development and how these might affect their communication, speech, language, and feeding needs.

Motor Development

Although the motor development of most young children occurs in an orderly, predictable sequence of events, the rate and age of motor skills vary from one child to the next. The process of motor development depends on the maturation of the central nervous system and muscular system. As these systems develop, a child's ability to move progresses. *Gross motor development* involves skills that require coordination of the large muscle groups (e.g., sitting, walking, rolling, standing) (Gonzalez et al., 2019). *Fine motor development* is concerned with the coordination of smaller muscles of the body, including the hands and face. Fine motor skills use the small muscles of both the hands and the eyes for performance. Changes in motor development support new learning opportunities for children to interact with objects, their environment, their parents, and caregivers (Gonzalez et al., 2019). Table 5–9 presents the milestones we should watch for as the infants and toddlers with whom we work grow and develop.

Table 5–9. Motor Milestones from Birth to 3 Years

Age at Which Skill Is Expected (90% of Children)	Milestone
Birth	<ul><li>Turns head easily from side to side</li><li>Moves head one way and then another when lying on the back</li><li>Comforts themself by bringing hands to their face to suck fingers or fist</li><li>Keeps their hands mostly closed and fisted</li><li>Blinks at bright lights</li></ul>
1 month	<ul><li>Raises their head slightly off the floor when lying on their stomach</li><li>Holds their head up momentarily when supported</li><li>Keeps their hands in closed fists when at rest</li><li>Continues to comfort by sucking on their fist or fingers</li></ul>

2 months	- Holds their head up and begins to push up with their arms when lying on their stomach - Makes smoother movements with their arms and legs - Moves both arms and both legs well - Brings their hands to their mouth
3 months	- Lifts their head and chest when lying on their stomach - Moves their arms and legs easily and energetically - Shows improved head control
4 months	- Holds their head steady without support - Grabs and shakes toys; brings toys to their mouth - Pushes down on their legs when their feet are placed on a hard surface - Pushes up to their elbows when lying on their stomach - Rocks from side to side and might begin to roll from stomach to back
6 months	- Rolls over in both directions - Begins to sit with minimal support - Supports their weight on both legs when standing; might begin bouncing - Rocks back and forth on their hands and knees; might begin to crawl backward
9 months	- Might creep or crawl (although not necessary for walking to develop) - Gets in and out of a sitting position; sits well without support - Pulls to stand - Stands while holding onto a sturdy surface - Begins to take steps while holding onto furniture (i.e., cruising)
12 months	- Pulls to stand and walks while holding onto furniture - Gets into a sitting position independently - Begins to stand alone - Begins to take independent steps

| 18 months | - Walks independently; begins to walk up the stairs and to run
- Walks backward while pulling a toy
- Feeds themselves with a spoon; drinks independently with a cup
- Helps dress and undress themselves |
|---|---|
| 24 months (2 years) | - Throws and kicks a ball
- Walks up and down stairs while holding onto the wall or a railing
- Stands on their tiptoes
- Begins to run
- Climbs on and off furniture independently
- Puts together simple puzzles |
| 36 months (3 years) | - Climbs and runs well
- Walks up and down stairs with one foot on each step
- Jumps with both feet; might hop on one foot
- Pedals a tricycle or three-wheel bicycle |

Note. Adapted from "Developmental milestones," by Centers for Disease Control and Prevention, 2022; "Mary Sheridan's from birth to five years 4th edition," by A. Sharma & H. Cockerill, 2014.

It is important that we, as SLPs, understand and are aware of the relationship between the development of motor skills. According to Gonzalez and colleagues (2019), both gross and fine motor skills help foster language development and are predictive of later language outcomes across early infancy and childhood. Recent studies suggest that co-occurring motor and language difficulties might have a common underlying genetic basis, with the genes that put a child at risk for communicative impairment also affecting motor development (Bishop, 2002; Iverson & Wozniak, 2007; Viholainen et al., 2006). As such, we must consider the connection between an infant or toddler's development of motor skills and their language development. New motor skills provide infants with opportunities to practice skills related to language development.

- Rhythmic hand and arm movements provide opportunities for infants to practice rhythmic, repetitive actions. Studies show that these hand and arm movements tend to emerge 2 or 3 weeks prior to an infant's use of reduplicated babbling (Iverson, 2010).

- Before children start to talk, they tend to take things apart (e.g., a sippy cup top and container). When infants and toddlers begin to use their first words, they tend to put things together more frequently. Children also begin to put objects together in different ways (e.g., putting a cracker inside the cup). As a child's vocabulary grows, children tend to make use of specific features of objects (e.g., putting a cracker in a bowl instead of the cup). This could reflect advances in a young child's cognitive development. It might also suggest that, as children develop motor skills, they are presented with more opportunities to attend to specific features of the toys and objects they are physically manipulating. As they make use of these features, they are also determining specific meanings of and for objects.

- When children are able to sit up on their own, they discover new possibilities for vocal production. They can make more sounds because sitting up increases lung capacity and repositions the lower jaw and tongue, both of which are relevant to consonant–vowel combinations (MacNeilage & Davis, 2000).

- Between 6 and 9 months of age, children tend to explore objects by putting them in their mouths. This period coincides with the development and use of consonants (which requires a degree of vocal tract closure). Mouthing objects can contribute to an infant's awareness of different postures with their teeth, lips, and tongue to produce new speech sounds (Fagan & Iverson, 2007).

- Research indicates that children who are walking at 13 months of age carry objects more frequently than those children who are still crawling. They are also more likely to share objects by moving to their mothers and holding the object out for inspection (Karasik et al., 2011). Walking also provides young children with greater opportunities to access things that are far away, to use their hands to carry objects, and to see and locate objects and people in their surroundings. Infants and toddlers are more likely to learn words when their attention is already focused on what they are naming (Tomasello & Farrar, 1986). Retrieving and sharing objects with parents and caregivers could provide expanded opportunities for a child to learn language.

The relationship between motor development and language development is complex. Motor skills have been found to play a role in language development, but meeting physical developmental milestones is not necessary for a young child to learn and use language. We also know that new motor skills can provide multiple opportunities for an infant or toddler to practice and refine skills important for language development (Iverson, 2010). As SLPs, we can support the children and families we serve in EI by being aware of the expectations related to physical development, monitoring delayed motor milestones as a risk factor for language delay, and consulting with our PT and OT team members as needed.

Oral Motor Development

The development of *oral motor skills* includes the use and function of the lips, tongue, jaw, teeth, and hard and soft palates. A child's development and ability to use these structures with coordinated patterns are necessary to produce speech sounds and engage in safe feeding and swallowing. The strength and coordination of these movements are foundational for feeding tasks, including tongue lateralization, sucking, munching, licking, and swallowing (Carruth & Skinner, 2002; Carruth et al., 2004). Oral motor skills also play a significant role in the development and use of facial expressions. Oral motor skills begin to develop before a child is even born and are expected to be completely functional between 3 and 4 years of age.

According to evidence presented by Carruth and their colleagues (Carruth & Skinner, 2002; Carruth et al., 2004), difficulties in the development of oral functions can lead to:

- Excessive drooling
- Difficulty with speech articulation
- Open-mouth posture
- Inconsistent eating habits
- Low range of motion in the tongue
- Difficulty sucking, swallowing, and chewing

Disorganized or dysfunctional patterns are often related to several diagnoses, including cerebral palsy and Down syndrome, and could also lead to delays in speech and language (Alcock, 2006). Alcock (2006) conducted several studies, determining that children who present limited oral motor movements before 2 years old tend to demonstrate poor language skills at the same age; children who present good oral motor skills could, however, present a range of language use. These results indicate that oral motor skills are a necessary, but not sufficient, prerequisite for good language skills (Alcock, 2006). Although we will examine the development and importance of oral motor skills in detail as they relate to feeding assessment and intervention of infants and toddlers in Chapter 11, we are also aware that the emergence of these skills affects the development of speech, language, and communication. Therefore, Table 5–10 offers an overview of the milestones expected between birth and 3 years associated with oral motor development and feeding.

Table 5–10. Oral Motor and Feeding Development

Age at Which Skill Is Expected	Milestone

Birth	- Reflexes that support eating are present:
	    ○ Swallow reflex
	    ○ Phasic bite reflex
	    ○ Palmomental reflex
	    ○ Transverse tongue reflex
	- Sucking is automatic.

2.5–3.5 months	- Volitional sucking emerges (and no longer relies on reflex).

| 4–6 months | - Rooting and phasic bite reflexes begin to integrate (2–6 months).
- Opens mouth when spoon approaches or touches the lips.
- Tongue used to move purees to back of mouth for the swallow.
- Munching (up and down) jaw movements.
- Lateral (side to side) jaw movements.
- Diagonal jaw movements (indicating the emergence of a more mature rotary chew).
- Lateral tongue movements (which support eating efficiency). |
|---|---|
| 7–8 months | - Moves upper lip down to draw food off of the spoon.
- Emergence of full lip closure.
- Consistent tongue lateralization occurs when various foods are presented to the sides of tongue.
- Active movement of foods from side of mouth to central tongue groove and back.
- Emergence of mature tongue lateralization.
- Diagonal rotary movements. |
| 8–10 months | - Emergence of circular rotary movements.
- Transition to slightly more texture (e.g., small bumps and thicker purees).
- Able to break off pieces of foods that dissolve in the mouth.
- "Chewing" (munching) of softer food. |
| 10–12 months | - Licking food off of lips emerges.
- Simple tongue protrusion may occur.
- More controlled biting (isolated from body movements).
- Complete transfer of foods from side to side in mouth with tongue (without difficulty).
- Emergence of rotary movements. |
| 12–14 months | - Chews and swallows firmer foods without choking.
- Chews foods that produce juice.
- Able to keep most bites in mouth while chewing. |
| 14–16 months | - Uses tongue to gather pieces of food.
- Sweeps pieces into a bolus with the tongue.
- Chews bigger pieces of soft table food.
- Working on chewing increasingly solid foods. |

18–24 months	<ul><li>Increasing speed and efficiency of eating.</li><li>Demonstrated improved chewing strength.</li><li>Better able to manage hard-to-chew foods.</li></ul>
24–26 months	<ul><li>Circulatory jaw movements improve.</li><li>Chews with lips closed.</li><li>Working further on increasing speed, strength, and efficiency with larger, solid pieces of food.</li></ul>
24–36 months (2–3 years)	<ul><li>Strong circulatory jaw rotations.</li><li>Eats wide range of foods, including all textures.</li></ul>

Note. Adapted from "Feeding behaviors and other motor development in healthy children (2-24 months)," by B. Carruth & J. Skinner, 2002; "Important developmental milestones relevant to feeding," by E. Toomey, 2016.

Sensory Development: Vision and Hearing

Although every one of our senses plays a role in early development, vision and hearing will most certainly affect the areas in which we focus with our families. When we consider infants interact with their environment, most of their engagement is related to seeing or hearing stimuli to which they respond. Early bonding with a parent or caregiver is related to the infant's ability to make eye contact and sustain a gaze with their parents, respond to their voices by gurgling and cooing, and receive comforting by the sight and sound of them. Infants will often attempt to move because they see or hear something that intrigues them. Infants learn that people and objects exist in the world primarily because they become aware of them in their environment. An infant's early development in all domains is typically linked to their vision and hearing abilities. When these senses do not develop as expected, all development is affected.

During the first 3 years of a child's life, major neural networks are being formed in the brain. Much of this development comes from the senses of vision and hearing, which allows them to formulate thoughts about people and objects in their environment, even when they are not physically able to touch them. After the first 3 years, development of these neural networks slows down. Skills that can be gained in EI cannot be made as quickly when the child is older. We know that even mild problems with these senses can have a major impact on a young child's ability to learn and their capacity to acquire skills in all areas of development. A mild hearing loss in a noisy home or day-care center can result in a child missing critical information. They might miss sounds that serve as the foundation for the development of normal language and speech sound development. They could miss information and instructions presented by their parents or caregivers and eventually become withdrawn because they are not sure what is expected of them. An infant or toddler with hearing or visual field loss will struggle with speech and language development; sensory, cognitive, social-emotional, and adaptive skills will be affected as well. As members of an EI team, it is our responsibility to be aware of and monitor the vision and hearing of the children we serve. Table 5–11 and Table 5–12 present age-related guidelines for vision and hearing to help us monitor the sensory development of the children we serve.

Table 5–11. Vision Milestones from Birth to 3 Years

Age at Which Skill Is Expected	Milestone
Birth	<ul><li>A newborn's eyesight is expected to be poor.</li><li>The infant will blink in response to bright light or someone touching their eye.</li><li>Their eyes are sometimes uncoordinated and might look cross-eyed.</li><li>They are able to stare at an object if it is held 8 to 10 inches away.</li><li>The infant initially fixes their eyes on a face or light before beginning to follow a moving object.</li></ul>
1 month	<ul><li>The infant looks at faces and pictures with contrasting black-and-white images.</li><li>They can follow an object up to 90 degrees.</li><li>They watch their parent or caregiver closely.</li><li>Tears begin to form at this age.</li></ul>
2–3 months	<ul><li>The infant begins to be capable of seeing an object as one image.</li><li>The infant can see and often look at their own hands.</li><li>The infant follows light, faces, and objects.</li></ul>
4–5 months	<ul><li>The infant is beginning to reach out their hands toward objects; they might bat at hanging objects with their hands.</li><li>They can stare at a block.</li><li>They recognize their bottle.</li><li>They will look at themselves in a mirror.</li></ul>
5–7 months	<ul><li>They now have full-color vision and are able to see from longer distances.</li><li>They can pick up a toy that has been dropped.</li><li>They will turn their head to see an object.</li><li>They like and respond to certain colors.</li><li>They will touch an image of themselves in a mirror.</li></ul>
7–11 months	<ul><li>They can stare at small objects.</li><li>Their depth perception is emerging.</li></ul>
11–12 months	<ul><li>They can watch objects that are moving fast.</li></ul>

18–24 months	• Toddlers at this stage are able to focus on both near and far objects. • They may imitate a drawing of a straight line or circle. • They can see and point to body parts (nose, hair, and eyes) when asked.
36–48 months	• They can copy shapes and clearly see colors. • Their vision is nearing 20/20 by this age range.

Note. Adapted from "Vision milestones," by Johns Hopkins Medicine, 2023b (htttps://www.hopkinsmedicine.org/health/wellness-and-prevention/vision-milestones).

Table 5–12. Hearing Milestones from Birth to 1 Year

Age at Which Skill Is Expected	Milestone
Birth–3 months	• The newborn reacts to loud sounds with startle reflex. • They are soothed and quieted by soft sounds. • They turn their head to an adult when they hear them. • They are easily awakened by loud voices and other sounds. • They begin to smile in response to certain voices.
4–6 months	• Infants look or turn toward a new sound. • They respond to "no" and change in tone of voice. • They enjoy rattles and other toys that make sounds. • They begin to respond to and repeat sounds (e.g., "ooh," "aah," and "ba-ba"). • They become scared by a loud voice or noise.
7–12 months	• The infant responds to their own name, the telephone ringing, or someone's (quiet) voice. • They make babbling sounds, even when alone. • They begin to respond to requests (e.g., "come here"). • They imitate simple words and sounds; they may use a few single words meaningfully.

Note. Adapted from "Milestones related to speech and hearing," by Johns Hopkins Medicine, 2023a(https://www.hopkinsmedicine.org/health/conditions-and-diseases/hearing-loss/ageappropriate-speech-and-hearing-milestones).

Summary

As SLPs in EI, it is not our responsibility to memorize all of the milestones presented throughout this chapter. To provide best practices in EI, however, it is our responsibility to be aware of and knowledgeable about the developmental expectations for the infants and toddlers we serve in all domains. We must be cognizant of a child's holistic development. In addition to speech, language, and communication, it is our responsibility to be knowledgeable about their cognitive development and executive functioning, play, self-help, motor, and social-emotional skills, as well as vision and hearing capabilities. We have now reviewed developmental milestones across each of these domains and have learned about how each relates and is connected to speech, language, and communication development. We understand how these domains intersect and affect all areas of a child's development.

Critical Thinking Questions

1. Why is it important that we have a solid foundation of knowledge regarding all early development domains in EI?

2. What are the areas associated with early communication development? Why do we need to have a strong understanding of the milestones related to these areas when providing EI services?

3. Present the basic expectations related to early communication development, receptive and expressive language development, and speech sound development.

4. Define the domains and concepts related to cognitive development and executive functioning, the development of play, social-emotional development, adaptive development, physical development including motor, oral motor, and sensory development in infants and toddlers.

5. Why is it important that we have access to the expectations and developmental milestones between birth to three years in the areas of cognition and executive functioning, play, social-emotional, adaptive, and physical development (including those related to motor, oral motor, vision, and hearing)?

6. Explain, as if to a parent or caregiver, how all developmental domains intersect and impact one another as a child learns and grows. Why is it so integral to our work as SLPs in EI that we need to consider all areas of development over time?

7. Consider and explain the influence of cultural and linguistic diversity on a young child's acquisition of knowledge and skills across all developmental domains.

References

Alcock, K. (2006). The development of oral motor control and language. *Down Syndrome Research and Practice*, *11*(1), 1–8. https://doi.org/10.3104/reports.310

American Speech-Language and Hearing Association. (2023). *Speech sound disorders—Articulation and phonology.* https://www.asha.org/practice-portal/clinical-topics/articulation-and-phonology/

American Speech-Language and Hearing Association. (n.d.) *Components of social communication.* https://www.asha.org/practice-portal/clinical-topics/social-communication-disorder/components-of-social-communication/

Barrera, M. E., & Mauer, D. (1981). The perception of facial expressions by the three-month-old. *Child Development, 52,* 203–206.

Bauer, P. (2002a). Early memory development. In U. Goswami (Ed.), *Handbook of cognitive development* (pp. 127-146). Blackwell.

Bauer, P. (2002b). Long-term recall memory: Behavioral and neuro-developmental changes in the first two years of life. *Current Directions in Psychological Science, 11*(4), 137–141.

Bauer, P. (2004). Getting explicit memory off the ground: Steps toward construction of a neuro-developmental account of changes in the first two years of life. *Developmental Review, 24,* 347–373.

Bernard, J. (1970). Mildred Parten Newhall, 1902–1970. *American Sociologist, 5*(4), 383. https://doi.org/https://www.jstor.org/stable/27701690

Bishop, D. V. M. (2002). Motor immaturity and specific speech and language impairment: Evidence for a common genetic basis. *American Journal of Medical Genetics (Neuropsychiatric Genetics), 114,* 56–63.

Bogartz, R. S., Shinskey, J. L., & Schilling, T. H. (2000). Object permanence in five-and-a-half-month-old infants? *Infancy, 1*(4), 403–428.

Bremner, J. G., Slater, A. M., & Johnson, S. P. (2015). Perception of object persistence: The origins of object permanence in infancy. *Child Development Perspectives, 9*(1), 7–13.

Capone, N. C., & McGregor, K. K. (2004). Gesture development: A review for clinical and research practices. *Journal of Speech, Language, and Hearing Research, 47,* 173–186.

Capone Singleton, J., & Saks, J. (2015) Co-speech gesture input as a support for language learning in children with and without early language delay. *Perspective on Language Learning and Education, 22,* 61-71. https://doi.org/10.1044/lle22.2.61

Carruth, B. R., & Skinner, J. D. (2002). Feeding behaviors and other motor development in healthy children (2–24 months). *Journal of the American College of Nutrition, 21*(2), 88–96.

Carruth, B. R., Ziegler P. J., Gordon A., & Henricks, K. (2004). Developmental milestones and self-feeding behaviors in infants and toddlers. *Journal of the American Dietetic Association, 104*(1, Suppl. 1), s51–56.

Centers for Disease Control and Prevention. (2022). *Developmental milestones.* https://www.cdc.gov/ncbddd/actearly/milestones/

Children's Behavioral Health Initiative. (2015). *Infant and early childhood mental health resources and services—A guide for early care and educational professionals.* MassHealth Publications.

Clements, D. H. (2004). Major themes and recommendations. In D. H. Clements and J. Samara (Eds.), *Engaging young children in mathematics: Standards for early childhood educators* (10-34). Lawrence Erlbaum Associates.

Coplan, R. J., Ooi, L. L, Kirkpatrick, A., & Rubin, K. H. (2015). Social and nonsocial play. In D. P. Fromberg & D. Bergen (Eds.), *Play from birth to twelve* (3rd ed., pp. 109–118). Routledge.

Crais, E., & Ogletree, B. (2016). Prelinguistic communication development. In D. Keen, H. Meadan, N. Brady, & J. Halle (Eds.), *Prelinguistic and minimally verbal communicators on the autism spectrum* (pp. 9–32). Springer. https://doi.org/10.1007/978-981-10-0713-2_2

Crowe, K., & McLeod, S. (2020). Children's English consonant acquisition in the United States: A review. *American Journal of Speech-Language Pathology, 29*(4), 2155–2169. https://doi.org/10.1044/2020_AJSLP-19-00168

Eliot, L. (1999). *What's going on in there? How the brain and mind develop in the first five years of life.* Bantam Books.

Fagan, M. K., & Iverson, J. M. (2007). The Influence of Mouthing on Infant Vocalization. *Infancy: the official journal of the International Society on Infant Studies, 11*(2), 191–202. https://doi.org/10.1111/j.1532-7078.2007.tb00222.x

Goldin-Meadow, S. (2015). Gesture as a window onto communicative abilities: Implications for diagnosis and intervention. *Perspectives on Language Learning and Education, 22,* 50–60.

Gonzalez, S., Alvarez, V., & Nelson, E. (2019). Do gross and fine motor skills differentially contribute to language outcomes? A systemic review. *Frontiers in Psychology, 10,* 1–16. https://doi.org/10.3389/fpsyg.2019.02670

Gordon Biddle, K., Garcia-Nevarez, A., Roundtree Henderson, W., & Valero-Kerrick, A. (2014). *Early childhood education: Becoming a professional.* Sage.

Gowen, J. W. (1995). Research in review: The early development of symbolic play. *Young Children, 50*(3), 75–84.

Gray, P. (2013). *Free to learn: Why unleashing the instinct to play will make our children happier, more self-reliant, and better students for life.* Basic Books.

Iverson, J. M. (2010). Developing language in a developing body: The relationship between motor development and language development. *Journal of Child Language, 37,* 229–261.

Iverson, J. M., & Wozniak, R. H. (2007). Variation in vocal-motor development in infant siblings of children with autism. *Journal of Autism and Developmental Disorders, 37,* 158–170.

Jarrold, C., Boucher, J., & Smith, P. (1993). Symbolic play in autism: A review. *Journal of Autism and Developmental Disorders, 23*(2), 281–307.

Johns Hopkins Medicine. (2023a). *Milestones related to speech and hearing.* https://www.hopkinsmedicine.org/health/conditions-and-diseases/hearing-loss/ageappropriate-speech-and-hearing-milestones

Johns Hopkins Medicine. (2023b). *Vision milestones.* https://www.hopkinsmedicine.org/health/wellness-and-prevention/vision-milestones

Joint Task Force on Social-Emotional Development. (n.d.). *Meeting the social-emotional development needs of infants and toddlers: Guidance for early intervention program providers and other early childhood professionals.* New York State Department of Health Early Intervention Program. https://www.health.ny.gov/publications/4226.pdf

Karasik, L., Tamis-LeMonda, C., & Adolph, K. (2011). Transition from crawling to walking and infants' actions with objects and people. *Child Development, 82*(4), 1199–1209.

Kid Sense Child Development Corporation. (2022). *Self care development chart.* https://childdevelopment.com.au/resources/child-development-charts/self-care-developmental-chart/

Levey, S. (2014). *Introduction to language development.* Plural Publishing.

Mangione, P. L., Lally, J. R., & Signer, S. (1992). *Discoveries of infancy: Cognitive development and learning.* Far West Laboratory and California Department of Education.

Mareschal, D., & French, R. (2000). Mechanisms of categorization in infancy. *Infancy, 1*(1), 59–76.

Mastrogiuseppe, M., Capirci, O., Cuva, S. & Venuti, P. (2015). Gestural communication in children with autism spectrum disorders during mother–child interaction. *Autism, 19*(4), 469–481.

MacNeilage, P. F., & Davis, B. L. (2000). On the origin of internal structure of word forms. *Science, 288*(5465), 527–531. https://doi.org/10.1126/science.288.5465.527

Meltzoff, A. N., & Moore, M. K. (1983). Newborn infants imitate adult facial gestures. *Child Development, 54*, 702–709.

Meltzoff, A. N., & Moore, M. K. (1989). Imitation in newborn infants: Exploring the range of gestures imitated and the underlying mechanisms. *Developmental Psychology, 25*(6), 954–962.

Michigan Department of Community Health. (2023). *Social and emotional health of children birth to age 8 fact sheet.* https://www.michigan.gov/-/media/Project/Websites/mdhhs/Adult-and-Childrens-Services/Children-and-Families/TTS/Social_Emotional_Health_Fact_Sheet.pdf?rev=bf25886f2ca741ae9e5cc88269107dad

Milteer, R. M., Ginsburg, K. R., Mulligan, D. A., Ameenuddin, N., Brown, A., Christakis, D., ... Swanson, W. S (2012). The importance of play in promoting healthy child development and maintaining strong parent–child bond: Focus on children in poverty. *Pediatrics, 129*(1), 204–213. https://doi.org/10.1542/peds.2011-2953

Mix, K., Huttenlocher, J., & Levine, S. (2002). *Quantitative development in infancy and early childhood.* Oxford University Press.

National Child Traumatic Stress Network (n.d.) *Families and trauma.* https://www.nctsn.org/trauma-informed-care/families-and-trauma

National Joint Committee on Learning Disabilities. (2023). *Early identification—Adaptive milestones.* https://www.ldonline.org/ld-topics/working-families/early-identification-adaptive-milestones

National Research Council and Institute of Medicine. (2000). *From neurons to neighborhoods: The science of early childhood development.* Committee on Integrating the Science of Early Childhood Development, National Academies Press.

O'Brien, M. (1997). *Meeting individual and special needs: Inclusive child care for infants and toddlers.* Brookes.

Owens, R. (2019). *Language development: An introduction* (10th ed.). Pearson Education.

Parten, M. (1932). Social participation among preschool children. *Journal of Abnormal and Social Psychology, 27*(3), 243–269. https://doi.org/10.1037/h0074524

Rossetti, L. M. (2005). *The Rossetti Infant Toddler Language Scale: A measure of communication and interaction.* Linguisystems.

Sharma, A., & Cockerill, H. (2014). *Mary Sheridan's from birth to five years: Children's developmental progress* 4th ed. Routledge.

Starkey, P., & Cooper. R. G. (1980). Perception of numbers by human infants. *Science, 210*(4473), 1033–1035.

Starkey, P., Spelke, E. S., & Gelman, R. (1990). Numerical abstraction by human infants. *Cognition, 36*(2), 97–128.

Sussman, F. (2016). *A closer look at social communication difficulties of children with Autism Spectrum Disorder.* The Hanen Centre. https://www.hanen.org/Helpful-Info/Articles/A-Closer-Look-at-Social-Communication-Difficulties.aspx

Tomasello, M., & Farrar, J. (1986). Joint attention and early language. *Child Development, 57*, 1454–1463.

Toomey, E. (2016). *Important developmental milestones relevant to feeding.* https://sosapproachtofeeding.com/wp-content/uploads/2019/02/Developmental-Milestones-Table.pdf

Ungerer, J. A., & Sigman, M. (1981). Symbolic play and language comprehension in autistic children. *Journal of the American Academy of Child Psychiatry, 20*, 318–337.

Viholainen, H., Ahonen, T., Lyytinen, P., Cantell, M., Tolvanen, A., & Lyytinen, H. (2006). Early motor development and later language and reading skills in children at risk of familial dyslexia. *Developmental Medicine & Child Neurology, 48*, 367–373.

Youngblade, L. M., & Dunn. J. (1995). Individual differences in young children's pretend play with mother and sibling: Links to relationships and understanding of other people's feelings and beliefs. *Child Development, 66*, 1472–1492.

ZERO TO THREE. (2009). *Laying the foundation for early development: Infant and early childhood mental health.* https://theartofchildhood.wordpress.com/2012/05/01/laying-foundation-for-earlydevelopment-policies-about-infant-and-earlychildhood-mental-health/

Chapter 6

Screening, Evaluation, and Assessment in Early Intervention

Learning Outcomes

When we have completed this chapter, we will be able to:

- Define screening, evaluation, and assessment under IDEA Part C and where each process fit within the supports and services pathway of EI.

- Present the DEC Recommended Practices in EI related to screening, evaluation, and assessment.

- List types of screening, evaluation, and assessment tools and techniques used by SLPs in EI.

- Describe how to choose tools and techniques to implement screening, evaluation, and assessment processes that effectively maximize both family and child outcomes through delivery of EI services.

- Recount observation techniques and the rationale for their use within EI assessment.

- Discuss the developmental domains, including specific skills, SLPs evaluate and assess in EI to ensure we obtain a holistic perspective of the young child's development.

- Define and describe augmentative and alternative communication (AAC) and role of the SLP to include AAC options within the EI assessment and intervention processes.

- Provide considerations related to cultural and linguistic responsiveness within screening, evaluation, and assessment processes.

What Will We Learn and How Can We Apply It?

When we work with young children with or are at risk for developmental delays or disabilities, it is important we implement evidence-based and recommended practices as we make our initial connection and engage effectively over time with their families. This process begins with screening, evaluating, and assessing the infants and toddlers who come to us for services. As SLPs in EI, we then embed these components within our practice to guide our decisions and inform our services. Therefore, this chapter focuses on how we can effectively implement screening, evaluation, and assessment to maximize both family and child outcomes through our delivery of EI services. First, we consider the DEC recommended practices that apply to our practice in screening, evaluation, and assessment. We then review the initial steps of the pathway through which families engage as they enter into and move through the EI system; in this chapter, we focus our attention on the components related to screening, evaluation, and assessment within the service pathway. We then examine key definitions and considerations related to the screening, evaluation, and assessment of infants and toddlers to ensure we understand the terms as they are presented within this arena.

We also address processes to guide our engagement, in addition to areas, methods, and tools used to evaluate and assess, and the interpretation of the evaluation and assessment results. Embedded within these sections, we explore strategies to effectively examine and respond to the strengths and needs of the children and families we serve. We focus on the inclusion of augmentative and alternative communication (AAC) within the assessment process, and present considerations related to cultural and linguistic responsiveness within the processes of screening, evaluation, and assessment.

Division for Early Childhood Recommended Practices in Assessment

As we learned in Chapter 1, the 2014 DEC Recommended Practices in EI/Early Childhood Special Education were developed to impart guidance to providers and families about the most effective ways to improve learning outcomes and promote the development of young children who have or are at risk for developmental delays disabilities. These practices are based on empirical evidence, as well as the experience of the professionals engaged in the field; as such, they serve as a guide for us to work with families to deliver the most effective services possible to infants, toddlers, and their families.

According to the DEC (2014), *assessment* is the generic term for the comprehensive process of gathering information to make informed decisions; they identify the purposes of assessment in EI as screening, determining eligibility for services, individualized planning, monitoring child progress, and measuring child outcomes. As such, the DEC (2014) recommended 10 EI practices related to these processes. Although IDEA Part C (2011) defines screening, evaluation, and assessment as distinct processes with different purposes, each of the following DEC (2014) recommendations support and guide these practices as we work with young children and their families and serve as a strong foundation for us as we dive into screening, evaluation, and assessment processes in EI.

- Providers work with the family to identify their preferences for assessment processes.

- Providers work as a team with the family and other professionals to gather assessment information. Providers use assessment materials and strategies, appropriate for the child's age and level of development, and accommodate the child's sensory, physical, communication, cultural, linguistic, social, and emotional characteristics.

- Providers conduct assessments that include all areas of development and behavior to ensure they are knowledgeable about the child's strengths, needs, preferences, and interests.

- Providers conduct assessments in the child's dominant language and in additional languages if the child is learning more than one language.
- Providers use a variety of methods to gather assessment information from multiple sources.
- Providers obtain information about the child's skills in daily activities, routines, and other natural environments.
- Providers use clinical reasoning in addition to assessment results to identify the child's current levels of functioning and to determine the child's eligibility and plan for instruction.
- Providers implement systematic and ongoing assessment to identify learning targets, plan activities, monitor progress, and revise intervention as needed.
- Providers use assessment tools with sufficient sensitivity to detect child progress.
- Providers report assessment results in a way that is understandable and useful to families.

Keeping these recommendations in mind as we engage and guide children and families will ensure we are implementing practices that are both evidence-based as well as effective.

Components Within the Early Intervention Pathway

As introduced in Chapter 1 and discussed in detail in Chapter 2, the fourth of five guiding principles presented by ASHA (2008a) states that the services we provide in EI should be "comprehensive, coordinated, and team-based." Regardless of state or local programming methods, all young children and their families follow the same basic steps, per IDEA (2004), as they enter and move through the EI system. The supports and services pathway begins with the referral for assessment and follows the child and family while they continue to receive services through the Part C program. This pathway consists of seven distinct components of service delivery: referral, intake, eligibility determination, assessment for service planning, IFSP development, implementation and reviews of the IFSP, and transition activities. Let's review the steps involved in referral, intake, and eligibility determination, and then focus on the details involved and implementation of the screening, evaluation, and assessment processes.

Referral

The first step in the pathway involves the referral of a child to the local EI system by a parent, pediatrician, or health department representative. The child might have a developmental delay or might need further assessment. Referral sources often have concerns based on observations, results of screenings, or a diagnosis indicating a potential delay. As long as we have secured parent or guardian permission, anyone in the community can make a referral of a child who might be eligible for Part C services. The local Central Point of Entry who receives the referral then collects the information and assigns a service coordinator to meet with the family. During the referral process, information regarding the local or statewide EI process is shared with the family, and initial information regarding the child and family is gathered. IDEA (2011) requires that providers (e.g., pediatricians) make referrals within 7 days after the infant or toddler has been identified as having a possible disability or delay. Once they have received a referral, the lead agency has 45 days to complete the intake or screening, initial evaluation, initial assessments, and initial team meeting to develop the initial IFSP for the child and the family (IDEA, 2011).

Intake

Intake involves face-to-face or phone meetings with the family to continue gathering information that will support the child's eligibility for EI services. This information includes developmental history, medical history and medical home information, family routines, schedules, and activities of interest, as well as the completion of a developmental screening, if and as needed.

Evaluation

An *evaluation* is defined by IDEA (2004) as "the procedures used by qualified personnel to determine a child's initial and continuing eligibility. An initial evaluation refers to the evaluation to determine his or her initial eligibility." This process may include the use of developmental checklists, standardized tests, objective, parent and caregiver report, a review of the child's medical records, and informed clinical opinion by the EI service providers. The evaluation must involve the parents or primary caregivers and be conducted by at least two qualified providers from different disciplines; one of the providers must be the service coordinator (IDEA 2004, §303.343(a)(1)(iv)). The multidisciplinary, or interprofessional, EI team then determines whether a child meets one or more of the criteria for eligibility. Part C of IDEA 2004 states that systems must serve any child "under 3 years of age who needs EI services" (IDEA 2004, §632(5)(A)) because the child "(i) is experiencing developmental delays, as measured by appropriate diagnostic instruments and procedures in one or more of the areas of cognitive development, physical development, communication development, social or emotional development, and adaptive development; or (ii) has a diagnosed physical or mental condition which has a high probability of resulting in developmental delay" (IDEA 2004, §632(5)(A)). Each state also has the option of serving children who show no delay but who are considered at risk for developmental challenges because of biological or environmental factors. If a child is not found eligible for Part C services, families could also choose to seek EI services through private or community resources and other federal or state-funded early childhood programs (e.g., Early Head Start).

Assessment for Service Planning

Assessment, as defined by Part C of IDEA, includes "the ongoing procedures used by qualified personnel to identify the child's unique strengths and needs and the EI services appropriate to meet those needs throughout the period of the child's eligibility" (IDEA 2011,

§303.321(a)(2)). We must remember the importance of going beyond the more formalized evaluation process to ensure we have a clear understanding of how each child is functioning, their strengths and needs, likes and dislikes, and priorities by the family. Assessment involves our use of observations, experiences and expertise, and conversations with the family and other caregivers to gather information about the child's interactions with and participation in family routines and everyday activities. The assessment process ensures the team has the opportunity to identify the EI supports and services that will effectively address the child's unique needs along with the family's priorities.

The Role of the Family

We have already identified family-centered practice as one of the most important foundations of effective EI services. When we engage in family-centered practice, we focus on the family's priorities and needs, as well as their capacity and ability to engage effectively with their own child(ren). We work with families to build their capacity to care for and optimize their child's development outcomes. The approach focuses on the important influence by the family on the child's development and is based on the belief that the best way to meet a child's needs is within their families and to engage in services that involve, strengthen, and support families. When family-centered practices are used in EI, we build on the strengths of the family, meet the family's changing needs, collaborate with the family, and support the family's ability to build partnerships with other people and organizations. In turn, the child benefits tremendously from the strong connection and sense of belonging through intentional engagement with their family. Family-centered practice is integrated into all of the steps in which we engage as SLPs in EI, including screening, evaluation, and assessment. With this in mind, there are several factors related to both the child and family that could affect the child's development and the family's response to our services. These include the child's developmental history and family background; environmental stressors affecting the family and child; language history and proficiency of the child and family; and the family's concerns, priorities, and resources. Table 6–1 presents these factors, along with discussion and strategies, to examine them within our practice.

Table 6–1. Family-Based Factors to Consider Within Screening, Evaluation, and Assessment

Factor	Considerations to Include in Process
Developmental history and family background	Gathering information about a child's birth, family, and medical history can help us identify risk and protective factors that can be useful in evaluation and assessment. This information should include the following: • A detailed review of the child's birth, medical history, developmental history, and potential risk factors (e.g., family history of disabilities, birth complications, genetic contributions).

	<ul><li>Examination and discussion regarding the family's protective factors (e.g., access to adequate medical care or family support).</li><li>A history of speech, language, and learning disabilities or related clinical diagnoses of parents and other family members that could be useful in evaluating a particular child's risk for communication deficits.</li></ul>
Environmental stressors	Environmental risk factors often co-occur and appear to have a cumulative effect; children who show greater numbers or higher levels of risk factors might be in greater need of intervention than children from more highly resourced backgrounds with the same level of disability. Therefore, it is important that we gather information about the following potential stressors:<ul><li>Social risk factors such as poverty, limited parent education, maternal depression, poor-quality child care, and adolescent or single parenthood.</li><li>Nontraditional family structures, including foster parents, adoptive parents, or grandparents who might not have complete information on the kinds of environmental stressors that could have affected the child, or who might know but choose not to share that information.</li><li>The family's access to housing, transportation, and food.</li></ul>
Language history and proficiency for children who are dual-language learners	The term 'dual-language learner' includes children who are exposed to two languages from birth or who receive sequential exposure to two languages (Crais, 2011). When we evaluate and assess young dual-language learners, we should inquire about the following information:<ul><li>Child and family language history.</li><li>Language(s) the family speaks predominantly at home and in the community.</li><li>Other languages spoken in the home.</li><li>The family's country of origin.</li><li>The length of time the family has been in the United States.</li><li>The child's age when first exposed to English.</li></ul>

	- The amount of English exposure.
- Who in the family speaks English or other languages (and how well).

It is also helpful to gather information about the family members' formal education and their perceptions of the child and disabilities in general, along with their previous experiences with health-care or child-care providers. This knowledge can help professionals adapt their interactions and the words they use with family members as well as gain a clearer understanding of the child and family's background. |
| Family concerns, priorities, and resources | IDEA (2004) requires us to offer all families the opportunity to identify their concerns, priorities, and resources related to enhancing their child's development. As such, we should consider the following outcomes to gather this information from the family:

- Identify the family's concerns and what family members hope to accomplish for the child.
- Determine how the family perceives the child's strengths and challenges in relation to its own beliefs, values, and everyday experiences.
- Identify the priorities of the family and how professionals can help with these priorities.
- Identify the family's existing resources related to their priorities. Resources should include both formal (e.g., social services, therapies) and informal (e.g., family members, neighbors, religious beliefs and affiliations) support systems.
- Identify the family's preferred roles in the service delivery process.
- Establish a supportive, informed, and collaborative relationship with the family. |

Note. Adapted from "Assessing family resources, priorities, and concerns," by D. B. Bailey, 2004; "Screening and assessment of young English-language learners," by National Association for the Education of Young Children, 2005; "Testing and beyond: Strategies and tools for evaluating and assessing infants and toddlers," E. Crais, 2011; "Understanding family, concerns, priorities, and resources," by P. Winton, 1996.

As presented in Table 6–1, there is a plethora of information that we can gather about a family and child that could add to the screening, evaluation, and assessment process. As EI SLPs, we need to work with each family to prioritize which types of information are most important to obtain, through what means, and how best to use the information we have received.

Definitions and General Considerations

Screening, evaluation, and assessment supplies us with valuable information about a child's interests, strengths, and needs. Screening a child gives us a snapshot of their development and whether it is on track. When screening indicates concern about a child's development, we conduct a comprehensive team-based evaluation to determine the child's needs, strengths, and ways in which we might support their development. Assessment is an ongoing process that includes observation and yields information about development over time. Systematic, ongoing assessment provides information regarding a child's development and learning. Assessment also helps us individualize services for every child and their family.

Screening

Screening refers to the process of identifying children who might need further evaluation to determine the presence of a developmental delay or disability. Under IDEA Part C (2004), screening is not mandatory; the process is, however, implemented at a state's discretion. If included in the state's post referral procedures, screening is conducted using selected instruments administered by trained providers in the lead agency or in an EI program. At any time during the screening, a parent or primary caregiver can request that we conduct an initial evaluation, even if the results of the screening do not indicate the need for further evaluation.

Screening is an important component of prevention, family education, and support that is particularly relevant for young children and their families. Screening results could lead to recommendations for monitoring and additional screening in the future or subsequent implementation of comprehensive assessments or referral for other examinations or services (ASHA, 2008b).

Speech, Language, Communication, and Swallowing Screening

As SLPs, we can screen for risk or presence of speech, language, communication, and feeding or swallowing difficulties using a variety of tools. We must select age-appropriate, culturally sensitive screening procedures conducted in the language(s) used by the child and family. A typical screening usually includes the following elements:

- Direct interaction with the child.

- Observation of interactions between child and parents or caregiver(s) in their natural environment.

- Interviews with family members or other caregivers (e.g., childcare provider) regarding concerns about the child's skills.

- Professionally administered and parent-completed tools (ASHA, 2008a, 2008b).

When evaluating screening results, we should consider whether responses by the child are indicative of a difference or a disorder. The differentiation between the two is critical when screening any child whose cultural or linguistic background, including English dialects, is different from that of the normative sample used in the screening tool (ASHA, 2008b). We discuss this consideration in greater detail in Chapter 8.

Recommendations and referrals for further evaluation and assessment of infants and toddlers are often based on developmental expectations. To evaluate whether a child is meeting these expectations, we need to determine if results of the screening are a valid reflection of the child's typical behavior (ASHA, 2008b). As noted earlier, the inclusion of families during the screening process is integral to ensure the child's responses are valid. Appendix A presents measures, several of which are available in multiple languages, we might use to screen the speech, language, communication, or swallowing skills of infants and toddlers.

Audiologic Screening

Hearing screening in EI is also within an SLP's scope of practice. Newborn hearing screenings have been the standard of care in hospitals in this country since 1999 (ASHA, 2008a). Infants who do not pass their newborn hearing screening are referred for medical and audiologic follow-up. Hearing screenings after the newborn period (0–6 months) are also important for early identification and management of the hearing status of an infant that might have been either missed during, or acquired after, the newborn period. Young children who are evaluated for EI services should receive a hearing screen as part of their comprehensive evaluation (ASHA, 2008a).

It is also important that we screen for vestibular disorders in the young children we serve. Vestibular system impairments in young children could present as developmental delays in activities such as walking. Children who have autism, brain injuries, reduced hearing, otitis media, and certain syndromes (e.g., Usher's syndrome, Waadenburg syndrome, Pendred syndrome, Alport's syndrome) might be at increased risk of vestibular disorders. We should be aware of related case history, gross motor milestones, balance, coordination, and parental concerns; if and when we have concerns about a child's vestibular system, we should refer for further evaluation and assessment by an audiologist (ASHA, 2008a; Doettl & McCaslin, 2017).

The Processes of Evaluation and Assessment

In some states, evaluation and assessment are separate processes. One team of professionals evaluates the child to determine eligibility; they then refer the child to another team for service coordination and assessment services. In other states, a single team might engage in a combined evaluation and assessment, and then provide service coordination and assessment planning services. Although there might be an overlap in the methods and teams that make up evaluation and assessment practices in EI, assessment usually encompasses more in-depth observations and information gathering than eligibility evaluations. Whereas the evaluation process is used to determine a child's eligibility for Part C services, assessment results are typically an integral part of intervention planning. In EI, it is not unusual for a larger team of providers to participate in the assessment process. Ongoing assessment by various team members also helps determine a child's response to treatment (ASHA, 2008a; Searcy, 2011).

IDEA (2004) specifies that both evaluation and assessment should be based on a variety of measures, including informed clinical opinion. The types of measures and activities used for both steps in the EI pathway can and often do include standardized tests as well as questionnaires, parent interviews and report forms, criterion-referenced tools, the use of play, dynamic procedures, and observational methods. When we engage in these practices, we should gather information from both direct interactions with the child and observation of the child in natural activities with parents and caregivers. IDEA (2004) also emphasizes that evaluation or assessment in EI requires us to use a range of tools in varied contexts; additionally, we should not make eligibility decisions based solely on the outcomes of standardized measures, but also include informed clinical opinion and information gathered from multiple sources across multiple contexts (ASHA, 2008b). Our role on the EI team, when engaged in both evaluation and assessment processes, is typically to measure and describe the child's communication and related behaviors, including feeding and swallowing; to share observations about the child's other developmental domains and how they might affect their overall learning; and to help in the decision-making process related to diagnosis, eligibility determination, and planning intervention and referrals for the child with the family (ASHA, 2008b).

Evaluation

Evaluation refers to the procedures used to determine a child's initial and continuing eligibility for EI services (DEC, 2014). As has been stated, no single procedure can be used as the sole criterion for determining a child's eligibility under Part C (IDEA, 2004). Part C of IDEA (2011) also requires a multidisciplinary team, including the parent and two or more individuals from separate disciplines or professions, with one of the individuals acting as the service coordinator. The multidisciplinary evaluation team typically includes at least two early childhood professionals who are appropriately qualified in their areas of expertise (i.e., SLP, occupational therapist, developmental specialist), at least one of whom is qualified in the primary area(s) of concern. The service coordinator works with the multidisciplinary evaluation team to facilitate evaluations. At a minimum, a multidisciplinary evaluation team gathers information from a review of pertinent records related to a child's current health status and medical history, family report, and the results of appropriate diagnostic methods. These methods might include additional reports from other sources, criterion-referenced instruments such as developmental checklists, a developmental history, language samples, criterion-referenced or norm-referenced instruments, observation of the child, play-based evaluations, and routine-based interviews. When we are working with families for whom English is not the native language or when there is a language barrier, an interpreter must be involved. The evaluation must be completed in the native language of the family or in the language(s) most likely to result in an accurate representation of the child's skills (DEC, 2014; IDEA, 2011).

Evaluation includes a comprehensive review of materials including medical and developmental reports, diagnostic reports, observations, and parent or caregiver interview and engagement. We now know that eligibility determination is based on the child's needs within their natural environment and that all areas of a child's development are considered to determine whether the child has a delay or differences that might make them eligible for Part C services. As such, "no single procedure may be used as the sole criterion for determining a child's eligibility" (IDEA 2011, §303.321(b)); these procedures must include administration of an evaluation instrument, an interview with the parent to gather the child's history, identification of the child's level of functioning in each of the developmental areas, a gathering of information from a variety of sources to understand the full scope of the child's individual strengths and needs, and a review of the child's medical, educational, and other records. As needed, our informed clinical opinion must also be considered in the process of determining eligibility (IDEA, 2011).

According to the IDEA (2011) regulations, evaluation considers data gathered from the following procedures:

1. Administering an evaluation instrument.

2. Taking the child's developmental and medical history (including interviewing the parent and family).

3. Identifying the child's level of functioning in each of the five developmental areas (cognitive, communication, physical, social or emotional, and adaptive).

4. Gathering information from other sources, such as caregivers, health care providers, and educators, to get a holistic view of the child's strengths and needs.

5. Reviewing medical, educational, or other records (IDEA, 2011).

Assessment

Assessment refers to the combination of formal and informal procedures used to identify a child's strengths and needs and determine the appropriate EI to meet those needs while they are involved in EI. Assessment in EI is an ongoing process. Culturally sensitive and linguistically appropriate assessments of both child and family occur to identify resources, priorities and concerns, and the supports and services necessary to enhance the family's capacity to meet the child's developmental needs (IDEA, 2011). Assessment is an integral part of the EI process, and many systems distinguish between two types of assessment.

- *Assessment for eligibility* might be offered if eligibility for EI services cannot be determined based on the intake process, in which a thorough review of the child's records, administration of a developmental screening tool, and family interview have been conducted.

- *Assessment for service planning* occurs once a child is found eligible for supports and services.

The assessment process yields valuable information that the EI team, including the family, uses to develop IFSP outcomes for the child and determine appropriate services to support families. This information is gathered using a functional assessment approach that explores a child's development in the context of their interactions with family, peers, and other caregivers while participating in the family's everyday activities and routines.

Although assessment tools might vary, ASHA (2008b) recommends combining formal and informal assessment tools that include both standardized and non-standardized measures to ensure the most comprehensive picture of the child is obtained. This combination of assessment tools provides information regarding the skills of the child in comparison to same-age peers. Conducting an assessment with a comprehensive battery is more conducive to encouraging family and team member participation and collaboration and to guide the IFSP development. Some local and statewide systems have implemented specific requirements regarding the choice and use of assessment tools for the purposes of both eligibility determination and assessment for service planning.

Evaluation and Assessment Tools and Techniques

Evaluation and assessment of infants and toddlers includes more than formal testing. A comprehensive set of activities are conducted to identify a child's strengths and challenges, address the family's priorities and concerns, and develop a plan for the next steps and opportunities to support the child and family (Crais, 2011; Raver & Childress, 2015).

Information gathered through the evaluation and assessment processes serves as the foundation on which the IFSP is developed; a plan for collaborative intervention is determined, initiated, and implemented; and desired outcomes are obtained (Dunst, 2017; McCormick et al., 2008; McWilliam, 2010a, 2010b, 2016; McWilliam et al., 2009; Searcy, 2018; Westby, 2009; Woods & Lindeman, 2008).

Standardized Assessments

Standardized assessments are tools that have been developed based on empirical data with established statistical reliability and validity. A standardized test requires all test takers to answer the same items or questions in the same way and is scored in a standard or consistent way. By maintaining consistent standards for administration, it is possible to compare the relative performance of individuals or groups of individuals. The two types of standardized assessment instruments include norm-referenced and criterion-referenced (ASHA, n.d.).

Norm-Referenced Tests

Norm-referenced tests are standardized tools designed to compare test takers in relation to one another. When we use a norm-referenced assessment tool, we can compare a child's score(s) with those of same-age peers who have already completed the test. A norm-referenced score is typically reported as a standard score or percentile ranking (ASHA, n.d.). Although this type of test measures a child's relative standing compared to a large population of children of the same age and is, therefore, valuable when we are determining eligibility for services, norm-referenced instruments offer us little value in measuring change and how a child is developing over time.

Criterion-Referenced Tests

Criterion-referenced tests are standardized tests that measure an individual's performance against a set of predetermined criteria or performance standards. In EI, these criteria include descriptions of what a child is expected to know or be able to do at a specific stage of development (ASHA, n.d.). Criterion-referenced assessments can be used during an observation to document a child's knowledge and functional use of speech, language, or communication skills within various routines or activities. We can also develop criterion-referenced procedures to informally address specific questions, observe skills embedded within play or other activities, and assess a child's response to intervention strategies (ASHA, n.d.).

Routines-Based Assessment

Routines-based assessment, which includes a description of a child's participation in family identified routines and activities, often begins with a family interview. We can ask the family to describe a typical day for and with their child. In addition to interviews, we can use observations, discussions, checklists, videos, and other methods to connect and collaborate with the family.

Engaging families as partners in their child's assessment includes gathering information from families about their child's strengths, interests, needs, and the ways in which they participate within daily routines. Gathering this information is critical for us to identify the child's strengths and needs and for making informed decisions about their goals and objectives. When we listen to family members, we need to encourage them to share their knowledge, and clarify their concerns, priorities, and goals for their child. During this process, we learn about a child's level of engagement, independence, and participation in familiar contexts as well as their communication, language, social, and play skills. Information gathered during the family interview gives us information related to opportunities throughout the natural course of the child's day that can serve as contexts for both assessment and intervention (Early Childhood Technical Assistance Center [ECTA], 2020a).

Play-Based Assessment

Play-based assessment focuses on child-directed activities. During a play-based assessment, children direct both interaction and experience, increasing the likelihood that we will observe behaviors in which they typically engage. In a play-based assessment, play serves as the primary context for observation and documentation of children's behavior as they interact with toys and people. Most play-based assessments include both free and structured play opportunities. Research supports that assessment processes embedded in play are perceived positively by both providers and families. EI providers also indicate play-based assessments can be completed in a significantly shorter time frame than traditional assessments, and the resulting reports tend to contain more useful information that can be directly translated into intervention (Crais, 2011; Owens, 2019).

When assessing how well an infant or toddler understands language, it is important to be sure that the child is responding to the words we are saying, rather than the nonverbal cues we might be providing within the structure of our play. For example, when we say to children, "give me the block," they might be responding to our outstretched hand as they hand the block to us; they might see the juice box we are getting out of the refrigerator rather than understand the question, "are you thirsty?" The same consideration should be incorporated into evaluation and assessment practices embedded within routines; children could also rely on the routine itself to follow directions or participate in everyday activities. For example, if a parent shares a snack at the table in the kitchen every morning, the child might follow the directions to "sit at the table" because they are associating the action with the snack that the parent is preparing rather than with the words "sit" and "table." To confirm valid evaluation and assessment results, we need to ensure the child is comprehending and responding to the language, rather than responding to their expectations based on a typical routine in which they engage every day.

Authentic and Functional Assessment

In EI, we are called upon to assess each child's knowledge and skills across environments, people, and time. The standardized, conventional testing tools and procedures that have been used in clinics or classroom-based programs are neither functional nor developmentally appropriate for the infants and toddlers we serve in EI. According to Bagnato and Ho (2006), *authentic assessment* is "the systematic recording of developmental observations over time about the naturally occurring behaviors and functional competencies of young children in daily routines" (p. 29) by their parents and those caregivers who know them best. Today, authentic and functional assessment is the recommended practice in EI by the DEC, the National Association for the Education of Young Children (NAEYC), and the National Association of Early Childhood Specialists in State Departments of Education (NAECS/SDE); as SLPs, we also recognize this process as best practice (ASHA, 2008b; Bagnato et al., 2014).

Authentic and functional assessment incorporates the observation and gathering of information about the young child's skills within everyday activities and routines (Macy et al., 2016). When using this approach, children do not have to score at a certain level or exhibit a certain type of behavior to achieve an acceptable score. Instead, the assessment process presents an ongoing opportunity for us to coach parents and caregivers to become aware of and appreciate their children's abilities and to consider how their knowledge, behaviors, and skills in one area affect their development in the range of developmental indicators (Hill et al., 2020). Functional assessment also helps us set goals with families. When we work together to document children's accomplishments while identifying areas that might need further development, we provide families with a vehicle to learn to observe their children and contribute to the evaluation of their learning and development. To honor family-centered and routines-based practices within our assessment process, we need to choose instruments considered authentic and functional. Appendix B imparts information about a selection of evaluation and assessment instruments that serve this purpose.

Strengths-Based Assessment

When we evaluate and assess an infant or toddler in EI, the strengths-based approach is used to identify children's interests and the abilities they use during their engagement in everyday activities and routines. *Strengths-based assessment* involves the collection of data about the things children like to do, the activities in which they participate, and the skills they have. This information then serves as our foundation for engaging children in everyday learning activities that focus on their strengths, supporting their participation in the activities, and interacting with them in a way that builds on their strengths to promote new learning (ECTA, 2020b).

To use the strengths-based approach within our assessment process, we need to embed authentic and functional strategies: These must include both family-centered and routines-based evaluation and assessment instruments. We can use various methods to gather information about a child's strengths. Table 6–2 offers suggestions for us to identify a child's abilities and interests when engaged in evaluation and assessment processes.

Table 6–2. Strategies to Identify a Child's Strengths and Abilities

Use a variety of methods to gather information about the child's strengths: • Observe them participating in everyday activities and routines. • Ask the parents and caregivers to complete a checklist that focuses on their child's personal interests, and behavioral as well as developmental strengths. • Interview parents and caregivers with open-ended questions about how the child expresses their abilities and interests every day.
When observing the child or administering assessment measures: • Notice the behaviors that keep the child engaged in various activities, identify the ways in which the child demonstrates curiosity, and observe how the child explores and uses objects and materials. • Identify how the child initiates and maintains interactions with parents, caregivers, or other adults and peers. Note the behaviors the child uses to respond to interactions with others. • Observe the ways in which the child expresses their needs, wants, and desires.
• Identify the objects, people, places, actions, activities, and events that get the child's attention and hold the child's interest. • Notice when the child indicates a like, preference, or choice. Observe those things that make the child smile, laugh, and show excitement.

Note. Adapted from "Identifying child strengths," by the Early Childhood Technical Assistance Center, 2020.

Dynamic Assessment

When we conduct a *dynamic assessment*, we test the child for a particular behavior, provide cues or models to facilitate the child's use of the behavior, and then test the child again. Feuerstein (1979) and Peña and Gillam (2000) identified dynamic assessment for SLPs as a tool used to determine skills a child presents independently versus skills a child demonstrates when an adult (or peer) serves as a facilitator. The results of this type of assessment offer us information about the child's strengths as well as current or potential barriers to success. This method can provide us with a measure of the child's stimulability; if we know a child is ready to learn a new skill based on how they respond to our cue or model, we can use this information to prioritize goals or identify intervention strategies. Although there are no published dynamic assessment tools specifically created for infants and toddlers, we can use most standardized tools intended for this age range and present the test items via a "dynamic" manner. As such, a test item that can be administered in a standardized way can be repeated with prompts or cues to determine if the child's performance improves (Crais, 2011).

Observation Techniques

Observation is a key component of assessment in EI (U.S. Department of Health and Human Services, 2019). Observation is one of the first steps in providing the kind of individualized, responsive care for infants and toddlers that builds relationships, supports attachment, and ensures we can measure and track children's progress in acquiring skills and concepts over time to ensure their development is on track (Jablon et al., 2007). As SLPs, when we are intentional about observing the children we serve and furnish coaching to the parents and caregivers to do the same, we are better able to understand how the children think, feel, and learn about the world around them. In turn, this helps us make more informed decisions about how to provide services to both the children and their families.

It takes practice to become a competent observer. Becoming an effective and accurate observer involves recognizing that what we notice and how we interpret our observations can be influenced by many variables. The U.S. Department of Health and Human Services (2024) notes that "culture, temperament, the presence of a delay or disability, personal experiences and relationships, professional knowledge, and even community values and messages in the media affect how we all see and experience children." Observing young children involves self-awareness, and we should expect our own awareness to develop with time and experience. In addition to practice, observations that produce useful information for both evaluation and assessment purposes involve multiple considerations. Table 6–3 presents several variables and strategies to conduct observations that support our evaluation and assessment processes in EI.

Table 6–3. Strategies to Engage in Effective Observations

Strategy	Considerations
Plan multiple opportunities to observe the child	To effectively capture the depth and breadth of a young child's skills, abilities, and interests, we should observe the child at different times of the day, and in different settings. Ideally, we want to observe children and their families: • Across locations (e.g., indoor and outdoor) and times of the day (e.g., morning, afternoon, evening) • Within routines (e.g., mealtimes, naptime, dressing diaper changing and toileting) • As they engage in play experiences and move from one play activity to another • As they interact with parents, caregivers, and other family members A single observation does not often provide enough information to observe the multiple layers, skills, and behaviors, including those that relate to cognitive, social and emotional, language, and approaches to learning. • A young child's behaviors are not usually consistent. Multiple considerations, including illness, lack of sleep, hunger, changes at home, changes in the daily schedule, and changes in staff, can influence what a child does and says from hour to hour and day to day. • One observation can, however, provide us with information about more than one area of development.
Involve families in the observation process	We should communicate with families about the importance of their role in observing their child between EI visits. We can support their observations through the following activities: • Provide them with relevant information, both verbally and written in their home language, about the development, skills, and activities their children might be demonstrating to ensure they have a clear understanding of what they are observing. • Encourage them to share what they observe about their children in person, in writing, or by showing us videos that they have recorded.

Plan spontaneous observation opportunities	Although this might sound like a contradiction, infants and toddlers often do and say things that are new and unexpected. The emergence of novel skills and behaviors can occur during unplanned observation times. We can prepare parents and caregivers to take note of these moments by: • Providing the family with materials on which to take notes (e.g., sticky notes, a small pad of paper).

Observation is one of the most powerful tools we have for building relationships with infants, toddlers, and their families. The process of observing allows us to truly see each child as a unique individual and a capable learner. Learning the art of observation and how it informs our practice takes time, effort, and awareness. The payoff, however, in regard to positive outcomes for the children and their families, as well as our own professional growth and development, is well worth the energy.

What Skills Are We Evaluating and Assessing?

As we discussed in Chapter 5, multiple domains contribute to the emergence of speech, language, and communication for both typically developing children and those who present with delays and disabilities (Calandrella & Wilcox, 2000; McCathren et al., 1999; Wetherby et al., 2002). Therefore, our evaluation and assessment of infants and toddlers should be focused on both their immediate abilities and needs, as well as on behaviors they present that could indicate long-term prognosis of the development of knowledge and skills. Embedded within our evaluation and assessment of a young child's comprehensive communication skills, several areas of development that produce a holistic perspective of the infant or toddler's knowledge and skills are worth noting. These include a young child's abilities related to function and means of communication; the relationship between the development of receptive language, grammar, and expressive language; and the child's engagement and levels of play.

Functions of Communication

We now know the ability of a young child to communicate with intent and use communication to engage with others is key to the development of higher-level communication skills (Brady et al., 2004). According to Bruner (1981), infants and toddlers should be using the following major communicative functions by 12 months of age:

- Social interaction includes initiating or sustaining a social game or routine, providing comfort, teasing, and showing off.

- Behavior regulation involves regulating the behavior of others to obtain an object, getting them to carry out an action, or stopping someone from doing something.

- Joint attention focuses on directing another's attention to comment on an object or event, providing information on an object or event, or acknowledging shared attention to an object or event.

Each of these skills was discussed in detail in Chapter 5, where we learned that the use of these specific types of communicative functions also plays a role in predicting children's later language skills; it is, therefore, important that we determine the functions of communication used by the infants and toddlers we assess in order to effectively plan intervention as and when needed in this area.

For prelinguistic children, interactive play contexts with caregivers and providers can serve as the foundation to sample the frequency, type, and variety of their intentional communication. During these interactions, we can watch for (and ask the caregiver about) the reasons the child communicates intentionally (e.g., to get something, to protest something). The SLP also can set up situations that encourage the child to communicate their needs. Use of tempting activities, such as starting a wind-up toy and letting it unwind or blowing bubbles and closing the lid, are examples of how we might use common toys to engage and prompt young children to demonstrate their use of communicative functions. For example, does the child communicate vocally or through eye gaze or gesture (e.g., reach, give it to us) to get the toy wound up? If not, what does the child do? Documenting the frequency, type, and variety of a child's communication is useful for assessing the child's current functioning and determining prognosis of communication skills for planning intervention (Crais, 2011).

Means of Communication

Means of communication used by young children include vocalizations, gestures, eye gaze, sentences, combinations of two or more prelinguistic means (e.g., eye gaze and gesture, gesture and vocalization), word approximations, words or signs, word combinations, and sentences. The ability of infants and toddlers to use these various means to communicate is strongly linked to their later language skills (McCathren et al., 2000; Zwaigenbaum et al., 2005).

When we assess the means by which a child communicates, we can use a variety of tools including observations, parent-report instruments, and standardized instruments. When we need to use formal methods for the purposes of eligibility, we could choose to supplement our process with informal measures as well, to ensure we have the opportunity to see the child's full repertoire of prelinguistic and linguistic means.

Receptive Language

Children typically demonstrate an understanding of language before they begin to use words to communicate. Deficits in language comprehension serve as a barrier for young children developing their use of language to express their needs and wants. These deficits also predict chronic language delays in toddlers who are late talking and children with autism spectrum disorders (Lyytinen et al., 2001; Paul, 2000a, 2000b; Wetherby et al., 2002; Wetherby et al., 2003). Comprehension also predicts language production in both speech and

AAC (Chapman et al., 2000) and the size of receptive vocabulary is a characteristic related to typical development in language skills among young children (Paul, 2000a). Finally, the research indicates that children with expressive language difficulties, but normal receptive language, are more likely to catch up expressively than those children with poor comprehension (Thal et al., 1997).

When we assess an infant or toddler, we should examine both nonlinguistic comprehension strategies, including their response to routines and interest in watching others, and linguistic comprehension skills. The ratio of words they produce to those they understand should be evaluated as a prognostic indicator of future expressive vocabulary (Owens, 2019).

Expressive Language

The expansion of vocabulary and grammatical structures is an important component of a child's overall development and is critical to both communication development and later academic success. A child's acquisition of new words is influenced not only by sensory and cognitive systems, but also by their experiences, the language they hear in their environment, and the sociocultural influences around the child.

Vocabulary

Although a traditional red flag for 24-month-old children has been the failure to have an expressive vocabulary of 50 words, no two-word combinations, or both (Paul, 1991; Rescorla, 1989), many of these late talkers perform at age level on standardized measures by 3 or 4 years of age (Paul et al., 1991; Thal et al., 1991; Whitehurst et al., 1992). Therefore, although vocabulary size is important, factors such as the rate of vocabulary growth; speech sound development, and social, cognitive, comprehension, gesture, play, emerging grammar, and imitative skills are also helpful variables to support our ability to differentiate between late talkers and children with language disorders. The diversity of word types (e.g., nouns, verbs, relational words) that a child verbalizes is a good indicator of the child's expressive language development.

Research by Schwartz and Leonard (1982) indicated that children are more likely to learn new words that include the sounds and syllable shapes already in their inventory. Therefore, once we have determined the child's expressive lexicon, we should categorize the words by both sound inventory and syllable shape. In addition, the rate of growth in the early years can be calculated and used in our clinical decision-making, as slow vocabulary growth might be a better indicator of risk in young children than vocabulary size (Hadley, 2006).

Most children begin to combine words when their vocabulary reaches between 50 and 100 words and word combinations typically emerge between 18 and 24 months of age (Fenson et al., 2007; Paul, 2007). By 24 months of age, most children are using a range of words per utterance (Fenson et al., 2007). The range of meanings expressed in early word combinations is also an important consideration, and we should consider intervention strategies that focus on enhancing word combinations by building on the ideas a child is attempting to express as well as on their word inventory. Therefore, vocabulary size and rate of growth, types of semantic relations expressed (e.g., agent-action, recurrence), and variety of word combinations are all elements of an evaluation or assessment of a young child's language skills (Crais, 2011).

Morphology and Syntax

When children add verbs to their lexicons, they also typically begin to form sentences; if we are working with a child who is not using any verbs by 24 months, or fewer than 20 verbs by 27 months, we should consider expansion of verbs in their vocabulary as a focus of our attention in intervention (Hadley, 2006). Klee and colleagues (2002) showed that 70% of children between 24 and 26 months of age used at least two subject–verb (e.g., baby cry) and subject–verb–object (e.g., I want snack) sentences. Therefore, the limited use of verbs and subject–verb sentences by 30 months indicates a risk for language impairment (Hadley, 2006). In addition, by 3 years of age, typically developing children had a diverse verb lexicon, produced frequent and diverse simple sentences, and demonstrated the onset of tense marking (i.e., use of morphological markers). We know the first tense morphemes usually emerge within sentences between 24 and 26 months and, despite some variability across children, all forms of tense morphemes are evident in most children by age 3 (Rispoli & Hadley, 2005). Therefore, absence of tense morphemes or limited productivity of tense morphemes at 36 months is an indication that a young child could be at risk for language impairment.

Most language measurement tools include items that tap into grammatical development. We might also consider collecting a language sample to confirm what grammatical structures, including use of verbs, morphological markers, and sentence combinations, a child is using.

Play

When we engage in evaluation and assessment, there are multiple advantages to examining a child's development of play skills. Play provides a nonlinguistic benchmark against which the child's linguistic performance can be compared when examining overall developmental level (Paul, 2007; Wetherby & Prizant, 2002). Profiling play skills with other developmental domains (e.g., communication, social, motor) also helps us identify the child's strengths and challenges across areas and can be useful in making diagnostic decisions as well as planning intervention with the family (Moon, 2019).

Although play skills, in and of themselves, are not considered prerequisites to specific language skills, relationships between play behaviors and other milestones at particular stages of development exist (Bates et al., 1980; Thal et al., 1991). In addition, the level of symbolic play exhibited by young children serves as a prediction of their later language skills (Lyytinen et al., 1999; Lyytinen et al., 2001). A child's play with, or interest in, objects might also affect the types of interactions and learning opportunities the child has (Pierce & Courchesne, 2001; Wetherby et al., 2003). When a child has fewer objects and actions about which to talk, and parents and caregivers are also constrained in their nonverbal and verbal attempts to engage in and facilitate the child's play and language, we will struggle to have content to support our intervention strategies. As suggested by Yoder and McDuffie (2006), facilitating the development of play skills ensures both children and their parents and caregivers, as well as us as their providers, have a greater variety of objects and actions to share in interactions, and serves as a context for enhancing the children's communication skills.

There are various ways to evaluate or assess a child's play. Informal approaches include observing the child while playing alone, or with a parent or caregiver, and identifying the type and complexity of play skills (Crais, 2011). Using play checklists could add more consistency to the process. Westby (1998) described seven stages of symbolic play that correspond to stages in children's language development. In a more recent play scale, Westby (2000) also integrated cognitive and communicative skills. We can also use more formal tools to assess a child's play.

When we assess a young child's play, we must remember that play skills and styles vary depending on several variables, including characteristics of play partners, type of toys available, and type of play in which the child is engaged (Cherney et al., 2003; Farver & Shin, 1997; Farver & Wimbarti, 1995). We should also consider cultural and linguistic differences within and among families. In some cultures, play is viewed as an avenue for learning; in others, play is considered entertainment. Additionally, parents in some cultures are more likely to label and describe their child's play, whereas those in other cultures might be more directive in play (Vigil, 2002). Therefore, young children's play interests and skills should be interpreted with these cultural and familial differences in mind.

Augmentative and Alternative Communication

ASHA (2023) defined AAC as an area of practice that supplements or compensates for impairments in speech-language production, comprehension, or both. AAC is considered augmentative when used to supplement existing speech, and alternative when used in place of speech that is absent or not functional (Elsahar et al., 2019).

Years ago, many SLPs believed that AAC should only serve as a last resort, if even an option at all, for young children with significant communication delays or disabilities. Research has been conducted and the evidence is now clear: All children with delayed communication should have access to AAC (Cress & Marvin, 2003; Romski & Sevcik, 2005; Romski et al., 2015; Wilkinson & Hennig, 2007). Additionally, access to the Internet, Wi-Fi, and mobile technologies have simplified our ability to assess and provide AAC options to the families we serve. With this access, we have seen many positive changes in overall awareness and use of AAC (McNaughton & Light, 2013). As SLPs, it is our responsibility in EI to determine whether the inclusion of AAC will support a young child's ability to communicate or facilitate the development of their speech and language skills. Although we do not go into great detail regarding the AAC assessment process in this textbook, a few key elements are worthy of our consideration at this time.

When working with young children and their families, AAC might involve the assessment of or use of a variety of techniques and tools to support an infant or toddler's ability to express their needs, wants, and feelings, including the following:

- Manual signs.

- Gestures.
- Finger spelling.
- Tangible objects.
- Line drawings.
- Picture communication boards and letter boards.
- Speech-generating devices.

Prior to selecting an AAC system, it is imperative that we assess the child's abilities in areas related to using AAC; these include language and communication, symbolic representation, and access (Beukelman & Mirenda, 2013). Assessment of a child's language and communication provides us with the knowledge we might eventually need to choose and organize an AAC system. Although standardized measures can be used to obtain preliminary information about a child's language and communication skills, the information provided by such tools is often limited when a child's expressive language, or concomitant physical impairments, impede the child's ability to respond to tasks using spoken responses or motor responses (Beukelman & Mirenda, 2013; Brady et al., 2012; Ross & Cress, 2006). In addition, these protocols do not provide the details we need regarding the child's comprehension or use of symbol representation, system organization, or vocabulary selection. Therefore, unstructured assessments, including interviews, checklists, and observational assessments, tend to provide us with greater details about the child's communication skills. Symbolic representation and access must also be assessed. Symbolic representation refers to the level of iconicity a child understands and can use to communicate a thought or a concept; access refers to the method through which the child uses a system (e.g., eye gaze, direct select, scanning). These elements of AAC assessment are most effectively assessed through a dynamic approach to identify what strategies, if any, the child currently uses to communicate, as well as which strategies the child is capable of learning (Beukelman & Mirenda, 2013).

Once we have determined that AAC is an appropriate choice to include in the child's EI services, evaluation of their needs and skills, daily activities, and capacity of parents and caregivers is necessary to select an appropriate system. Feature matching is an assessment model that involves collaborative decision-making in which the EI team determines which key features a child needs in an AAC system (Costello et al., 2013; Glennen & DeCoste, 1997). Within this process, we introduce AAC systems to the child and observe their skills with different features (e.g., symbol sets, system organization, voice output, keyboard layouts, alternative access methods). Based on our observations with different systems, we can compare features to determine which AAC system will best support the child's communication needs.

To successfully engage in assessment, system selection, training, and use of an AAC system for a young child, it is imperative we ensure family-centered practices are infused in each of these stages. We now know how important a family-centered approach is in EI. Providing the family with choices, identifying their strengths, and addressing their needs through individualized services is also necessary when assessing a child's need for or potential use of an AAC system.

Collaborating With Families

Evaluation and assessment can take many forms, and we can use a variety of methods, tools, and measures to consider, and content areas to examine, infants and toddlers in EI. As SLPs, we can work together with each family to determine the most appropriate and accessible options for identifying each child's strengths and challenges, acknowledging the priorities, needs, and opportunities for the family.

Gathering and Sharing Information With Families

As we know, families serve a central role in EI and we must consistently engage in family-centered practice to serve as effective SLPs. Because this approach focuses on the important influence of the family on the child's development, it is imperative that we include families in service pathways related to evaluation and assessment. When family-centered practices are used within these processes, we build on the strengths of the family, collaborate with the family, and support the family's ability to build partnerships with us and their EI team. This requires full family participation throughout the process to ensure that our observations and interpretations of their child's knowledge and skills are a meaningful reflection of the family's perspective.

Significant evidence supports parents and caregivers as reliable informants who are able to offer accurate descriptions of their children's abilities and development (Crais et al., 2004; Fenson et al., 2007; Squires et al., 1998). Because parents are able to observe large samples of their children's behavior in natural environments and within their own routines and daily activities, their input can enhance the validity and reliability of our evaluation and assessment outcomes (Fenson et al., 2007; Simeonsson et al., 1995). When parents are asked to observe and rate their child's behaviors, the results can also help parents and providers integrate their views of the child and accurately determine the child's strengths and challenges (Bricker & Squires, 1999; LaRocque et al., 2001; Squires et al., 1998). We should, therefore, ensure families have every available opportunity to contribute to evaluation and assessment processes both with and for their own children.

With family-centered practice in mind, an important component of our comprehensive evaluation or assessment for program planning for the child we serve is the parent or caregiver or family interview. We have not necessarily been trained to connect with and interview family members, yet we are expected to be prepared to gather a solid foundation of information as we partner with the families we serve in EI. Table 6–4 includes a list of helpful and important questions we can ask when we meet with a young child's family. These questions serve as a strong starting point for learning about infants, toddlers, and families to prepare ourselves to meet their needs.

Table 6–4. Family-Based Interview Questions

Questions regarding family composition
- Please share with us who your family members are and their relationship to one another.
- Where do you and your family members live?
- What are the major roles of each of your family members?
- Which family members serve as the primary caregivers for your children?
- Do you and your family members make decisions together or does one member make the major decisions?
    - Who makes the decisions about child-rearing goals?
    - Who makes decisions about disciplinary standards?
    - Who makes decisions related to health issues and treatment?
- Who and how are other family members or caregivers included in your family's circle of support?

Questions related to family culture, ethnicity, and language
- With which cultural, ethnic, and linguistic groups does your family identify with?
- What languages do family members speak in the home?
- What is your language of preference when you communicate with us?
- Is an interpreter needed for communication with us?
- Do family members prefer written materials or information through another medium (e.g., in a conversation) instead?
- Would you like written materials to be translated into a preferred language?

Questions related to family preferences and customs
- How would you and your family members prefer to be greeted?
- Are we, as EI service providers, invited into the family's home? Where and when would you prefer to meet for our visits?
- What are your family's customs in the home (e.g., removal of shoes when entering the home, shaking hands or not touching family members unless invited to do so)?
- What are your hopes and dreams for your family and children?

Questions related to child-rearing and child development
- What is your understanding of and beliefs related to child development?
    - Your expectations related to your child's developmental milestones (e.g., toileting, feeding, caring for self)?
    - Your goals for your child's development?
- What are your family mealtime practices? Do any of you have any dietary preferences or restrictions?
- Who is responsible for feeding the children? What are the mealtime practices in which you engage?
- What are your child's sleeping arrangements and routines?

- What are your family's beliefs about behavior and discipline?

Questions related to education, health care, and support services
- What are your beliefs and perceptions about the development of your child?
- What are your family's beliefs and approach to early intervention and health care?
- What are your beliefs about the education of your child (e.g., school readiness)?
- What education and treatment approaches does your family use?
- Does your family seek help from other family members or individuals?
- Does your family receive or seek support from any other formal agencies, organizations, or community services? For what services?
  - Do you and your family members agree about the use of these services and supports and the approaches they use?
  - What are your feelings and your family members' feelings about seeking help, and your degree of comfort in doing so?

Questions about routines and everyday activities
- What are your main concerns for your child and family?
- What does a typical day look like for your child? For your family? (Walk the parent or caregiver through the activities of the day, prompting as needed with "What's next?").
  - Can you describe what wake-up time is like?
  - What do mealtimes like?
  - How does getting dressed go?
  - How do things go when you are getting ready to go somewhere with your child?
  - What does your family do when you are relaxing at home?
  - What is bath time like?
  - How does bedtime go?
  - How are trips to the grocery store (or other errands)? Do you bring your child with you?
  - Does your family spend much time outdoors? If so, where and what do you do?
- When you lie awake at night worrying, what is it you worry about?
- If you could change anything about your life, what would it be?
- How is sleep going for your child? How is sleep going for you (i.e., the parents or primary caregivers)?

Parent and caregiver evaluation and assessment measures also include rating scales, checklists, inventories, and questionnaires completed by family members or caregivers, teacher, or individual. Findings from these sources can then be compared and included in a comprehensive profile of the child's communication skills. Table 6–5 provides us with suggestions about how we can connect with families during the evaluation and assessment processes.

Table 6–5. Considerations to Connect With Families During the Evaluation and Assessment Process

• Families have varying knowledge about EI. They might feel apprehensive sharing input about the assessment. They might feel anxious if or when more information is shared than they are ready to hear. We need to meet families where they are, follow their lead, and provide information as often, and as repeatedly, as needed (Caicedo, 2014; Raver & Childress, 2015; Searcy, 2011).
• The type and amount of information we share and the way we share can affect how families feel about the assessment process and the decisions we make regarding referral, intervention, and eventual transition (Crais, 2011).
• We need to present families with complete and unbiased information in terms they can understand. They can only make informed decisions and actively participate in conversations regarding planning and implementation of services when they feel comfortable with the information they have received.
• Before discussing results, we should ask families to share their impressions of the evaluation and assessment activities, any concerns they have, and what they see as their child's strengths and needs (Woods & Lindeman, 2008).
• Evaluation or assessment findings could sometimes be unexpected or difficult for families to hear. They might be overwhelmed, grieving, or even in denial. It is important to address the emotional responses of parents and caregivers within the evaluation, assessment, and intervention process (Bhat, 2017; Caicedo, 2014; Raver & Childress, 2015; Searcy, 2011; Searcy & Hughes, 2015).

Considerations Related to Cultural and Linguistic Diversity

Children and families who receive EI supports and services are increasingly diverse, representing different cultures, ethnicities, traditions, values, and belief systems. As we have already discussed, the second guiding principle that reflects current best practices for SLPs engaged in the EI arena is the assurance to families of infants and toddlers that they will have access to, and receive, culturally and linguistically responsive and competent services (ASHA, 2023; IDEA, 2011). This means we effectively interact with and support people of different cultures by understanding, including, and valuing the diversity of the families, while seeking further knowledge regarding their culture and language (Hopf et al., 2021). We must be culturally humble and responsive by engaging in a team approach that involves both self-reflection and collaboration with the families we serve; we listen and remain open to understanding their perspectives (Hopf et al., 2021). As SLPs we must, therefore, be willing to demonstrate humility to be culturally and linguistically responsive across the EI supports and services pathway. Screening, evaluation, and assessment services are no exception and must be provided to families in their native language (IDEA, 2011). In the case of a child, that means the language normally used by the child's parents. When conducting an evaluation and assessment, however, it might be developmentally appropriate to use the language(s) typically used by the child (which might be different from that of the parents). These processes should be conducted in the language(s) most likely to yield an accurate picture of the child's skills (DEC, 2014; IDEA, 2011). In addition, standardized tests should be culturally and linguistically appropriate. Standard scores should not be determined if the norming sample does not adequately represent the child being assessed. We must consider the language spoken or dialect used by the child before selecting a standardized assessment. For parents or caregivers who speak a language other than English in the home, we need to gather detailed information about their use of the primary language and English. When possible, checklists should be made available in the family's native language to obtain the most accurate information about the child we are serving. It is also imperative that we refrain from making assumptions about parents, caregivers, or families as a whole based on any cultural, linguistic, or other variables they might present to us.

We expound on inclusive practices in Chapter 8, where we examine and discuss details regarding variables to ensure our services in EI are culturally competent, humble, and responsive for the families we serve.

Summary

This chapter addressed the processes and best practices involved in screening, evaluation, and assessment within the EI arena. We have discussed how and why these processes are such critical components when we serve young children and their families in EI because they guide our decisions and inform our services. Each time we welcome children and their families into our EI caseloads and into our hearts, we are presented with a unique opportunity and challenge. Screening, evaluating, assessing infants and toddlers, and engaging parents and caregivers within the process, will look different with every family. Behavior, play, routines, everyday activities, timelines, priorities, and parent–caregiver interactions will vary from one child and family to another. Throughout this chapter, we reviewed the options and the opportunities to embed family-based practice, routines- and strengths-based approaches, and authentic, functional processes within the evaluation and assessment components of EI. Armed with this knowledge, we are able to effectively follow the lead and the needs of the children and families we serve to see who they truly are and the skills of which they are capable. In Chapter 7, we focus our attention on the next steps in the EI pathway, including practices involved in determining a child's eligibility, developing the IFSP, monitoring progress, and measuring outcomes.

Critical Thinking Questions

1. Define screening, evaluation, and assessment under IDEA Part C. What are the differences between each of these processes and where does each one fit within the supports and services pathway of EI?

2. Why is it important that we are familiar with the Division for Early Childhood (DEC) Recommended Practices in EI related to screening, evaluation, and assessment?

3. What are the various types of screening, evaluation, and assessment tools we use as SLPs in EI? What are some of the variables we might consider to effectively maximize both family and child outcomes as we choose the tools to screen, evaluate, and assess each child?

4. What is the difference between assessment for eligibility and assessment for service planning? How might we describe these two types of assessment to a parent or caregiver?

5. Why is authentic and functional assessment considered best practice in EI? How do we engage in this type of assessment to ensure we honor family-centered and routines-based practices within this process?

6. Describe effective observation techniques and the rationale for their use within an EI assessment.

7. What are the developmental domains, including specific skills, we evaluate and assess in EI to ensure we obtain a holistic perspective of the young child's development?

8. Define augmentative and alternative communication (AAC) and describe our role to include AAC options within the EI assessment and intervention processes.

9. How and why should we consider cultural and linguistic responsiveness within our screening, evaluation, and assessment processes?

References

American Speech-Language-Hearing Association. (2008a). *Core knowledge and skills in early intervention speech-language pathology practice.* https://doi.org/10.1044/policy.KS2008-00292

American Speech-Language-Hearing Association. (2008b). *Roles and responsibilities of speech-language pathologists in early intervention: Guidelines.* https://doi.org/10.1044/policy.GL2008-00293

American Speech-Language-Hearing Association. (2023). *Augmentative and alternative communication practice portal.* https://www.asha.org/Practice-Portal/Professional-Issues/Augmentative-and-Alternative-Communication/#collapse_3

American Speech-Language-Hearing Association. (n.d.). Assessment tools, techniques, and data sources. https://www.asha.org/practice-portal/clinical-topics/late-language-emergence/assessment-tools-techniques-and-data-sources/

Bagnato, S. J., Goins, D. D., Pretti-Frontczak, K., & Neisworth, J. T. (2014). Authentic assessment as "best practice" for early childhood intervention: National consumer social validity research. *Topics in Early Childhood Special Education, 34,* 116–127.

https://doi.org/10.1177/0271121414523652

Bagnato, S. J., & Ho, H. Y. (2006). High-stakes testing with preschool children: Violation of professional standards for evidence-based practice in early childhood intervention. *KEDI International Journal of Educational Policy, 3*(1), 22–43. http://eng.kedi.re.kr

Bailey, D. B. (2004). *Assessing family resources, priorities, and concerns*. In M. McLean, M. Wolery, & D. Bailey (Eds.), Assessing infants and preschoolers with special needs 3rd ed. (pp. 172–203). Upper Saddle River, NJ: Pearson Merrill Prentice Hall.

Bates, E., Bretherton, I., Snyder, L., Shore, C., & Volterra, V. (1980). Vocal and gestural symbols at 13 months. *Merrill-Palmer Quarterly, 2*, 407–423.

Beukelman, D., & Mirenda, P. (2013). *Augmentative and alternative communication: Supporting children and adults with complex communication needs* (4th ed.). Brookes.

Bhat, V. (2017). Family centered developmental care as early intervention for children with special needs. *International Educational Applied Scientific Research Journal, 2*, 26–28.

Brady, N. C., Fleming, K., Thiemann-Bourque, K., Olswang, L., Dowden, P., Saunders, M. D., & Marquis, J. (2012). Development of the communication complexity scale. *American Journal of Speech-Language Pathology, 21*(1), 16–28.

Brady, N., Marquis, J., Fleming, K., & McLean, L. (2004). Prelinguistic predictors of language growth in children with developmental disabilities. *Journal of Speech, Language, and Hearing Research, 47*, 663–677.

Bricker, D., & Squires, J. (1999). *Ages and stages questionnaires (ASQ): A parent-completed child-monitoring system* (2nd ed.). Brookes.

Bruner, J. (1981). The social context of language acquisition. *Language and Communication, 1*, 155–178.

Caicedo, C. (2014). Families with special needs children. *Journal of the American Psychiatric Nurses Association, 20*, 398–407.

Calandrella, A., & Wilcox, J. (2000). Predicting language outcomes for young prelinguistic children with developmental delay. *Journal of Speech, Language, and Hearing Research, 43*, 1061–1071.

Chapman, R., Seung, H., Schwartz, S., & Bird, E. (2000). Predicting language production in children and adolescents with Down syndrome: The role of comprehension. *Journal of Speech, Language, and Hearing Research, 43*, 340–350.

Cherney, J. D., Kelly-Vance, L., Glover, K. G., Ruane, A., & Ryalls, B. O. (2003). The effects of stereotyped toys and gender on play assessment in children aged 18–47 months. *Educational Psychology, 23*(1), 95–106.

Costello, J. M., Shane, H. C., & Caron, J. (2013). *AAC, mobile devices, and apps: Growing pains with evidence-based practice.* http://www.vantatenhove.com/files/papers/AACandApps/CostelloShaneCaron-WhitePaper.pdf

Crais, E. (2011). Testing and beyond: Strategies and tools for evaluating and assessing infants and toddlers. *Language, Speech, and Hearing Services in Schools, 42,* 341–364.

Crais, E., Douglas, D., & Campbell, C. (2004). The intersection of the development of gestures and intentionality. *Journal of Speech, Language, and Hearing Research, 47,* 678–694.

Cress, C. J., & Marvin, C. A. (2003). Common questions about AAC services in early intervention. *Augmentative and Alternative Communication, 19*(4), 254–272.

Division for Early Childhood. (2014). *DEC recommended practices in early intervention/early childhood special education 2014.* http://www.dec-sped.org/recommendedpractices

Doettl, S. M., & McCaslin, D. L. (2017, July). How young is too young to evaluate children for dizziness? As our knowledge of childhood vestibular disorders grows, so do calls for audiologists to test for dizziness and recommend treatment. *The ASHA Leader, 22,* 18–20.

Dunst, C. J. (2017). Family systems early childhood intervention. In H. Sukkar, J. Kirby, & C. J. Dunst (Eds.), *Early childhood intervention: Working with families of young children with special needs* (pp. 36–58). Routledge.

Early Childhood Technical Assistance Center. (2020a). *Engaging families as assessment partners* [Assessment Practitioner Practice Guide 2 of 5]. http://ectacenter.org/decrp

Early Childhood Technical Assistance Center. (2020b). *Identifying child strengths.* https://ectacenter.org/~pdfs/decrp/PG_Asm_IdentifyingChildStrengths_prac_print_2017.pdf

Elsahar, Y., Hu, S., Bouazza-Marouf, K., Kerr, D., & Mansor, A. (2019). Augmentative and alternative communication (AAC) advances: A review of configurations for individuals with a speech disability. *Sensors, 19*(8), 1911. https://doi.org/10.3390/s19081911

Farver, J. M., & Shin, Y. L. (1997). Social pretend play in Korean- and Anglo-American pre-schoolers. *Child Development, 68,* 544–556.

Farver, J. M., & Wimbarti, S. (1995). Indonesian children's play with their mothers and older siblings. *Child Development, 66,* 1493–1503.

Fenson, L., Marchman, V. A., Thal, D., Dale, P., Reznick, J. S., & Bates, E. (2007). *The MacArthur-Bates communicative development inventories: User's guide and technical manual* (2nd ed.). Brookes.

Glennen, S., & DeCoste, D. (1997). *Handbook of augmentative and alternative communication.* Singular Publishing.

Hadley, P. A. (2006). Assessing the emergence of grammar in toddlers at-risk for specific language impairment. *Seminars in Speech and Language, 27*, 173–186.

Hill, C. F., Children, D. C., Terry, L. M., & Brager, A. M. (2020). Implementing recommended assessment practices in early intervention. In Division for Early Childhood (Ed.), *Assessment recommended practices for young children and families* (pp. 41–52). Division for Early Childhood of the Council for Exceptional Children.

Hopf, S. C., Crowe, K., Verdon, S., Blake, H., & McLeod, S. (2021). Advancing workplace diversity through the culturally responsive teamwork framework. *American Journal of Speech-Language Pathology, 30*(5), 1949–1961.

Individuals With Disabilities Education Improvement Act of 2004, Pub. L. No. 108-446, § 632, 118 Stat. 2744 (2004). http://idea.ed.gov/

Individuals With Disabilities Education Improvement Act. (2011). Part C Final Regulations. 34 C.F.R. §§ 303 (2011). https://www.gpo.gov/fdsys/pkg/FR-2011-09-28/pdf/2011-22783.pdf

Jablon, J. R., Amy L. D., & Dichtelmiller, M. L. (2007). *The power of observation for birth through eight* (2nd ed.). Teaching Strategies and National Association for the Education of Young Children.

Klee, T., Gavin, W., & Letts, C. (2002, June). *Development of a reference profile of children's grammatical development.* Poster presented at the International Congress for the Study of Child Language/Symposium for Research on Child Language Disorders, Madison, WI.

LaRocque, M., Brown, S. E., & Johnson, K. L. (2001). Functional behavioral assessments and intervention plans in early intervention settings. *Infants and Young Children, 13*, 59–68.

Lyytinen, P., Laakso, M., Poikkeus, A.& Rita, N. (1999). The development and predictive relations of play and language across the second year. *Scandinavian Journal of Psychology, 40*, 177–186.

Lyytinen, P., Poikkeus, A., Laakso, M., Eklund, K., & Lyytinen, H. (2001). Language development and symbolic play in children with and without familial risk of dyslexia. *Journal of Speech, Language, and Hearing Research, 44*, 873–885.

Macy, M., Bagnato, S. J., & Gallen, R. (2016). Authentic assessment: A venerable idea whose time is now. *Zero to Three, 37*(1), 37–43.

McCathren, R. B., Yoder, P. J., & Warren, S. F. (1999). The relationship between prelinguistic vocalization and later expressive vocabulary in young children with developmental delay. *Journal of Speech, Language, and Hearing Research, 42,* 915–924.

McCathren, R. B., Yoder, P. J., & Warren, S. F. (2000). Testing predictive validity of the communication composite of the Communication and Symbolic Behavior Scales. *Journal of Early Intervention, 23*(3), 36–46.

McCormick, K. M., Stricklin, S., Nowak, T. M., & Rous, B. (2008). Using eco-mapping to understand family strengths and resources. *Young Exceptional Children, 11,* 17–28.

McNaughton, D., & Light, J. (2013). The iPad and mobile technology revolution: Benefits and challenges for individuals who require augmentative and alternative communication. *Augmentative and Alternative Communication, 29,* 107–116. https://doi:10.3109/07434618.2013.784930

McWilliam, R. A. (2010a). *Routines-based early intervention: Supporting young children and their families.* Baltimore, MD: Brookes.

McWilliam, R. A. (2010b). Assessing families' needs with the routines-based interview. In R. A. McWilliam (Ed.), *Working with families of young children with special needs* (pp. 27–60). Guilford Press.

McWilliam, R. A. (2016). The routines-based model for supporting speech and language. *Revista de Logopedia, Foniatría y Audiología, 36,* 178–184.

McWilliam, R. A., Casey, A. M., & Sims, J. L. (2009). The routines-based interview: A method for assessing needs and developing IFSPs. *Infants & Young Children, 22,* 224–233.

Moon, K. (2019). *The reliability of early language assessment tools.* University of the Pacific. https://core.ac.uk/download/478081995.pdf

National Association for the Education of Young Children. (2005). *Screening and assessment of young English-language learners* [Supplement to the NAEYC position statement on early childhood curriculum, assessment, and program evaluation].

Owens, R. (2019). *Language development: An introduction* (10th ed.). Pearson Education.

Paul, R. (1991). Profiles of toddlers with slow expressive language development. *Topics in Language Disorders, 11*(4), 1–13.

Paul, R. (2000a). Predicting outcomes of early expressive language delay: Ethical implications. In D. V. M. Bishop & L. B. Leonard (Eds.), *Speech and language impairments in children: Causes, characteristics, intervention, and outcome* (pp. 195–209). Psychology Press.

Paul, R. (2000b). Understanding the "whole" of it: Comprehension assessment. *Seminars in Speech and Language, 21*(3), 10–17.

Paul, R. (2007). *Language disorders from infancy through adolescence: Assessment and intervention* (3rd ed.). Mosby.

Peña, E. D., & Gillam, R. B. (2000). *Dynamic assessment of children referred for speech and language evaluations*. In C. Lidz & J. Elliott (Eds.), Dynamic assessment: Prevailing models and applications (Vol. 6, pp. 543–575). Elsevier Science.

Pierce, K., & Courchesne, E. (2001). Evidence for a cerebellar role in reduced exploration and stereotyped behavior in autism. *Biological Psychiatry, 49*, 655–664.

Raver, S. A., & Childress, D. C. (2015). *Family-centered early intervention: Supporting infants and toddlers in natural environments*. Brookes.

Rescorla, L. (1989). The language development survey: A screening tool for delayed language in toddlers. *Journal of Speech and Hearing Disorders, 54*, 587–599.

Rispoli, M., & Hadley, P. (2005, June). *The acquisition and automaticity of finiteness marking* [Poster presentation]. Symposium on Research in Child Language Disorders, Madison, WI.

Romski, M., & Sevcik, R. A. (2005). Augmentative communication and early intervention: Myths and realities. *Infants & Young Children, 18*(3), 174–185.

Romski, M., Sevcik, R. A., Barton-Hulsey, A., & Whitmore, A. S. (2015). Early intervention and AAC: What a difference 30 years makes. *Augmentative and Alternative Communication, 31*(3), 181–202.

Ross, B., & Cress, C. J. (2006). Comparison of standardized assessments for cognitive and receptive communication skills in young children with complex communication needs. *Augmentative and Alternative Communication, 22*, 100–111.

Schwartz, R., & Leonard, L. (1982). Do children pick and choose? Phonological selection and avoidance in early lexical acquisition. *Journal of Child Language, 9*, 319–336.

Searcy, K. L. (2011). *Here's how to do early intervention for speech and language: Empowering parents*. Plural Publishing.

Searcy, K. L. (2018). Funding and documentation for early intervention (0 to 3 years). In N. Swigert (Ed.), *Documentation and reimbursement for speech-language pathologists: Principles and practice* (pp. 251–291). Slack Incorporated.

Searcy, K. L., & Hughes, D. M. (2015, November). *A collaborative framework for early intervention services: Redefining natural environments* [Paper presentation]. American Speech-Language-Hearing Association Annual Convention, Denver, CO.

Simeonsson, R., Edmondson, R., Smith, T., Carnahan, S., & Bucy, J. (1995). Family involvement in multidisciplinary team evaluation: Professional and parent perspectives. *Childcare, Health, and Development, 21*(3), 199–215.

Squires, J. K., Potter, L., Bricker, D., & Lamorey, S. (1998). Parent-completed developmental questionnaires: Effectiveness with low and middle income parents. *Early Childhood Research Quarterly, 13*(2), 345–354.

Thal, D. J., Bates, E., Goodman, J., & Jahn-Samilo, J. (1997). Continuity of language abilities: An exploratory study of late- and early-talking toddlers. *Developmental Neuropsychology, 13*(3), 239–273. https://doi.org/10.1080/87565649709540681

Thal, D., Tobias, S., & Morrison, D. (1991). Language and gesture in later talkers: A 1-year follow-up. *Journal of Speech and Hearing Research, 34*, 747–753.

U.S. Department of Health and Human Services, Administration for Children and Families, Office of Head Start. (2024). *Identifying the lenses through which staff and families observe children.* https://eclkc.ohs.acf.hhs.gov/child-screening-assessment/child-observation-heart-individualizing-responsive-care-infants-toddlers/identifying-lenses-through-which-staff-families

U.S. Department of Health and Human Services, Administration for Children and Families, Office of Head Start. (2019). *Ongoing child assessment: A guide for program leaders.*

Vigil, D. C. (2002). Cultural variations in attention regulation: A comparative analysis of British and Chinese-immigrant populations. *International Journal of Language and Communication Disorders, 37*, 433–458.

Westby, C. (1998). *Social–emotional bases of communication development.* In W. Haynes & B. Shulman (Eds.), Communication development: Foundations, processes, and clinical applications 2nd ed. (pp. 165–204). Williams & Wilkins.

Westby, C. E. (2000). *A scale for assessing development of children's play.* In K. Gitlin-Weiner, A. Sandgrund, & C. E. Schaefer (Eds.), Play diagnosis and assessment 2nd ed. (pp. 15–57). Wiley.

Westby, C. (2009). Considerations in working successfully with culturally/linguistically diverse families in assessment and intervention of communication disorders. *Seminars in Speech and Language, 30,* 279–289.

Wetherby, A., Allen, L., Cleary, J., Kublin, K., & Goldstein, H. (2002). Validity and reliability of the Communication and Symbolic Behavior Scales Developmental

Profile with very young children. *Journal of Speech, Language, and Hearing Research, 45,* 1202–1218.

Wetherby, A., Goldstein, H., Cleary, J., Allen, L., & Kublin, K. (2003). Early identification of children with communication disorders: Concurrent and predictive validity of the CSBS Developmental Profile. *Infants & Young Children, 16,* 161–174.

Whitehurst, G., Fischel, J., Arnold, D., & Lonigan, C. (1992). Evaluating outcomes with children with expressive language delay. In S. F. Warren & J. Reichle (Eds.), *Causes and effects in communication and language intervention* (Vol. 1, pp. 277–313). Brookes.

Wilkinson, K. M., & Hennig, S. (2007). The state of research and practice in augmentative and alternative communication for children with developmental/intellectual disabilities. *Mental Retardation and Developmental Disabilities, 13,* 58–69.

Winton, P. (1996). Understanding family concerns, priorities, and resources. In P. McWilliam, P. Winton, & E. Crais (Eds.), *Practical strategies for family-centered early intervention* (pp. 31–53). Singular Publishing.

Woods, J. J., & Lindeman, D. P. (2008). Gathering and giving information with families. *Infants & Young Children, 21,* 272–284.

Yoder, P., & McDuffie, A. (2006). Teaching young children with autism to talk. *Seminars in Speech and Language, 27,* 161–172.

Zwaigenbaum, L., Bryson, S., & Rogers, T. (2005). Behavioral manifestations of autism in the first year of life. *International Journal of Developmental Neuroscience, 23,* 143–152.

Chapter 7

Eligibility Determination and Development of the Individualized Family Service Plan

Learning Outcomes

When we have completed this chapter, we will be able to:

- Present eligibility determination, established criteria for eligibility, and the requirements related to this step of the EI supports and services pathway under IDEA Part C.

- Define late language emergence and describe the characteristics, related factors, and risk factors for young children with this diagnosis.

- Review and recount the role of informed clinical opinion by the service providers on the EI team to establish eligibility of services.

- Discuss the required components of the IFSP and the initial steps taken to develop this document.

- Provide the elements involved in writing functional IFSP outcomes with a focus on working with parents and caregivers to support the entire family in the process.

- Describe details and strategies to implement McWilliam's family-focused Routines-Based Interview and how to include and document these interview outcomes within the IFSP.

- Present the roles and responsibilities of the SLP to support the family and their decision-making process in completing each step within the EI supports and services pathway.

What Will We Learn and How Can We Apply It?

In this chapter, we continue to follow along and learn about the essential steps of the supports and services pathway children and their families follow when engaged in the EI system. In Chapter 6, we focused on the initial steps in program delivery, including referral, intake, evaluation, and assessment for service planning. In this chapter, we revisit eligibility determination and discuss, in greater detail, how this significant step leads to the initial development of the IFSP. We dive deeply into eligibility categories and considerations specific to our SLP role and responsibilities, including a thorough discussion of the variables related to developmental delay and the determination of a diagnosis of late language emergence. We also ensure we understand the IDEA expectations regarding IFSP timeline, implementation, and review.

We know supporting the family of the infant or toddler lends itself to supporting the child and their development; an effective EI program, therefore, requires that we develop the IFSP with input from and including features designed to support the entire family. This chapter also provides the information we need to effectively include parents and caregivers in these steps of the EI pathway. We discuss details to support our use of McWilliam's (2010) family-focused Routines-Based Interview and spend some time determining how to include and document these interview outcomes within the IFSP. Once we have gathered information from parents and caregivers regarding their concerns, resources, and priorities, we work with the EI team to create functional family and child-focused outcomes that can be addressed within natural environments and embedded within everyday activities and routines. The elements of, and steps to, writing functional IFSP outcomes are discussed to ensure we know how to complete this integral step to facilitate the development of the children and families we serve. We examine the final components of the IFSP as well, including the determination of services, ongoing assessment and monitoring of progress, updating the IFSP, and transition planning to Part B services. We consider our roles and responsibilities within each step of the supports and services pathway to support the family and their decision-making process.

The Role of Eligibility Within the Early Intervention Pathway

Chapter 6 focused on the processes required for referral, intake, evaluation, and assessment for service planning in EI. Before conducting our assessment for service planning, however, the EI team must first determine whether a child is eligible for services. As a member of the team, we work with other service providers to meet and review all of the data, results, and reports collected and related to the assessment and evaluation processes. We then connect with parents and caregivers to determine whether their child meets the criteria under IDEA and state policy for having a developmental delay, having a diagnosed physical or mental condition, or being at risk for having a substantial delay.

Determination of Eligibility

Eligibility determination is the process of establishing whether a child meets the system's eligibility criteria to receive EI services. As presented in Chapter 6, the eligibility process includes the evaluation of the child's skills and needs through the review of information, including medical and developmental reports, assessment reports, observations, and parent report. Eligibility determination is based on the infant's or toddler's needs within their natural environment, which could include the home or any community setting in which children without disabilities participate (e.g., child-care centers or public playgrounds). All areas of a child's development are considered to determine whether they present a delay or differences in development that might make them eligible for Part C services.

When determining a child's eligibility for services, Part C of IDEA (2011) requires a multidisciplinary composition of the team, including the parent and two or more individuals from separate disciplines or professions, with one of the individuals serving as the service coordinator. The multidisciplinary evaluation team typically includes at least two early childhood professionals who are appropriately qualified in their areas of expertise (i.e., SLP, occupational therapist, developmental specialist), at least one of whom is qualified in the primary area(s) of concern. The service coordinator also works with the multidisciplinary evaluation team to facilitate the evaluations, ensuring that all of the appropriate procedures are completed and properly documented. At a minimum, a multidisciplinary evaluation team gathers information from a review of pertinent records related to a child's current health status and medical history, family report, and the results of appropriate diagnostic methods. These methods might include additional reports from other sources, criterion-referenced instruments such as developmental checklists, a developmental history, language samples, criterion-referenced or norm-referenced instruments, observation of the child, play-based evaluations, and routine-based interviews. As needed, our informed clinical opinion must also be considered in the process of determining eligibility (IDEA, 2011). When we are working with families for whom English is not the native language or when there is a language barrier, an interpreter must also be involved. The evaluation must also be completed in the native language of the family or in the language(s) most likely to result in an accurate representation of the child's skills (DEC, 2014; IDEA, 2011).

It is important to note that although IDEA is a federal law, each state implements its own EI programs. Because specific regulations and procedures vary from state to state in regard to eligibility, we must become familiar with the guidelines in the state in which we practice. Each state's definition of an infant or toddler with a disability (IDEA, 2004, 34 CFR §303.21) must include an infant or toddler with:

- A developmental delay.

- A diagnosed physical or mental condition with a high probability of resulting in developmental delay.

States receiving Part C funds are required to develop a clear definition of developmental delay, which specifies the level of delay in functioning that constitutes a developmental delay (34 CFR §303.111). Each state can also choose to serve infants and toddlers at risk, defined as those children under 3 years old who are at risk of experiencing a substantial developmental delay if EI services are not provided. Eight states currently serve infants and toddlers at risk (ECTA, 2023).

If we have done our job well, we have gathered developmental information about the child beyond just the standardized testing of their ability to perform structured tasks. We have included opportunities for functional and authentic assessment through which we observed and assessed the child within the routines and activities that are part of their everyday life; we have gathered information from the parents and caregivers who know the child best. At a minimum, we have noted the natural interactions that take place during all encounters with the child and family. This approach creates an opportunity to combine formal developmental evaluation information with functional application. The type and amount of information needed for the EI team to make an eligibility determination varies depending on the circumstances of each individual child. All of these results are then reviewed by the EI team, who then determines whether the child meets one or more of the established criteria for eligibility. If a child is not found eligible for Part C services, families could choose to seek EI services through private or community resources and other federal or state-funded early childhood programs (e.g., Early Head Start). If a family continues to have concern about their child's need for EI, they can request a reevaluation through their Part C program at a later date.

Developmental Delay

Each state can determine the criteria for developmental delay in its own way. Many states determine criteria quantitatively, including (a) the difference between chronological age and actual performance level expressed as a percentage of chronological age, (b) delay expressed as performance at a certain number of months below chronological age, or (c) delay as indicated by standard deviation below the mean on a norm-referenced instrument. There is wide variability in the type of quantitative criteria states use to describe developmental delay, and there also is a wide range in the level of delay states require for eligibility. Common measurements of the level of delay are 25% delay or 2 *SD* below the mean in one or more developmental areas, or 20% delay or 1.5 *SD* in two or more areas. Traditional assessment instruments, yielding scores in standard deviations or developmental age in months, might not adequately address some developmental domains or might not be comparable across developmental domains or age levels (Benn, 1994; Brown & Brown, 1993). For this reason, some states have included qualitative criteria for determining developmental delay. Qualitative criteria include delay indicated by atypical development or observed atypical behaviors. Currently, 25 states include two eligibility criteria required to determine developmental delay in their policies; 17 states include one eligibility criterion in their policies; and 15 states include three, four, five, or six eligibility criteria in their policies (ECTA, 2023).

Late Language Emergence

It is worth noting that one of the most common diagnoses we encounter, under the umbrella of developmental delay, as SLPs in EI is *late language emergence* (LLE). We often see young children who were referred to services because, according to their parents or caregivers, they "are not talking yet." Approximately 10% to 20% of 24-month-old children demonstrate a delay in expressive vocabulary of unknown origin (Collisson et al., 2016; Zubrick et al., 2007). Young children who exhibit delays in spoken word use compared with age-expected norms are often referred to as "late talkers" (Rescorla & Dale, 2013). Children with LLE might also exhibit delays in receptive vocabulary, gesture use, or play skills (Olswang et al., 1998); use fewer speech sounds for their age; and exhibit atypical speech error patterns (Hodges et al., 2017). Children with expressive delays present delayed vocabulary acquisition and often exhibit delayed development of their sentence structure and articulation. Those with LLE are at higher risk of exhibiting poor socioemotional development, more frequent and more severe tantrums (Manning et al., 2019), and difficulties with parent–child and peer relationships (Irwin et al., 2002). Some of these young children demonstrate language skills at age expectation by the time they are school age; however, they might continue to show a language weakness compared with peers without a history of late talking (Marchman & Fernald, 2013; Rescorla, 2009). It is, therefore, imperative that we address the needs of children with LLE, and ensure they receive adequate support and services through evidence-based EI.

Some researchers distinguish a subset of children with LLE as "late bloomers;" these are children with LLE who catch up to their peers (ASHA, n.d.). Because this distinction can be made only after the fact, it is difficult for us to differentially diagnose children with LLE when we are conducting an initial evaluation. Some research, however, suggests there might be some early differences between young children who have LLE and those who will most likely develop their expressive language skills within several years. Table 7–1 provides us with the evidence-based speech and language differences we tend to see between children who are late bloomers and those who are diagnosed with LLE. It is essential we review these variables at regular intervals (e.g., every 6 months) to assess the development of a child's language and support our determination of diagnosis and need for services (ASHA, n.d.).

Table 7–1. Speech and Language Differences Between Children Who Are Late Bloomers and Children with Late Language Emergence

Children Who Are Late Bloomers	Children With Late Language Emergence
Use more communicative acts and gestures	Use fewer communicative acts and gestures
More likely to meet developmental expectations for receptive language milestones	More likely to demonstrate receptive language delay
Demonstrate higher levels of symbolic play and combinatorial play	Demonstrate decreased levels of symbolic play and combinatorial play
Present more mature syllable structures	Present less mature syllable structures including lower percentage of accurately produced consonants and limited speech sound inventories

Note. From "Communicative gestures in children with delayed onset of oral expressive vocabulary," by D. J. Thal & S. Tobias, 1992; "Language and gesture in late talkers: A 1-year follow-up," by D. J. Thal, S. Tobias & D. Morrison, 1991; "Phonetic skills and vocabulary size in late talkers: Concurrent and predictive relationships," by J. Mirak & L. Rescorla, 1998.

Related Factors of Late Language Emergence. When assessing the emergence of expressive language with a young child in EI, it is also important to consider related factors, including rate of vocabulary development, speech sound development, emerging grammar, language comprehension, social language skills, use of gestures, and symbolic play behaviors (ASHA, n.d.; Olswang et al., 1998; Wetherby et al., 2002). Additional research suggests that delays and differences in babbling before the age of 2 years are predictors of later delays in expressive vocabulary, limited phonetic repertoire, and use of simplified syllable shapes (Fasolo et al.,

2008; Oller et al., 1999; Stoel-Gammon, 1989). Compared to toddlers of the same age who demonstrate typical language development, children with LLE can present with the following:

- delayed comprehension and use of symbolic gestures for communication (Thal et al., 2013).

- Use of shorter and less grammatically complex utterances (Thal et al., 2013).

- Comprehension of fewer words (Thal et al., 2013; Thal et al., 1991).

- Phonological differences once they do produce their first words, including less complex or mature syllable structures, lower percentage of consonants correct, and smaller consonant and vowel inventories (Mirak & Rescorla, 1998; Paul & Jennings, 1992; Rescorla & Ratner, 1996).

Although many children with LLE present expressive and receptive language skills within the normal range by kindergarten (Ellis Weismer, 2007; Rescorla, 2000, 2002), their scores on such measures continue to be lower than those of children, matched for socioeconomic status, with a history of typical language development (Paul, 1996; Rescorla, 2000, 2002).

Risk Factors of Late Language Emergence. We do not know the cause of LLE in otherwise healthy children. There are, however, several child- and family-based risk factors of which we should be aware when evaluating young children. The research supports early identification and intervention to mitigate the impact of these factors (Guralnick, 1997, 1998; National Research Council, 2001; Thelin & Fussner, 2005); it is, therefore, imperative that as SLPs, we recognize the following risk factors when identifying LLE and when we are considering service delivery options.

- Boys are at higher risk for LLE than girls (Collisson et al., 2016; Horowitz et al., 2003; Klee et al., 1998; Rescorla, 1989; Rescorla & Achenbach, 2002; Rescorla & Alley, 2001).

- Children with LLE tended to have delayed motor development (in the absence of disorders or syndromes associated with motor delays) when compared with typically developing children (Klee et al., 1998; Rescorla & Alley, 2001).

- Children born at less than 85% of their optimal birth weight or earlier than 37 weeks gestation were at higher risk for LLE (Zubrick et al., 2007).

- Children with LLE are more likely to have a parent with a history of LLE (Collisson et al., 2016; Ellis Weismer, 2007; Paul, 1991; Rescorla & Schwartz, 1990).

- Lower maternal education and lower family socioeconomic status are associated with greater risk for LLE (Fisher, 2017; Zubrick et al., 2007).

Atypical Development

Children are considered to have *atypical development* if they demonstrate abnormal or questionable sensorimotor responses or have an identified affective disorder (IDEA, 2004). Atypical or questionable sensorimotor responses might include abnormal muscle tone, limitations in joint range of motion, abnormal reflex or postural reactions, poor quality of movement patterns or quality of skill performance, and oral-motor skills dysfunction, including feeding difficulties. Atypical or questionable social-emotional development could include delay or abnormality in achieving expected emotional milestones, persistent failure to initiate or respond to most social interactions, and fearfulness or other distress that does not respond to comforting efforts provided by caregivers. Young children who present with atypical or questionable behaviors that interfere with the acquisition of developmental skills, as well as impairment in social interaction and communication skills along with restricted and repetitive behaviors, are also often eligible for EI services. We work together with our interprofessional team to determine the needs and eligibility of children who present with atypical development.

Physical or Mental Condition

A child who has a diagnosed physical or mental condition that has a high probability of resulting in a developmental delay is automatically eligible for EI services. These conditions might include chromosomal abnormalities; genetic or congenital disorders; severe sensory impairments; inborn errors of metabolism; disorders reflecting disturbance of the development of the nervous system; congenital infections; disorders secondary to exposure to toxic substances, including fetal alcohol syndrome; and severe attachment disorders (IDEA, 2004). Each state has the option to include language within their eligibility policies that goes beyond this description in Part C of IDEA (ECTA, 2023; IDEA, 2004). It is important, therefore, that we are knowledgeable regarding the diagnoses and established conditions for which children in our own state are automatically eligible for EI services.

As a group, children with established diagnoses or conditions are easier to identify; we also know they are at greatest risk for developmental difficulties. There are disorders in this category that are more common than others; we tend to work with these children more frequently because of their anticipated needs related to the development of communication, speech, language, and feeding. These diagnoses include the following:

- Autism spectrum disorders.
- Cerebral palsy.
- Down syndrome.
- Fetal alcohol spectrum disorders.
- Intellectual disabilities.
- Organic disorders such as cleft lip and palate.
- Preterm and low birth weight.

- Sensory and perceptual disorders including hearing loss and visual disabilities.
- Traumatic brain injury.

We spend considerable time addressing evidence-based and best practices when working with children who have been diagnosed with these physical or mental conditions in Chapter 12.

At Risk and Established Risk

An at-risk infant or toddler is defined under Part C as "an individual under 3 years of age who would be at risk of experiencing a substantial developmental delay if EI services were not provided to the individual" (IDEA, 2004, §632(1)). Although many states are interested in serving children at risk, they also fear increasing the numbers of eligible children because of escalating costs. At this time, only eight states have criteria established to serve infants and toddlers in the EI system who are considered at risk (ECTA, 2023).

Two categories of risk frequently described by the states that serve these children include conditions of biological or medical risk and environmental risk. The most common categories related to eligibility for children who are considered at risk of experiencing a significant development delay include the following:

- Low socioeconomic status of the family.
- Maltreatment and neglect.
- Prenatal substance exposure including neonatal abstinence syndrome.
- Preterm and low birth weight (in those states in which this is not considered a diagnosed physical or mental condition).

Many states consider some or all of these conditions as *established risk;* this means the state recognizes the child is at high risk for experiencing a substantial developmental delay if EI services are not provided. In these states, infants and toddlers who face these conditions are automatically eligible to receive EI services. When diagnostic assessment tools do not establish eligibility, the state lead agency must ensure that informed clinical opinion is independently considered to establish eligibility of services for children who are considered at risk (IDEA, 2011). States that do not serve children at risk under their guidelines for eligibility typically indicate they will monitor the development of these children and refer them for EI services when delays are manifested (ECTA, 2023). Regardless of whether the state in which we work as SLPs serves children who are considered at risk, it is important that we should be aware of best practices in monitoring and implementing intervention to support their development.

In Chapter 12, we focus our attention on infants and toddlers who present these conditions of biological, medical, and environmental risk. We review the evidence-based literature to ensure we have the knowledge to implement best practices when serving these children and their families.

Informed Clinical Opinion

On occasion, intake information and eligibility evaluation are not sufficient for determining a child's eligibility. When the diagnostic evaluation or assessment tools we have used do not establish eligibility, the state lead agency must ensure that the informed clinical opinions of the service providers on the EI team are considered to establish eligibility of services for children who are considered at risk (IDEA, 2011). The use of informed clinical opinion serves as a necessary safeguard against eligibility determination based on isolated information or test scores alone and allows us to use both qualitative and quantitative information to form a determination regarding those aspects of current developmental status that may otherwise be difficult to measure, as well as the potential need by a child for EI. Appropriate training, previous experience with evaluation and assessment, sensitivity to cultural needs, and the ability to elicit and include family perceptions are all important elements of informed clinical opinion. As such, both parents and service providers contribute information needed in this decision-making process. We consider using informed clinical opinion as a basis for determining eligibility, under the category of developmental delay, when:

- Team members believe that the child's performance on standardized measures is at odds with their own observations and judgments about the child.
- The child's capabilities are demonstrated at extremely low frequencies or are inconsistently exhibited and, therefore, negatively affect the child's functioning.

To reach an informed clinical opinion about the development of a particular infant or toddler, multiple procedures and sources of information must be used, including the following:

- Review of a child's developmental history.
- Interviews with parents (including taking the child's history).
- Observation of the child at play and in various settings.
- Observation of parent–child interaction.
- Information gathered from family members, other caregivers, medical providers, social workers, and educators.
- Review of medical, educational, or other records.
- Neurodevelopmental or other physical examinations.
- Use of an evaluation instrument.
- Identification of a child's level of functioning (and needs) in each developmental area.

The EI team, including family members, then synthesizes and interprets all available information about the child and family, integrating observations, impressions, and evaluation findings to discuss and consider eligibility and the development of the IFSP. When using informed clinical opinion to determine a child's eligibility for EI services, we must clearly document the process to ensure we have an established baseline against which to measure the progress and changing needs of the child and family over time. Additionally, assessment and subsequent eligibility determination is an ongoing process that could require IFSP modifications over time. The perceptions and impressions of individual EI providers might also change over time. Documentation of the individual and team findings can facilitate transition when families move, change service providers, or enter additional or new service delivery systems.

Documentation of the sources and use of informed clinical opinion also brings forth information to ensure that procedural safeguards were presented in the evaluation and assessment process as well as the process in which we determined eligibility for EI services. This documentation should include the following information:

- Providing information about who was involved in the team and in gathering information.

- Describing the procedures used and in which settings.

- Summarizing the information and describing the functioning of the child in each developmental area.

- Stating the decision of the team and rationale for concluding that the child is eligible.

When handled effectively, informed clinical opinion ensures the EI team implemented a dynamic assessment approach, supported and encouraged the acquisition and interpretation of multiple sources of information as part of the evaluation and assessment process, and ensured greater compatibility between a child and family's needs and the provision of services (ECTA, 2023).

Eligibility of Children With Linguistic Diversity

Under Part C (IDEA, 2004), young children who are English language learners with typical development do not qualify for EI services. Dual-language learners who present with difficulties in developing their native language and a second language, however, might be eligible for services. We explore these considerations in depth in Chapter 8.

Developing the Individualized Family Service Plan

Once a child has been determined to be eligible for EI services, we work with our interprofessional team and the family to develop an individualized plan of action for the child and family. This IFSP is a written document that outlines the EI services that the child and family will receive. We have learned that an integral guiding principle of EI is that the family is a child's greatest resource; as such, a young child's needs are closely tied to the needs of the family. The best way to support children and meet their needs, therefore, is to support and build on the individual strengths of their family. The IFSP focuses on the family as a unit, and the parents serve as major contributors in its development. The level of involvement by other team members depends on what the child needs. These other team members might include medical specialists, child development specialists, social workers, and others. As SLPs, we often engage on the EI team as primary providers; we might even find ourselves in the role of service coordinators.

Based on the eligibility assessment for service planning, the IFSP is developed. The IFSP provides the foundation for EI supports and services. The IFSP is developed through a collaborative process that includes the child's family as the most important members of the intervention team. A well-developed IFSP is individualized to each child and family's specific routines, activities, strengths, and needs and reflects the family's priorities for the child's development. Information about the child's development, outcomes and goals, supports and services, and the transition plan that will be implemented to support the child and family as they exit the EI system is included in each IFSP.

The IFSP is a written plan for providing EI services to eligible children and their families. The plan is developed jointly by the family, the service coordinator, ourselves, and other providers who might also be supporting the child and family. The IFSP is based on the multidisciplinary evaluation and assessment of the child and the assessment of the resources, priorities, and concerns of the child's family. The plan includes outcomes, strategies, and services necessary to enhance the development of the child and the capacity of the family to meet the special needs of the child (IDEA 2004, §303.340(2)). To review, the following information must be included in the IFSP:

- Family's resources, priorities, and concerns related to the child with a disability.
- Child's developmental status or present levels of development.
- Measurable outcomes expected to be achieved for the child and the family.
- Specific services necessary to meet the needs of the child and the family.
- Natural environments in which services will be implemented.
- Dates of initiation of services and the anticipated length, duration, and frequency of services.
- Identification of the provider who will act as the family's service coordinator.
- Steps to plan and support the transition of the toddler with a disability to preschool or other appropriate services.

Table 7–2 offers additional details for us to consider when addressing and gathering the data for these required components.

Table 7–2. Required Components of the IFSP

Statement of the child's present levels of development based on objective criteria. • Physical development (including fine motor, gross motor, vision, hearing, and health status) • Cognitive development • Communication development • Social-emotional development • Adaptive (self-help) development This information must be presented in the IFSP as an age level or age range.
Statement of the family's resources, priorities, and concerns as they relate to the development of the child who will be receiving EI services. • Resources include people in the family's life on whom they rely and with whom they interact. • Priorities can include the hopes and dreams of the family for their child. • Information about how the family would like their child to participate in family and community activities can be included. The family must grant their permission, in writing, to include this information in the IFSP.
Statement of the measurable results or outcomes expected to be achieved by the child and their family including the criteria, procedures, and timelines to determine the degree to which progress is made toward achieving the results or outcomes. • Any modifications or revisions of the results or outcomes or services that might be necessary should be included. • Outcomes should be individualized for each child and family, relevant to the family, and focused on the whole child and their participation in routines and everyday activities. • The statement should include developmentally appropriate emergent literacy and language skills for the child.

Statement of specific EI services necessary to meet the unique needs of the child and family.<ul><li>The statement should include the frequency, intensity, and method of delivering the services.</li><li>Supports and services should be individualized. EI services include, but are not limited to, service coordination, speech-language therapy, physical therapy, occupational therapy, special instruction, and assistive technology.</li><li>All children must receive service coordination.</li><li>Additional services are dependent on many variables and often change over the course of the child's involvement in EI.</li></ul>
Statement of the natural environments in which services will be provided. If the services are not established in a natural environment, justification must be included in the statement.
Projected dates of initiation of services and the anticipated length, duration, and frequency of the services.
Identification of the service coordinator from the profession most immediately relevant to the child's or family's needs (or who is otherwise qualified to carry out all applicable responsibilities).<ul><li>All families have a service coordinator who is responsible for overseeing the IFSP, ensuring that all IFSP services are delivered, and seeing that changes in the IFSP are made when necessary.</li></ul>
Steps that will be taken to support the transition of the child with a disability, at the appropriate age, to preschool or other appropriate services.<ul><li>The transition plan must be individualized for each child.</li></ul>

Note. Adapted from "Agreed upon practices for providing early intervention services in natural environments," by the Workgroup on Principles and Practices in Natural Environments, OSEP TA Community of Practice: Part C Settings, 2011 (http://www.ectacenter.org/~pdfs/topics/families/AgreedUponPractices_FinalDraft2_01_08.pdf1); "Individualized family service plan process guidance handbook," Early Childhood Technical Center, 2014 (https://ectacenter.org/eco/assets/pdfs/EDISIFSPProcess-GuidanceHandbook.pdf); "Part C Final Regulations," of the Individuals with Disabilities Education Improvement Act, 2004, 2011. (https://www.gpo.gov/fdsys/pkg-/FR-2011-09-28/pdf/2011-22783.pdf).

Part C of IDEA mandates that the IFSP meeting is conducted in settings and at times convenient for the family. The meeting and the documents must also be in the native language of the family. An interpreter must be involved if the native language of the family is not English. We must work collaboratively with the interpreter to ensure that families fully understand their rights and role in the EI system. We take a closer look at working with an interpreter in Chapter 8.

Identifying the Family's Resources, Priorities, and Concerns

When working with young children, we know how important it is to connect with the family members as equal partners of our team, particularly when making decisions, developing the IFSP, and discussing plans for intervention. We are also now well aware that EI involves activating a system of supports to scaffold a family's capacity to help their children grow, learn, and develop. To do this, we must first learn about their existing supports. The information we gather from and about the family while engaging in the IFSP process serves as a foundation to planning and guiding intervention. As we gather information from the parents and caregivers, special attention should be paid to the details they share about what is working well and what is challenging for their child and their family. When paired with our knowledge regarding developmental expectations and the evaluation and functional assessments the EI team has conducted across multiple situations and settings, what we learn from talking with the family yields all the information we need to develop high-quality, child- and family-centered outcomes.

Before inquiring about family and child strengths and resources, we must let the family know that the information they choose to share is voluntary, that this information is gathered to support everyone who will be supporting their child and family, and that all information is kept confidential. We want to be sure they understand that EI is a collaborative process in which they are equal partners. For us to effectively support the child and family over time, it is important to be aware of and understand their strengths, resources, needs, and concerns at this stage in the IFSP process. We also want to be sure families know their rights, effectively communicate their child's needs, and help their child develop and learn. We must be aware of and address the family's priorities, needs, and choices to focus on skills within activities and routines both familiar and comfortable to the parents and caregivers (Crawford & Weber, 2014; McWilliam, 2010). It is important to work collaboratively with families and engage them in intentional conversations about their values, principles, priorities, and practices (DEC, 2014). The question remains this: How do we effectively and efficiently gather this information?

The Routines-Based Interview

Gathering information about parent and caregiver interests facilitates an understanding of the family and possible cultural and community influences that could affect the EI services they receive and in which we engage. Learning about the family's interests provides us with information about activities they find enjoyable and consequently make time for in their day. These interests could serve as valuable opportunities for learning, as it is within their activities that we will coach the families to facilitate and embed strategies to support their child's development.

The Routines-Based Interview is an assessment used by EI service providers to connect with families and ensure the IFSP outcomes are functional and child- and family-centered (McWilliam et al., 2009; McWilliam, 2010). By focusing on the everyday activities of the family, the inclusion of the Routines-Based Interview during the early stages of the IFSP development ensures the priorities are chosen by the family and are meaningful to them. This process gives us a tool to encourage the family to think in terms of their own routines and activities in preparation for developing outcomes and strategies. It also allows the family an opportunity to see that the focus of early intervention extends beyond the child to include the greater context of the family (ECTA, 2023).

When introducing the Routines-Based Interview to the parents and caregivers, it is helpful for us to reinforce how the information will help the team gain an understanding of the child's functional skills across family routines and activities. This information is added to what we already know, based on the evaluation and assessment processes and the conversations in which we have engaged to determine their eligibility. The interview process involves our EI team and the family engaging in dialogue about their everyday activities, including what is going well and what is challenging for their child and the family as a whole. This approach gives the family an opportunity to share information they feel is relevant, rather than answering questions that might be intrusive or irrelevant. It facilitates a collaborative relationship between the EI service providers and the members of the family and puts the focus of the IFSP development on the family's natural settings, routines, and everyday activities. Our understanding of the family's routines promotes the identification of functional outcomes and ensures the services and subsequent intervention we implement make sense within the life of the family (ECTA, 2023; McWilliam, 2010).

Using the Routines-Based Interview, we are able to determine what is working, what is not working, and what a typical day is like for the family; subsequently, this exchange of information facilitates collaborative discovery of the family's concerns, priorities, and resources. Understanding the child in the context of the family facilitates a holistic perspective that emphasizes functionality, rather than a focus on development deficits in specific areas. As a result, IFSP outcomes become both functionally important and contextually relevant. This in turn promotes identification and enhancement of children's learning opportunities within family and, as appropriate, community routines and activities. There are several interview conversation starters, presented in Table 7–3, that we might consider to facilitate our discussion and to support our gathering of information with the family during the interview. We know that each family is unique; therefore, a single set of questions that must be asked are not expected within the interview process. These questions could, however, serve as a starting point when we are initiating a Routines-Based Interview. Additionally, the questions we ask, and the depth of the parent's or caregiver's responses will vary from one family to the next. We should invite families to share only what they wish (ECTA, 2023; McWilliam, 2010).

Table 7–3. Conversation Starters When Engaged in the Routines-Based Interview

Questions to facilitate our discovery of information about the family and their support systems
- Who lives at home with you and your child?
- What about other extended family? Are there grandparents or other relatives with whom you are in close contact?
- Tell me about your family. Where do they live? How often are you able to get together or talk with friends?
- Tell me about community services your family can access. What kind of support do they offer?
- Are there any weekend or evening activities or groups in which you participate?
- How about work colleagues? How, if at all, are they involved with or do they support your family?
- Who do you contact when something really good happens?
- Who do you contact if something difficult has happened?

Questions to facilitate our understanding of what the family enjoys doing at home and in the community
- What do you enjoy doing with your child?
- What are the fun parts of the day for you and your child?
- Does your family have a favorite restaurant? Do you tend to eat out or do you order delivery to your home?
- Do you have favorite shows or videos you like to watch together?
- Are there tasks in which the whole family is involved?

Questions to identify and discover information about the family's routines and everyday activities
- On a typical day, who usually wakes up first? How does that go? Are you happy with the way this time of day goes?
- What happens after your child wakes up?
- Tell me about getting your child dressed. How much can your child do on their own? How does your child communicate during dressing? Is there anything that would make this process easier?
- What about breakfast? How much can your child do on their own? How does your child let you know when they are done eating or want more? Does your child have favorite foods or do they eat most of the food you offer? How about lunch? Is there anything that would make these meals easier? What do

- you think your child is ready for next with regard to eating and mealtime activities?
- What about playing at home? What does your child like to do? How well does your child play with toys by themselves or with others? How do you tend to be involved? What are the other family members doing? Is there anything that would make this easier?
- What about getting ready to go outside of the home? Who helps your child get ready? How does your child handle this transition or other transitions?
- What about time in the evening? Is the evening meal different than breakfast? What does your child typically do during this activity?
- What typically happens in the evening? How and what does your child do in the evening? What is their energy like? How would you describe this window of time?
- What about bath time? Describe a typical bath routine. How involved is your child in bath time? How much play time is there? How enjoyable is bath time for you and for your child?
- What about bedtime? What typically happens before bedtime? Is there anything you would change about bedtime or your child's sleeping routine?
- What does your family tend to do on the weekends when you do not have any planned activities?
- Does your child attend day care? If so, full time or part time? How do you feel about the care they receive there?
- Is there anything else you would like to share about your family activities at this time?

Questions to gather information about each routine in which the family and child engage

- When engaged in this (particular) routine, what is everyone else doing?
- When engaged in this (particular) routine, what is the child doing?
- In what ways does the child participate in this routine?
- How independent is the child when engaged in this routine?
- What kind of social interactions does the child engage in through this routine?
- How well is the routine working for you, the child, and the family as a unit?

Note. Adapted from "Individualized family service plan process guidance handbook," by the Early Childhood Technical Center, 2014 (https://ectacenter.org/eco/assets/pdfs/EDISIFSPProcessGuidanceHandbook.pdf); "Routines-based early intervention: Supporting young children and their families," by R. A. McWilliam, 2010.

We hope that, at the end of a comprehensive interview with the family, we have identified 10 or more possible concerns the parents or caregivers want to address with the assistance of the EI team. In accordance with IDEA (2004), these concerns should be focused, family-related, and child-specific. It is important to note, however, that the list of concerns generated during the interview are not yet IFSP outcomes. Instead, they are merely a list of the contextually identified concerns discovered through the Routines-Based Interview process. The family's identified concerns, and subsequent hopes for their child, should serve as the springboard for writing functional and measurable outcomes and criteria. In addition to our discovery of family concerns, we gain a clear understanding of those routines that are going well. This information is as important as consideration of the issues that could arise within everyday activities, as these present as natural learning opportunities that we might highlight and expand on when implementing intervention strategies (McWilliam, 2010; Rush & Shelden, 2020).

Documenting the Child's Present Levels of Development

Documenting information in the IFSP about the child's present levels of development is not only needed to guide eligibility determination, but also necessary to facilitate a shared understanding of the child within and across EI team members. Our written descriptions of present levels of development should be comprehensive and reflect the child's abilities, interests, strengths, and needs. They should not be a reiteration of the results of the evaluation tools and protocols; instead, we should provide a holistic picture of the child's skills and functional abilities within naturally occurring routines and activities. Documentation of the child's development status is based on descriptive results from evaluation, observation of their spontaneous behaviors, and reports from parents and caregivers who are most familiar and engaged with the child. Information gathered during the Routines-Based Interview should also be included in this section of the IFSP to ensure that it provides a holistic picture of the child (ECTA, 2023; McWilliam, 2010).

What Is a Functional Outcome?

One of the most important components of the IFSP is the section in which we present the outcomes we expect the child and family to achieve while they are engaged in EI services. The key to supporting the development of high-quality, functional outcomes is creating a clear and deliberate link between every step of the EI process, beginning with our interactions with the family during initial contact and referral and continuing throughout the development of the IFSP. Critical to this process is our fundamental belief that children learn best through their participation in everyday activities and routines with familiar people. As SLPs in EI, it is important we possess the following knowledge and skills to ensure we maintain this link (Lucas et al., 2014):

- The ability to effectively gather information from families throughout the IFSP and EI process.

- The ability to conduct a functional assessment that gives us, and our EI team, a clear picture of the child's abilities and needs in their natural, everyday settings, activities, and routines.

- The ability to use the information we have gathered to develop functional child- and family-based outcomes.

As we gather information from our families through assessment, observation, and the Routines-Based Interview, we should pay special attention to the information they share about what is working well for them and what is challenging to and for them. Between the knowledge we have about the family's strengths, needs, and priorities, the EI team's knowledge of early development, and the results of the evaluation and assessment processes, through which we have gathered data regarding the child's current developmental levels, we are ready and able to develop the IFSP outcomes.

Each IFSP outcome is a statement of the measurable results expected to be achieved for or by the infant or toddler and the family. Ultimately, outcomes are statements about what the family wants its child to learn or do. Each statement should include emergent literacy and language skills developmentally appropriate for the child. It should also include the criteria, procedures, and timelines we will use to determine the degree to which progress toward achieving the outcome is being made. Any modification or revision of the outcomes or services that might be necessary should be included. An IFSP outcome might focus on the child learning to sit at the table with the family at dinner and eat with a spoon, walk around the block to the playground with the family in the evening, or say new words to tell the family what toys the child wants. Outcomes should be individualized for each child and family. As such, each outcome should be contextualized, functional, and discipline-free. Outcomes should be relevant to the family and focused on the whole child and their participation in activities and within settings important to the family (IDEA, 2004, 2011).

Criteria of Quality and Functional Outcomes

Based on a review of both expert-generated and evidence-based resources, the National Early Childhood Technical Assistance Center identified the following six criteria to define IFSP outcomes that are functional and of high quality (Lucas et al., 2014):

- The outcome statement is necessary and functional for the child's and family's life.
- The statement reflects real-life contextualized settings.
- The wording of the statement is jargon-free, clear, and simple.
- The outcome is not linked to a specific discipline.
- The statement uses active words.
- The wording emphasizes the positive.

When the child's contextual information is available (e.g., evaluation and assessment information, other components of the IFSP), the following criteria should also be included:

- The outcome is based on the family's priorities and concerns.

- The outcome describes both strengths and needs of the child based on the information from the initial evaluation or ongoing assessment.

Table 7–4 presents additional information related to each of these criteria to support our involvement in and development of quality IFSP outcomes with our families.

Table 7–4. Components of a High-Quality, Functional Child or Family Outcome

Quality Component: The Outcome Statement Is …	Description
Necessary and functional within the life of the child and family.	• The outcome is based on the family's priorities both with, and for their child. • The statement focuses on ways in which the child and parents or caregivers participate in their community and family life.
Reflects real-life contextual settings.	• The outcome reflects how the family would like their child to function within their own routines and everyday activities.
Worded with language that is free of jargon, clear, and simple.	• The language is parent friendly and contains no clinical terms or discipline-specific jargon.
Integrates developmental domains and is not linked to a specific discipline.	• The outcome reflects the integration of functional skills and abilities across developmental domains. • The statement is written to describe the child's participation in routines and everyday activities that can be addressed by any member of the EI team.
Uses active words.	• Words that encourage the active participation of the child and family are used. • These include verbs that are measurable and observable and that all members of the EI team, including the family members, will recognize when the goal has been achieved. • Passive verbs that reflect a state of being (e.g., understand, tolerate) or a change or lack of change in performance (e.g., improve, maintain, increase, decrease) should be avoided.
…emphasizes the positive.	• The outcome builds upon the child's strengths and states what the child and/or family will do, rather than what they will not do or stop doing.

	• Negative words and phrases (e.g., not, no longer) should be avoided.

Note. Adapted from "Enhancing recognition of high quality, functional IFSP outcomes," by A. Lucas, K. Gillaspy, M. L. Peters, & J. Hurth, 2014; "Routines-based early intervention," by R. A. McWilliam, 2010.

Developing Functional Outcomes With a Child and Family Focus

There is a clear connection between outcomes that focus on the child and those that address the needs of the family. A positive outcome experienced by the family serves to promote their child's needs; likewise, outcomes achieved by the child will benefit the family. Writing strong, effective functional IFSP outcomes, however, is easier said than done. How do we ensure the entire EI team, including the parents and caregivers, understand the purpose of and ways in which to include the components we just discussed to develop meaningful and quality functional outcomes?

According to McWilliam (2010), there are multiple steps we can take to ensure everyone who is developing and writing the outcomes understands the context in which the skill is needed should come first. By focusing on what the author termed *participation-based outcomes*, the entire EI team recognizes the desired behavior (i.e., the target skill) is not meaningful by itself; rather, it is how the behavior supports the child's engagement and participation in their natural environments that brings meaning to the skills and subsequent outcomes (McWilliam, 2010; Wilson et al., 2004).

Additionally, by focusing on a child's participation in their home and community, parents and caregivers are naturally prompted to work toward the outcome within the routines and everyday activities in which the skill is needed. The following steps include those we can take as an EI team to ensure we develop functional, participation-based outcomes that focus on the priorities for the child and of the family (Lucas et al., 2014; McWilliam, 2010):

- With the family, we review and assess the results of the Routines-Based Interview and the functional assessment we conducted of the child. Determine when the child most needs to be engaged, independent, or social within their routines and everyday activities.

- Determine which routines should be involved in each outcome. Again, by focusing on the family interview and functional assessment, the needs of the child and the routines in which those needs are most needed should emerge.

- Begin writing the statement. Start with "who." This is typically the name of the child, although it could include the parent or family.

- Determine the "will do what" element. This is what the child or family will learn to do. Be sure to use jargon-free, clear, simple, and active language.

- Include a "measure of success." This element includes how the members of the EI team, including the parents or caregivers, will know that the outcome has been met;

this portion of the statement should also be observable. This is the criterion specifying the amount of time over which the behavior or skill needs to be demonstrated (i.e., how often, how much, how long, or how well).

- Add a "routine or activity" to the statement. This includes events that occur typically during the child's day and are individualized by the family's environment or culture.

- The next element is "under what condition." This is a specific situation or adaptation that the child might need to support their achievement of the outcome. This is an optional component, as the child might not require any assistance or adaptation.

- The final element of the outcome statement is the "so what" phrase. Why does the family want to focus on this skill? What is the reason for targeting this action?

Individualizing outcomes, measuring them, taking the time to make sure they are meaningful and reflect the family's priorities, and trying to write them so that they will meet requirements are all important, yet challenging, aspects of outcome development. We often struggle with families to determine which outcomes to write, what words to use, how to describe the context, and how to measure them. We know the IFSP belongs to the family. Outcomes should, therefore, be written so that the parents and caregivers will know when and feel confident that the goal is met. We know to ask the family the questions, "What would you like for your child to be able to do?" or "What are your goals for your child?" These questions elicit broad dreams or specific milestones, depending on the parent's priorities and how we facilitate the conversation. Parents will often reply with a response similar to "I just want them to communicate with me!" For the purpose of writing the IFSP outcomes, however, which need to be functional, measurable, and reflect everyday activity or a routine that is natural for the child and family, there is an additional question we can ask the family: "What would it look like when they are communicating?" This question, as simple as it seems, could help us and the EI team, including the parents and caregivers, think through the elements that need to be included in each outcome and how to determine when the child or family has met their goal. Table 7–5 presents these elements in a template, along with several examples, to ensure our outcomes are child- and family-focused, participation-based, and functional.

Table 7–5. Elements and Examples of Comprehensive Participation-Based Outcomes

IFSP Outcome Statement Template
_____ + _____ +   Who   Will Do What
_____ + _____ +   Routine or Everyday Activity   Measure of Success
_____ + _____ .   Under What Condition (optional)   So That/In Order To … (optional)
Example 1   August will make sounds to participate in library story time for 15 minutes one time per week, while sitting with his parent(s).

Example 2
Bailey will feed herself using her fingers and thumb to pick up food during her family's dinner meal every night over the course of 1 week.
Example 3
Olive will use a two-word phrase to tell her parents what she wants to eat (e.g., want cookie, more milk) during snack time for at least 10 afternoons during a 2-week period.

Note. Adapted from "Enhancing recognition of high quality, functional IFSP outcomes," by A. Lucas, K. Gillaspy, M. L. Peters, & J. Hurth, 2014; "Routines-based early intervention," by R. A. McWilliam, 2010.

Determining Early Intervention Services

Once the EI team develops and writes the outcomes in the IFSP, we talk with the family about which services will effectively support the child to accomplish their goals. With the team, we talk with the parents and caregivers about the different providers and who will best support and assist the child and family to meet their needs. Services must also honor the values and beliefs of the family. As we discussed in Chapter 1, these services could include any or all of the following:

- Assistive technology devices and assistive technology services.
- Counseling.
- Early identification, screening, and assessment services.
- Family training.
- Health services necessary to enable the child to benefit from EI services.
- Medical services only for diagnostic or evaluation purposes.
- Occupational therapy.
- Physical therapy.
- Psychological services.
- Service coordination services
- Sign language and cued language services.
- Social work services.
- Special instruction.
- Speech-language pathology and audiology services.
- Transportation and related costs necessary to enable the child and their family to receive services.
- Vision services (IDEA, 2011).

Families must be offered a choice of programs and services for their child. If the appropriate choice does not exist, the EI team must work together to create an option or opportunity. Each service plan should be individualized and created to meet the family's needs and priorities. It is important we ensure families understand the decision regarding EI services is their own. As service providers, we provide parents and caregivers with information to support the decisions they make; ultimately, however, families have the option to use some services offered and to refuse others. Once services are established and confirmed by the family in the IFSP, the EI team will set timelines:

- When can the family expect services to start?

- How often and where will they be delivered?
- How long will they last?
- When does the team anticipate the child and family will achieve the outcomes that have been determined?
- When will the team meet again to review the plan?

Only after the outcomes are determined should these decisions about the services and supports needed to meet those outcomes be made. The IFSP must include length, duration, frequency, intensity, and method of delivering each service; each of these considerations must be based on the amount of support the parents or caregivers need to effectively engage with their child throughout everyday routines and activities in their natural environments (Dunst, 2002; Jung, 2003). To clarify further, according to IDEA (2004):

- *Frequency* and *intensity* indicate the number of days or sessions that a service will be provided, as well as whether the service is delivered on an individual or group basis.
- *Method* refers to how a service is bestowed.
- *Length* is the extent of time the service is provided during each session.
- *Duration* is a projection of how long the service will be needed (including start and end dates).

As we have discussed in earlier chapters, each family will also be assigned a service coordinator. The service coordinator could also be the child's primary service provider. The role of the service coordinator is to keep the IFSP process flowing smoothly by arranging meetings and communicating with team members. They will also support the family by connecting them with community resources, information, and other services that will facilitate and support the needs of the family and their child. The service coordinator also assists with and ensures the child and family receive the rights, procedural safeguards, and services authorized under the state EI program.

Individualized Family Service Plan Implementation and Review

Implementation and review of the IFSP involves the coordination and monitoring of the delivery of IFSP supports and services. The IFSP must be developed within 45 days from the date of referral. EI services must begin within 30 days of the IFSP being written and agreed on by the multidisciplinary team. Periodic reviews are held to facilitate IFSP changes as necessary. These changes can reflect the child's development and any changes, including those that might be medical in nature, that occur regarding a family's priorities and concerns. IFSP reviews must take place at least once every 6 months or each time a child has either achieved a documented outcome or presents a new area of need. Annual reviews must be completed within 365 days of the initial or previous annual IFSP meeting (IDEA, 2004).

Individualized Family Service Plan Periodic Review and Annual Evaluation

Once the family signs the IFSP, EI services will begin at once. According to IDEA (2004), the EI team will engage in an annual evaluation of the IFSP. More frequent periodic reviews must also be conducted at least once every 6 months. Depending on the needs of the child and their family at any given time, a periodic review must be completed by the family and the service coordinator; as needed, additional members of the EI team might become involved in a periodic review. The purpose of this review is to assess the progress made by the child and family toward their outcomes. We should keep in mind that the family will play an integral role in determining whether, and at what time, changes need to be made in regard to the IFSP outcomes or services.

Ongoing Assessment and Monitoring of Progress

Ongoing assessment in EI includes observing the child engaged in everyday activities with parents and caregivers who are typically present in these activities to address current IFSP outcomes or determine the need for a new IFSP outcome and reviewing the strategies and supports that will promote the child's participation in natural settings to achieve their IFSP outcomes. As needed, we can make modifications to strategies and supports based on the data we obtain through this review. When services and supports are provided in natural environments, the child's daily activities serve as the basis for ongoing assessment and intervention. These activities can occur simultaneously or be repeated multiple times within different settings, as needed, to maximize child learning and development opportunities. When we view ongoing assessment as a form of planning, this process occurs continuously and in the context of the child's capacity within everyday activities and routines. We use this information to inform our periodic reviews and annual IFSPs (Early Intervention-Early Childhood Professional Development Community of Practice, n.d.; IDEA, 2004).

We engage in ongoing family assessment in the same way we attend to ongoing child assessment. Ongoing assessment of the family assists us with planning changes to intervention or determining when alternative or additional supports are needed; this process helps us determine progress toward family-focused IFSP outcomes. Continuing to gather information from families regarding their interests, priorities, concerns, and everyday routines and activities is important for ongoing assessment of the family. We can effectively gather this information through conversations with the parents and caregivers. This information is critical for the EI team to develop meaningful family outcomes and to design intervention strategies that build on a family's strengths and capacity. Over time, parents and caregivers often want to participate in new activities or add community resources to their portfolios; they might need our help to include their child. Accompanying the family on an outing and problem-solving in the new setting are strategies we can use to help the family engage in new activities that will lead to natural learning opportunities for their child. Ongoing family assessment also includes our continuous support of the family as their child grows and learns through their transition out of EI (Early Intervention-Early Childhood Professional Development Community of Practice, n.d.; IDEA, 2004).

Updating the Individualized Family Service Plan

Families can request to change or update the IFSP at any time while they are receiving EI services. The IFSP can be revised any time there is a need to do so and should be flexible enough to adjust as the child grows, learns, and develops, and as the family's needs, priorities, and resources change (Early Intervention-Early Childhood Professional Development Community of Practice, n.d.; IDEA, 2004).

It is important to ensure we check in with the parents or caregivers on a continuous basis to determine when and if they have any concerns related to the routines and activities in which we are engaging with their child. Because not every skill or strategy might fit into a set time or activity within the day, discussing the outliers to routines could lead to conversations about other important events or issues that might be effectively addressed as well (McWilliam, 2010; Rush & Shelden, 2020). At this stage in the IFSP development, we know to ask parents and caregivers specific questions to clarify how each routine or activity works within the dynamics of their own unique family. At this time, we might want to review the questions presented in Table 4–4 and Table 7–3 with the families to support the continued focus of our practice on their routines and everyday activities.

Transition Planning

To wrap up our discussion regarding the development and implementation of the IFSP, we must be clear about our role and responsibilities regarding a child's transition from EI (IDEA Part C) services to early childhood (IDEA Part B) services. Transition planning is an integral component of the IFSP and must be included and discussed with the family when developing the very first IFSP for a child and their family. The IFSP must contain a transition plan to help the child and family transition from Part C services. Transition planning should begin at least 90 days before the child's third birthday, or, at the team's discretion, up to 6 months before the child's third birthday. This timeline supports a seamless move from an EI program to a preschool or other community program. If a child qualifies, an Individualized Education Program (IEP) signed by the parents must be in place by the child's third birthday (IDEA, 2004, 2011).

When a child turns 3 years old, all special education and related services must be provided in the least restrictive environment possible. With this policy in mind, when planning for a child's transition to preschool, the EI team should consider whether or not the child could make appropriate progress in an inclusive environment if they did not receive supports and services. Possible preschool programs might include public or private preschools, as well as Head Start centers. Should the team determine the most appropriate educational services for a child need to be offered in a segregated setting, we must justify this decision in writing (IDEA, 2004, 2011).

Individualized Family Service Plan Timeline, Implementation, and Review

Once a referral about a child with a suspected disability or developmental delay is received by an intake coordinator in the EI system, the clock starts ticking. According to IDEA (2004), the IFSP must be developed within 45 days from the date of referral. Prior to the creation of the IFSP, this timeline includes completion of the screening, comprehensive evaluation, and initial assessment of the child and family. Services must be initiated within 30 days after the EI team agrees on supports and services and the family signs the IFSP. Implementation and review of the IFSP involves the coordination and monitoring of the delivery of IFSP supports and services. Periodic reviews are held to facilitate IFSP changes, if and as necessary. These changes might reflect the child's development and any changes that occur in regard to a family's priorities and concerns. IFSP reviews must take place at least once every 6 months or each time a child has either achieved a documented outcome or presents a new area of need. Annual reviews must be completed within 365 days of the initial or previous annual IFSP meeting (IDEA, 2004).

Summary

To ensure we are addressing and implementing evidence-based best practices in EI, we must consider the involvement and ownership of the family within each step of the process. By intentionally involving and collaborating with the parents and caregivers, including determination of their child's eligibility for services and the development of the IFSP, we establish a foundation to ensure we are embarking on a family- and routines-based journey.

This chapter also focused on the steps involved in developing the IFSP. IDEA Part C eligibility categories were presented and explored, particularly those that tend to result in communication, speech, language, and feeding impairments. We know supporting a young child's family lends itself to supporting the child and their development. As SLPs on the EI team, we dove further into our roles and responsibilities when determining the concerns, resources, and priorities of the family; our attention was on the strategies we can use to encourage and gather input from and with the family through the use of McWilliam's (2010) Routines-Based Interview. We learned the importance of gathering information from the parents and caregivers to create functional, family- and child-focused outcomes that can be addressed within natural environments and embedded within the child's everyday activities and routines. We then discussed the elements and steps involved in writing functional IFSP outcomes to ensure we provide evidence-based, child- and family-focused intervention that facilitates the development of the children and supports the families we serve. We wrapped up by considering the final components of the IFSP and recognized our responsibilities when guiding the family and their decision-making process in preparation for and throughout the transition out of EI services.

Critical Thinking Questions

1. Define eligibility determination and the established criteria for eligibility, and describe the requirements related to this step of the EI supports and services pathway under IDEA Part C.

2. What is late language emergence? What are the characteristics, related factors, and risk factors for young children with this diagnosis…and why is it important we have a clear understanding of these considerations when working with infants and toddlers?

3. Describe the role of informed clinical opinion by the service providers on the EI team.

How does informed clinical opinion relate to the process of establishing a young child's eligibility for services?

4. Present the required components of the Individualized Family Service Plan (IFSP) and the initial steps taken to develop this document.

5. With a focus on working with the parents and caregivers to support the entire family, how would you explain the elements involved in writing functional IFSP outcomes?

6. Discuss the strategies we might incorporate when conducting McWilliam's family-focused *Routines-Based Interview*. How might we include and document the information we gather from the interview within the IFSP?

7. How can we support a family and their ability to make decisions while completing each step within the EI supports and services pathway? What are our roles and responsibilities within the process?

References

American Speech-Language-Hearing Association. (n.d.). *Late language emergence [Practice Portal]*. https://www.asha.org/practice-portal/clinical-topics/late-language-emergence/

Benn, R. (1994). Conceptualizing eligibility for early intervention services. In D. M. Bryant & M. A. Graham (Eds.), *Implementing early intervention* (pp. 18–45). Guilford Press.

Brown, W., & Brown, C. (1993). Defining eligibility for EI. In W. Brown, S. K. Thurman, & F. Pearl (Eds.), *Family-centered EI with infants and toddlers: Innovative cross-disciplinary approaches* (pp. 21–42). Brookes.

Collisson, B. A., Graham, S. A., Preston, J. L., Rose, M. S., McDonald, S., & Tough, S. (2016). Risk and protective factors for late talking: An epidemiologic investigation. *The Journal of Pediatrics, 172*, 168–174. https://doi.org/10.1016/j.jpeds.2016.02.020

Crawford, M. J., & Weber, B. (2014). *Early intervention every day! Embedding activities in daily routines for young children and their families*. Brookes.

Division for Early Childhood. (2014). *DEC recommended practices in early intervention/early childhood special education 2014*. http://www.dec-sped.org/recommendedpractices

Dunst, C. J. (2002). Family-centered practices: Birth through high school. *Journal of Special Education, 36*(3), 139–147. https://doi.org/10.1177/00224669020360030401

Early Childhood Learning & Knowledge Center. (2018). *Readiness and relationships: Issues in assessing young children, families, and caregivers*.

https://eclkc.ohs.acf.hhs.gov/child-screening-assessment/article/readiness-relationships-issues-assessing-young-children-families-caregivers

Early Childhood Technical Assistance Center. (2014). *Individualized family service plan process guidance handbook.* https://ectacenter.org/eco/assets/pdfs/EDISIFSPProcessGuidanceHandbook.pdf

Early Childhood Technical Assistance Center. (2023). *Summary of state and jurisdictional eligibility definitions for infants and toddlers with disabilities under IDEA Part C.* https://ectacenter.org/topics/earlyid/state-info.asp

Early Intervention-Early Childhood Professional Development Community of Practice. (n.d.) *Authentic assessment in early intervention.* http://universalonlinepartceicurriculum.pbworks.com/w/page/79638626/Universal%20Online%20Part%20C%20EI%20Curriculum

Ellis Weismer, S. (2007). Typical talkers, late talkers, and children with specific language impairment: A language endowment spectrum. In R. Paul (Ed.), *The influence of developmental perspectives on research and practice in communication disorders: A festschrift for Robin S. Chapman* (pp. 83–102). Erlbaum.

Fasolo, M., Majorano, M., & D'Odorico, L. (2008). Babbling and first words in children with slow expressive development. *Clinical Linguistics & Phonetics, 22*(2), 83–94. https://doi.org/10.1080/02699200701600015

Fisher, E. (2017). A systematic review and meta-analysis of predictors of expressive-language outcomes among late talkers. *Journal of Speech, Language, and Hearing Research, 60,* 1–14. https://doi.org/10.1044/2017_JSLHR-L-16-0310

Guralnick, M. J. (1997). *The effectiveness of early intervention.* Brookes.

Guralnick, M. J. (1998). Effectiveness of early intervention for vulnerable children: A developmental perspective. *American Journal of Mental Retardation, 102*(4), 319–345. https://doi.org/10.1352/0895-8017(1998)102%3C0319:EOEIFV%3E2.0.CO;2

Hodges, R., Baker, E., Munro, N., & McGregor, K. K. (2017). Responses made by late talkers and typically developing toddlers during speech assessments. *International Journal of Speech-Language Pathology, 19,* 587–600. https://doi.org/10.1080/17549507.2016.1221452

Horowitz, S. M., Irwin, J. R., Briggs-Gowan, M. J., Bosson Heenan, J. M., Medoza, J., & Carter, A. S. (2003). Language delay in a community cohort of young children. *Journal of the American Academy of Child & Adolescent Psychiatry, 42*(8), 932–940. https://doi.org/10.1097/01.CHI.0000046889.27264.5E

Individuals With Disabilities Education Improvement Act of 2004, Pub. L. No. 108-446, § 632, 118 Stat. 2744 (2004). http://idea.ed.gov/

Individuals With Disabilities Education Improvement Act. (2011). Part C Final Regulations. 34 C.F.R. §§ 303 (2011). https://www.gpo.gov/fdsys/pkg/FR-2011-09-28/pdf/2011-22783.pdf

Irwin, J. R., Carter, A. S., & Briggs-Gowan, M. J. (2002). The social-emotional development of "late-talking" toddlers. *Journal of the American Academy of Child & Adolescent Psychiatry, 41*(11), 1324–1332. https://doi.org/10.1097/00004583-200211000-00014

Klee, T., Carson, D., Gavin, W. J., & Hall, L. (1998). Concurrent and predictive validity of an early language screening program. *Journal of Speech, Language, and Hearing Research, 41*(3) 627-641. https://doi.10.1044/jslhr.4103.627

Lucas, A., Gillaspy, K., Peters, M. L., & Hurth, J. (2014). *Enhancing recognition of high quality, functional IFSP outcomes.* http://www.ectacenter.org/~pdfs/pubs/rating-ifsp.pdf

Manning, B. L., Roberts, M. Y., Estabrook, R., Petitclerc, A., Burns, J. L., Briggs-Gowan, M., ... Norton, E. S. (2019). Relations between toddler expressive language and temper tantrums in a community sample. *Journal of Applied Developmental Psychology, 65,* 101070. https://doi.org/10.1016/j.appdev.2019.101070

Marchman, V. A., & Fernald, A. (2013). Variability in real-time spoken language processing in typically developing and late-talking toddlers. In L. A. Rescorla & P. S. Dale (Eds.), *Late talkers: Language development, interventions, and outcomes* (pp. 145–166). Brookes.

McWilliam, R. A. (2010). *Routines-based early intervention: Supporting young children and their families.* Brookes.

McWilliam, R. A., Casey, A. M., & Sims, J. L. (2009). The Routines-Based Interview: A method for assessing needs and developing IFSPs. *Infants & Young Children, 22,* 224–233.

Mirak, J., & Rescorla, L. (1998). Phonetic skills and vocabulary size in late talkers: Concurrent and predictive relationships. *Applied Psycholinguistics, 19*(1), 1–17. https://doi.org/10.1017/S0142716000010559

National Research Council. (2001). *Educating children with autism.* National Academies Press.

Oller, D. K., Eilers, R. E., Neal, A. R., & Schwartz, H. K. (1999). Precursors to speech in infancy: The prediction of speech and language disorders. *Journal of Communication Disorders, 32*(4), 223–245. https://doi.org/10.1016/S0021-9924(99)00013-1

Olswang, L. B., Rodriguez, B., & Timler, G. (1998). Recommending intervention for toddlers with specific language learning difficulties: We may not have all the answers, but we know a lot. *American Journal of Speech-Language Pathology, 7*(1), 23–32. https://doi.org/10.1044/1058-0360.0701.23

Paul, R. (1991). Profiles of toddlers with slow expressive language development. *Topics in Language Disorders, 11*(4), 1–13. https://doi.org/10.1097/00011363-199111040-00003

Paul, R. (1996). Clinical implications of the natural history of slow expressive language development. *American Journal of Speech- Language Pathology, 5*(2), 5–21.

Paul, R., & Jennings, P. (1992). Phonological behavior in toddlers with slow expressive language development. *Journal of Speech and Hearing Research, 35*(1), 99–107. https://doi.org/10.1044/jshr.3501.99

Rescorla, L. A. (1989). The language development survey: A screening tool for delayed language in toddlers. *Journal of Speech and Hearing Disorders, 54*, 587–599.

Rescorla, L. A. (2000). Do late-talking toddlers turn out to have reading difficulties a decade later? *Annals of Dyslexia, 50*(1), 85–102. https://doi.org/10.1007/s11881-000-0018-2

Rescorla, L. A. (2002). Language and reading outcomes to age 9 in late-talking toddlers. *Journal of Speech, Language, and Hearing Research, 45*(2), 360–371. https://doi.org/10.1044/1092-4388(2002/028)

Rescorla, L. A. (2009). Age 17 language and reading outcomes in late-talking toddlers: Support for a dimensional perspective on language delay. *Journal of Speech, Language, and Hearing Research, 52*(1), 16–30. https://doi.org/10.1044/1092-4388(2008/07-0171)

Rescorla, L. A. (2013). Late-talking toddlers: A 15-year follow-up. In L. A. Rescorla & P. S. Dale (Eds.), *Late talkers: Language development, interventions, and outcomes* (pp. 219–239). Paul H. Brookes Publishing Co.

Rescorla, L. A., & Achenbach, T. M. (2002). Use of the Language Development Survey (LDS) in a national probability sample of children 18 to 35 months old. *Journal of Speech, Language, and Hearing Research, 45*(4), 733–743. https://doi.org/10.1044/1092-4388(2002/059)

Rescorla, L. A., & Alley, A. (2001). Validation of the Language Development Survey (LDS): A parent report tool for identifying language delay in toddlers. *Journal of Speech, Language, and Hearing Research, 44*(2), 434–445. https://doi.org/10.1044/1092-4388(2001/035)

Rescorla, L. A., & Ratner, N. B. (1996). Phonetic profiles of toddlers with specific expressive language impairment (SLI-E). *Journal of Speech and Hearing Research, 39*(1), 153–165. https://doi.org/10.1044/jshr.3901.153

Rescorla, L. A., & Schwartz, E. (1990). Outcome of toddlers with specific expressive language delay. *Applied Psycholinguistics, 11*(4), 393–407. https://doi.org/10.1017/S0142716400009644

Rush, D. D., & Shelden, M. L. (2020). *The early childhood coaching handbook* (2nd ed.). Brookes.

Stoel-Gammon, C. (1989). Prespeech and early speech development of two late talkers. *First Language, 9*(6), 207–223. https://doi.org/10.1177/014272378900900607

Thal, D. J., Marchman, V. A., & Tomblin, J. B. (2013). Late-talking toddlers: Characterization and prediction of continued delay. In L. A. Rescorla & P. S. Dale (Eds.), *Late talkers: Language development, interventions, and outcomes* (pp. 169–201). Brookes.

Thal, D. J., & Tobias, S. (1992). Communicative gestures in children with delayed onset of oral expressive vocabulary. *Journal of Speech and Hearing Research, 35*(6), 1281–1289. https://doi.org/10.1044/jshr.3506.1289

Thal, D. J., Tobias, S., & Morrison, D. (1991). Language and gesture in late talkers: A 1-year follow-up. *Journal of Speech and Hearing Research, 34*(3), 604–612. https://doi.org/10.1044/jshr.3403.604

Wetherby, A., Allen, L., Cleary, J., Kublin, K., & Goldstein, H. (2002). Validity and reliability of the Communication and Symbolic Behavior Scales Developmental Profile with very young children. *Journal of Speech, Language, and Hearing Research, 45*(6), 1202–1218. https://doi.org/10.1044/1092-4388(2002/097)

Wilson, L. L., Mott, D. W., & Batman, D. (2004). The asset-based context matrix: A tool for assessing children's learning opportunities and participation in natural environments. *Topics in Early Childhood Special Education, 24*, 110–120.

Workgroup on Principles and Practices in Natural Environments. (2011). *Agreed upon practices for providing early intervention services in natural environments.* http://www.ectacenter.org/~pdfs/topics/families/AgreedUponPractices_FinalDraft2_01_08.pdf1

Zubrick, S. R., Taylor, C. L., Rice, M. L., & Slegers, D. W. (2007). Late language emergence at 24 months: An epidemiological study of prevalence, predictors, and covariates. *Journal of Speech, Language, and Hearing Research, 50*(6), 1562–1592. https://doi.org/10.1044/1092-4388(2007/106)

Chapter 8

Culturally and Linguistically Responsive Practices in Early Intervention

Learning Outcomes

When we have completed this chapter, we will be able to:

- Present current data related to equity in EI, access to services, and disparities in screening, referral, and identification for services of young children who are culturally and linguistically diverse.

- Describe policies presented within IDEA that specifically focus on and emphasize culturally and linguistically responsive services.

- Define inclusion, cultural and linguistic diversity, and culturally and linguistically responsive practices as they relate to EI.

- Reflect on our roles and responsibility to reduce barriers, embrace challenges, and seek opportunities to engage in EI practices that respect and support the cultural and linguistic diversity of different families.

- Discuss best practices when working with an interpreter to support EI services.

- Share the existing evidence with families and colleagues related to young children acquiring two languages, including those with speech and language disorders.

- Describe evaluation and assessment considerations and strategies when working with culturally and linguistically diverse families.

- Present intervention strategies, including the use of coaching, to effectively work with children and families who are culturally and linguistically diverse.

What Will We Learn and How Can We Apply It?

ASHA guides us to provide young children and families engaged in EI with services that are inclusive and address culturally and linguistically responsive and competent practices (ASHA, 2023). IDEA (2004) requires that EI teams consider a child's English language proficiency status as well as their family's experiences and cultural background when providing services. The DEC of the Council for Exceptional Children (CEC) emphasizes the need for service providers to recognize and address the effects that culture, language, and other variables have on assessment and intervention to ensure our processes are culturally responsive (Mongomery, 2001). All of these expectations compel us to competently and effectively interact with and support children and families of different cultures. Throughout the previous chapters and within various contexts in this textbook, we have referred to each of these principles, noting we would learn about how to address each in detail in this chapter. It is time to focus on the knowledge and skills needed, as EI SLPs, to engage in inclusive practice. To recognize and implement inclusive practices that address the unique differences of each family we serve, we must first embrace the definitions, challenges, and opportunities to develop the skills that will support effective collaboration with each of the infants, toddlers, parents, and caregivers we serve. We dive into these considerations to ensure our hearts, our minds, and our EI practices are truly inclusive.

The Facts About Equity in Early Intervention

We have learned that children who have access to EI services are more likely to have better outcomes compared to those who do not receive services (ECTA, 2023). Immediate benefits of EI for children include cognitive, language, motor, and social emotional development; improvements were evident for the child's family members as well (Camilli et al., 2010; Casto & Mastropieri, 1986; Karoly et al., 2005). Regardless of these outcomes, however, there is no doubt there are disparities regarding access by families to EI screening, identification, and referral. Children who are culturally or linguistically diverse also disproportionately live in poverty (DeNavas-Walt & Proctor, 2015). In 2016, 34% of American Indian children, 34% of Black children, 28% of Hispanic or Latino children, and 12% of Asian or Pacific Islander children lived in families with incomes below the federal poverty level (Kids Count Data Center, 2018). With these data in mind, evidence-based, family-centered intervention for young children who are culturally or linguistically diverse is clearly a growing need.

Despite the growing need to provide services to these children, the evidence indicates racial disparities in developmental screening and EI referral and identification, and these disparities only become larger over time. The *Zero to Three State of Babies Yearbook* (Keating et al., 2021) presents data showing the national average for toddlers between the ages of 9 to 35 months who have received a developmental screening in the past year is 32.5%. When presented by race, the data show the following statistics of toddlers who have participated in a developmental screening:

- 35.7% are White families.
- 27.9% are Hispanic families.
- 27.2% are Black families.
- 26.1% are Asian families.

Of families living above low income (based on 200% of the federal poverty level), 36.0% reported their child had received a developmental screening in the past year (ECTA, 2023); only 27.2% of families with low income reported their child had participated in a screening process in the past year (Keating et al., 2021). The research also indicates that Black children are less likely than their White and higher income counterparts to be referred for EI services

(McManus et al., 2020). It is important for us to consider that, although the population of infants and toddlers served in EI mirrors the population of the United States in terms of race and ethnicity, White children are slightly more likely to receive services than other children; Black children are slightly less likely to receive services (U.S. Department of Education, Office of Special Education Programs, 2020). State and local data and national surveys also present disparities in service access, based on children's racial and ethnic background and type of community in which they live (Khetani et al., 2017). Children found eligible for EI services in neighborhoods that are low-income communities of color are, in fact, least likely to receive services. Even in neighborhoods where higher rates of eligible children receive services, Black children are less likely to receive services than White children (Khetani et al., 2017).

The evidence is clear: Many young children with delays, disorders, and disabilities and their families face issues in accessing and participating in EI services. Current research presents key information and evidence that supports these disparities and inequities in the access and implementation of EI services. With this in mind, we also know IDEA (2004) requires that states prioritize measurement of performance in the areas of racial and ethnic groups in EI and related services. Each state that receives funding for EI must examine their data to determine if significant disproportionality based on race and ethnicity is occurring in the state with respect to identification of children receiving services (IDEA, 2004; O'Hara & Bollmer, 2021). IDEA (2011) also supports program delivery in EI that recognizes and addresses cultural and linguistic diversity to ensure we provide all children and their families with inclusive services.

Defining Inclusion and Inclusive Practice

The DEC and the National Association for the Education of Young Children (NAEYC) define *inclusion* in EI as providing appropriate accommodations and support for each child to participate to the fullest of their developmental abilities. The DEC and NAEYC also note that inclusion requires acceptance, compassion, and a commitment to creating a culture of belonging for all children and their families (DEC & NAEYC, 2009). This definition is aligned with Part C of IDEA (2004), which states providers are required to provide EI services and supports in natural environments, including both home and community settings, where children would be participating if they did not have any disabilities.

There are many ways to support children and their families within inclusive environments and learning experiences. We can begin to demonstrate our support by developing a collaborative relationship with each family. These relationships are initiated by meeting the child and their parents or caregivers where they are; learning about their culture, language, and family practices; and accepting them for who they are and how they connect with one another. We begin to build these relationships by first embracing and celebrating each child's uniqueness, treating every child and family equally and with respect, and providing the family with resources that reflect the background of their child. As we learn more about the family and move forward on the EI pathway, we continue to engage in inclusive practices by learning about and honoring their ethnicity, culture, language, gender, socioeconomic background, and the experiences in which the family chooses to engage.

IDEA Part C Regulations Related to Cultural and Linguistic Diversity

IDEA (2004, 2011) includes language that specifically focuses on and emphasizes the importance of culturally and linguistically responsive services in all of the arenas in which we provide services. As EI providers, we need to be particularly aware of the language associated with IDEA Part C.

- All families of infants or toddlers with a disability must be provided with access to "culturally competent services within their local geographical areas" (§303.227).

- Procedural safeguards state that prior written notice must be "provided in the native language ... of the parent or other mode of communication used by the parent, unless it is clearly not feasible to do so" (§303.421(c)).

- Part C regulations define native language as the "language normally used by that individual, or in the case of a child, the language normally used by the parents of the child" (§303.25(a)(1)).

- Evaluations and assessments should be conducted in "the language normally used by the child, if determined developmentally appropriate for the child by qualified personnel conducting the evaluation or assessment." This definition allows for the consideration of the child's total language system in a way that permits qualified service providers to assess a child who typically uses more than one language and supports culturally competent service delivery for customization of the language(s) for assessment and evaluation as appropriate for each child (§303.25(a)(2)).

- All evaluations and assessments of a child must be conducted in the native language of the child unless it is clearly not feasible to do so; when needed, an on-site or telephonic interpreter should be included in the process (§303.321(a)(5); §303.321(a)(6)).

- Each family must be involved in the assessment process and services are expected to be relevant and culturally competent. An assessment must include a description of the family's resources, priorities, and concerns related to enhancing the child's development (§303.321(c)(2)(i-iii)).

As SLPs, it is our responsibility to be cognizant of and to embed these policies into our practice. This requires us to learn about and honor the diverse experiences and expectations of each family to provide the highest quality of services possible.

Defining Cultural Diversity and Culturally Responsive Practice

It is critical that we recognize everyone belongs to and represents a culture. Some of the cultural variables that might influence our perceptions and behaviors are age, disability, gender, occupation, religious beliefs, race, sexual orientation, socioeconomic status, and ethnicity (ASHA, 2023). Children and families receiving EI supports and services are increasingly diverse, and represent different cultures, ethnicities, traditions, values, and belief systems. We know now that cultural responsiveness involves our understanding, including, and responding to these variables, in addition to valuing the diversity of and seeking further knowledge about a family's culture and language (Hopf et al., 2021). Cultural responsiveness is also necessary to ensure our success, and the success of the child and family, in every step of the EI process. Culture influences how a family defines and structures itself, family functions, the family life cycle, and events that are viewed by the family as stressors (Wayman & Lynch, 1991). Cultural perspectives can also relate to and affect in which services a family chooses to participate (Hanson & Lynch, 1990; Peredo, 2016).

In Chapters 1 and 2, we introduced the concepts of cultural responsiveness and humility, and our responsibility, as EI providers, to engage in these practices. Cultural responsiveness is a complex process in which we engage in ongoing self-assessment and continuous cultural education, are willing to share our own values and beliefs, and are open to the values and beliefs of others (Hopf et al., 2021). Cultural humility is a dynamic concept that represents the need for lifelong learning and the recognition of biases and power differentials within the health-care system (Agner, 2020). The concept of cultural humility incorporates mutual respect and a validation of the inequalities that families with cultural and linguistic diversity face. Culturally responsive practice requires us to engage in both self-reflection and collaboration with the family, emphasizing an openness and ability in order to listen to understand the perspectives of the families (Hopf et al., 2021). We must be willing to demonstrate humility to provide culturally responsive services to the children and the families we serve.

As SLPs, we interact with families of many different cultures. Our awareness and ability to engage in cultural responsiveness when providing EI services affects our ability to respond to demographic diversity; understand and respond to social determinants of health and health-related disparities as they affect the families with whom we work; provide services that will improve the quality of services and outcomes; and meet accreditation, legislative, and regulatory mandates (ASHA, 2021). We must be aware of the different cultural dimensions and the unique influences of each family's cultural background to ensure we are using effective clinical approaches within our services. Different cultural dimensions can also influence a family's level of engagement and their decisions regarding EI services and supports. By becoming more culturally competent and responsive, we reduce our own cultural biases and recognize the cultural issues important to each family.

Framework to Meet the Needs of Culturally Diverse Children and Families

One goal of SLPs in EI is to effectively serve families in ways that respect their culture and individuality. To provide culturally responsive services to families, we need to consider those factors that affect families' perspectives as well as those considerations that might relate directly to services. Bradshaw (2013) provided a framework for EI service providers to meet the needs of the culturally diverse children and families they serve. The framework was created to organize existing research and literature on cultural responsiveness in a way that fits the unique context of EI and synthesizes both knowledge and best practices into the following four guiding principles (Bradshaw, 2013):

1. *Examining one's own culture* encourages us, as EI providers, to take an in-depth look at our own cultural values and beliefs.

2. *Acquiring knowledge of family cultures* highlights the importance of finding out about the cultures of the families we serve.

3. *Building culturally responsive practices* actively engages us in developing and implementing culturally responsive practices to respond to the unique strengths, needs, and desires of different families.

4. *Reflecting and evaluating practices* encourages us, as SLPs in EI, to reflect often on our practices to identify our most and least effective practices with families of cultures different from our own.

By following this framework, we engage in active listening and learning about the family's own systems. During the initial assessment for the program planning process, we ask questions and listen to the family members discuss their needs and concerns. Based on their feedback and by collaborating with family members, we develop outcomes that are aligned with family culture, values, needs, and priorities. Because intervention activities are built directly into family routines that already exist, the routines-based approach builds on the strengths that are inherent to individual family systems, eliminating cultural mismatches (Raver & Childress, 2015). By determining optimal routines and empowering parents to incorporate opportunities into their own everyday activities, we are able to provide effective services while respecting and considering every family's culture as well as value system (Bradshaw, 2013; Peña & Fiestas, 2009).

Defining Linguistic Diversity and Linguistically Responsive Practice

Linguistic diversity refers to the different ways people speak and communicate with each other. According to ASHA (2023), the linguistic diversity of individuals can affect aspects of communication, such as vocabulary, dialect, and literacy. As SLPs, we often work with families who speak a language different from our own and we know there are a limited number of bilingual SLPs in the field (ASHA, 2021).

To effectively support families, it is necessary that we develop a heightened level of awareness and sensitivity to the influences that linguistic identity brings to the family system (McManus et al., 2020; Peredo, 2016; Segal & Beyer, 2006). When providing linguistically responsive services, we must consider both the native and home language(s) as well as acquisition of the language needed for the child's academic success. This can present differently, depending on the services and supports each family is receiving. We need to conduct our evaluation and assessments in the family's native language and should teach parents and caregivers how to implement strategies in their home language to maximize comprehension and carryover of both knowledge and skills (Peredo, 2016). We frequently work with interpreters to honor the needs of the child and family and engage in linguistically responsive EI services. We further explore each of these considerations throughout this chapter.

Involving Families

As SLPs, we have the opportunity to reduce barriers that families could experience regarding access to effective EI services and improve the satisfaction of services experienced by families who are culturally and linguistically diverse by supporting the culture and home language of the children, parents, and caregivers through family-centered, routines-based services. We must be authentic, open-minded, and flexible in our approaches and demonstrate respect for the family's priorities and needs. Although their perspectives and opinions might differ from our own, when we take the time to learn about a family's culture, routines, and everyday activities, while also being respectful of their choices, we will successfully collaborate with parents and caregivers to best serve their children and their own needs (Rush & Shelden, 2020). There are multiple strategies we can incorporate into our practice to ensure that this connection is made.

Respecting and Supporting the Family's Culture

When we use the approaches considered best practice in EI with culturally and linguistically diverse families, there are strategies of which we should be aware of, and in which we should engage to ensure we connect and respond both appropriately and effectively. First, we must be open to understanding and learning about family perspectives, choices, and lifestyles. We could find ourselves in situations in which we have had no prior experience; we might have difficulty understanding or even valuing a family's position or decision regarding their child's services or their own parenting styles. In some cultures, families might view developmental delays and disabilities differently. Additionally, guided by different cultural and spiritual beliefs, families could have a different understanding of what happens to children and how they are viewed if they are diagnosed with a disability. In some cultures, a disability is viewed as a gift from a higher power, and an opportunity for the parent or caregiver to compensate as a means of demonstrating their love for both their child and the higher power. Beliefs differ across and within cultures; even families with similar cultural backgrounds can hold very diverse views on disability.

We must also remain open-minded and flexible about a family's styles, preferences, and routines. Each family with whom we work will present unique differences between their everyday activities, the routines as well as the various ways in which they engage in their routines, and their perspectives about how they interact with and respond to their child's needs. As EI providers participating in coaching with a family, particularly those who present cultural and linguistical differences from our own, it is imperative that we are able to embrace the family's differences and consider the opportunities for everyone to support and maximize the child's development and learning (Rush & Shelden, 2020).

Understanding Our Own Values and Biases

Earlier in this chapter, we reviewed the strengths-based approach as a way in which we can facilitate our connection with each family's cultural and linguistic perspectives, priorities, and everyday activities. This approach also requires that we, as EI providers, engage in a more reflective practice, examine our own values and professional practice, and determine how these could affect each child's learning and development. By developing a reflective stance toward our practice, we are better positioned to develop the skills, knowledge, and approaches necessary for achieving the outcomes that will be most successful and most appropriate for each child and family (McCashen, 2017).

When we work with culturally and linguistically diverse families, it is important that we understand our own cultural values and biases (Bradshaw, 2013). Families from different cultural communities could have vastly different expectations regarding development milestones and priorities for their child's development (Rogoff, 2003). When we understand our own biases, it is easier to overcome them and work with families in a more empathetic way. As EI providers, we need to recognize and come from the viewpoint that most parents and caregivers want what is best for their child. If it is not a functional need or goal for the family, and is not harmful to the child, there is no reason to push a culturally inconsistent goal on a family simply based on our own culture's developmental expectations.

Learning About the Family's Values and Priorities

The best way to understand how a parent or caregiver thinks or feels is to ask them. One way to understand family values, parenting practices, and cultural expectations of their children is through the Routines-Based Interview (McWilliam, 2010), which we learned about in Chapter 7. This process gives us a medium through which to encourage the family to think in terms of their own routines and activities in preparation for developing outcomes and strategies. It also allows the family to see that the focus of EI extends beyond the child to include the greater context of the family (ECTA, 2023). Table 8–1 presents conversation starters we might consider facilitating our discussion with a family and encourage the parents and caregivers to share information from a holistic perspective. As such, we might want to include questions about a family's values, priorities, practices, and expectations as they relate to the cultural and linguistic differences. Table 8–1 offers additional questions to engage a family in conversation to develop our relationship with the family; gain a stronger understanding of their values, parenting practices, and the role of caregivers; learn about family and child strengths; and serve as a platform for setting functional goals and intervention planning. If we are genuine with the children, parents, and caregivers, asking them questions and listening to their responses for the sake of learning more about them, our relationships will emerge seamlessly, and we will enjoy the connections we make with our families.

Table 8–1. Questions to Ask Families About Their Values and Priorities

Family Composition
- Name the members of your family (identify all family members and their relationship to one another).
- Who lives in the home with [child]?
- Tell me about your immediate and extended family.
- Are there any other children in the family?
- Where does [child] fall in the birth order?
- Are family members employed outside the home?
- Who participates in parenting or caregiving [child]?
- Who do you go to when you want or need parenting advice?

Family Customs and Preferences
- How do you and your family members prefer to be greeted (e.g., formally or informally; by name or role)?
- Are service providers invited into your home?
- What are the customs or preferences in your home (e.g., removal of shoes when a visitor enters the home, shaking hands, greeting with touch or not touching unless invited to do so)?
- Where and when would you prefer to meet or discuss issues?
- What are your hopes and dreams for the family and children?

Family Culture, Ethnicity, and Language
- With which cultural, ethnic, and linguistic groups does your family identify?
- What is your language of preference in communication with professionals?
- Do you believe an interpreter is needed for us to communicate?
- Do you or other family members prefer written materials or information that is shared in a specific way (e.g., written or verbal)?
- Do written (or other) materials need to be translated into the family's preferred language?

Family Support System
- What other family members or friends are included in your circle of support? How are these other individuals included?
- In addition to those individuals you just named, are there other friends or individuals who have been supportive?
- Are there other programs or systems that provide your family with support?

Child-Rearing Practices
- What are your beliefs about child development? Your child/ren's developmental milestones (e.g., toileting, feeding, caring for self)?
- What are family mealtime practices? Are there dietary preferences or restrictions?
- What are your beliefs about parenting infants and young children?
- How do you think [child] should behave at home?
- How should [child] behave in the community?
- What are your expectations for [child] regarding eating and feeding? Napping and bedtime? Potty training? Playing?
- What are your beliefs regarding standards of behavior and discipline?

Education, Health Care, and Seeking Help and Support
- What are your beliefs about the development or health conditions of your child or other members of your family?
- What is your approach to health care and/or healing?
- What are your beliefs about the education of the children (e.g., readiness for school, academic goals, and outcomes)?
- Do you seek help from any formal agencies, organizations, or community services? If so, for what services?
- Do you agree with other family members about the use of services and supports and the approaches you use?

Other Goals, Needs, and Priorities
- Besides some of the things we talked about regarding your family's activities, what are some of your other goals for [child]?
- What would you like to get out of participating in early intervention?
- If there was one thing you could change to make your life easier or better, what would it be?
- What have been some successful strategies for you with [child]?
- Is there anything else we have not talked about that you would like to share?

Note. Adapted from "A framework for providing culturally responsive early intervention services," 2013, by W. Bradshaw; "Routines-based early intervention," by R. A. McWilliam, 2010; "Supporting culturally and linguistically diverse families in early intervention," by T. N. Peredo, 2016.

Every family is unique; cultural considerations add a layer of complexity to the different perspectives, priorities, and resources within each family. Some of the questions we might need to consider asking when meeting with a family should focus on the following cultural differences in expectations about roles and responsibilities throughout the EI process.

- As EI providers and SLPs, we will be viewed by some families as the professionals and they may consider it disrespectful to argue or state their opinion even if it differs from ours (Agazzi et al., 2010; Fadiman, 1998).

- Parents and caregivers want the best for their children. If strategies and goals are not being addressed between sessions, however, they might not fit with the family's parenting practices or everyday activities (Westby, 2009).

- In many families, there are multiple caregivers who contribute to and make decisions about child-rearing and who participate in everyday activities. These family members likely include individuals who are not the child's biological parents. To successfully communicate and collaborate with each family, we need to ensure we are aware of all caregivers identified by the family as important, and to include them in the EI process (Peredo, 2016).

- One of the challenges we often face when working with culturally and linguistically diverse families is presenting the evaluation and assessment results in a meaningful way that is jargon-free, family-friendly, and sensitive. Sharing the results of a child's delay with any family is difficult in most circumstances. Adding to that the different verbal and body language the families and EI providers might use, as well as the possible use of an interpreter, often presents further challenges (Banerjee & Guiberson, 2012).

Using Interpreters to Support Our Services

Ideally, as EI SLPs, we will speak the family's home language. However, given that there are not enough EI providers who speak languages other than English (Caesar, 2013), the more likely scenario is that we will need to teach the parent or caregiver how to support their child's language development and acquisition in a language we do not speak. At the very least, we should educate ourselves on how the family's home language is structured and ask for the family's input about what would be natural for us to model within their culture and language.

When we do not speak the family's home language, the next best practice is to find a bilingual SLP who speaks the language; this scenario is also often not possible. When this is the case, locating and collaborating with an interpreter is the best option. We will often find the use of an interpreter helpful to bridge and adapt language teaching strategies into the home language. It can be challenging to connect with and coach a family when there is a language barrier, but a good interpreter can help us overcome that challenge. An experienced interpreter offers a bridge for communication and, at the same time, is invisible as an outside contributor to the interaction. The interpreter should be sure that every individual fully understands each other without adding extraneous information or taking over the interaction. Although this is a difficult task, remaining in the role of the invisible bridge is important to ensure the interpreter does not instead become a roadblock in the relationship-building process between the EI providers and the family. Table 8–2 offers us additional strategies to ensure we connect effectively with parents and caregivers while using the services of an interpreter.

Table 8–2. Strategies to Connect With Families When Using an Interpreter

Speak with the interpreter prior to the session with the family. • Introduce and get to know each other. • Explain what will happen on the visit. • Review the purpose of the meeting, as well as roles and responsibilities during the EI session. • Share any guidelines from the Part C program, if applicable, regarding inclusion of an interpreter in EI sessions.
Allow for additional time. • Plan ahead for the first EI session with the family and interpreter and add an extra 15-30 min for the session. We want to be sure to have enough time for the extra communication involved.
Sit in a circle. • The SLP should face the parent or caregiver. • The interpreter should sit in a location in which they can see and speak with both the SLP and the parent or caregiver.
Always look at and speak directly to the parent. • This suggestion can feel a bit awkward, but the SLP should be sure to look at the parent or caregiver when speaking to them. Remember the interpreter's role is to serve as the invisible bridge between the EI provider and parent. • If the SLP speaks or looks directly at the interpreter, they are no longer invisible.
Keep statements and questions short and remember to pause. • This one is also difficult because shortening our sentences and remembering to pause might not be how we normally talk to other adults. • An intentional and mindful approach to communication is important because it makes it easier for the interpreter to accurately share everything we are saying.

Establishing a connection and collaborating with an interpreter takes time. Once we have established this relationship, however, we will have an essential partner to support us in helping the children and families we serve.

Language and Communication Skills of Dual-Language Learners

As the percentage of families with cultural and linguistic diversity continues to grow in the United States, the number of bilingual children on our EI caseloads will also continue to expand. As SLPs, we need to understand the benefits of a child's use of their home language and bilingual language development and be able to clearly articulate these benefits to families. To effectively empower parents and caregivers to make decisions regarding the use of their home language, we must also provide them with accurate information (Peredo, 2016). It is therefore imperative that we have accurate information regarding the language development of the bilingual infants and toddlers we serve. Several evidence-based conclusions have been confirmed over the past decade that can and should inform our practice in EI with children and their families from bilingual environments. Keeping in mind that this information is primarily focused on children who are *simultaneous bilinguals* (i.e., exposed to two languages from birth and living in a home in which two languages are spoken on a daily basis), Hoff and Core (2015) examined empirical findings and presented us with the following conclusions related to bilingual development:

- Young children can learn two languages at the same time and dual-language input will not confuse children.

- Although there might be influences of each language on the other, infants are actually good at distinguishing one language from another and develop two separate phonological, lexical, and grammatical systems (Hoff & Core, 2015).

- Children who are exposed to dual languages build two separate linguistic systems. Bilingual children often understand and use words in both languages for the same object; they also use different phonological and grammatical structures, appropriate to the language they are using at any given time (Core et al., 2013; Meisel, 1989; Pearson et al., 1993; Werker, 2012).

- Bilingual children tend to code-switch; they will move from one language to another and might use words from both languages in a single sentence. They tend to use code-switching as an intentional strategy when they do not find a word they need in the language they are speaking (Genesee, 2007).

- Parents and caregivers do not need to be advised that their two languages be kept separate in their children's experience to avoid confusion.

- It is much more natural for many parents and caregivers who are bilingual and live in bilingual communities to use both of their languages (Hoff et al., 2013; Place & Hoff, 2011).

- There is no research to support the concept that each parent or family member should "choose and use" only one language.

- Learning two languages takes longer than learning one; bilingualism does not, however, slow overall language development (Hoff & Core, 2015).

- Bilingual children tend to fall behind monolingual children in the stages of early language development in single language comparisons. It is important to note, however, that although their rate of single language growth might fall behind that of monolingual children, the rate of total vocabulary growth by bilingual children is equal to or greater than the rate of monolingual children (Bosch & Ramon-Casas, 2014; Hoff et al., 2012).

- Phonological skills and higher-level narrative skills of bilingual children are often similar to these skills for monolingual children (Oller et al., 2007; Paradis & Kirova, 2014); early receptive language skills might be stronger than their early expressive language skills (Ribot & Hoff, 2014).

- In a comprehensive meta-analysis of studies of bilingual language development, which included 64 studies and a sample of 1,906 children, Kohnert and Medina (2009) concluded that exposure to two languages does not cause delays in language development. When language outcomes are measured appropriately and account for all of a child's linguistic systems (i.e., measures skills in both languages), bilingualism does not slow overall language growth (Mancilla-Martinez & Vagh, 2013; Moore & Pérez-Méndez, 2006).

- Both quantity and quality of input in each language influence the bilingual child's rates of development in each language.

- The research consistently supports the finding that children develop their skills more rapidly in the language they hear more (Hoff et al., 2012; Pearson et al., 1997; Place & Hoff, 2011).

- The quality of the language input bilingual children receive also affects the rate of development. The same quality indicators that apply to monolingual input apply to input of two languages, including use of vocabulary, syntax, decontextualized speech, and book reading (Hoff, 2006; Huttenlocher et al., 1991; Patterson & Pearson, 2004; Rowe, 2012; Song et al., 2012).

- Bilingual environments vary significantly in the support they provide for each language; as a result, bilingual children vary significantly in their dual-language skills.

- Bilingual children can have different strengths in each language (Hoff & Core, 2015).

- Determining how proficient a bilingual child is in both languages is complex. They might have different experiences in and with their two languages; these differences could affect their level of proficiency or the patterns they present in regard to their strengths and weaknesses in the components of each language (Bialystok & Peets, 2010; Hoff & Core, 2015).

- Immigrant parents should not be discouraged from speaking their native language to their children (Hoff & Core, 2015).

- Children in families who can speak their family's native or home language have stronger relationships and ethnic identities (Oh & Fuligni, 2010; Tseng & Fuligni, 2000).

- Parents and caregivers might be more capable of providing cognitively stimulating input to their children in their native, versus second, language (Winsler et al., 2014).

- When the choice has been to develop only one of a child's languages, research has demonstrated these children experience irreversible negative effects in their overall development (Moore & Pérez-Méndez, 2006).

- Loss of home language and bilingual development of languages by a young child can result in the loss of the cognitive benefits of bilingualism, loss of psychosocial supports and protective factors associated with a bicultural identity, and loss of family connections as children lose the ability to communicate with some family members, and eventually, reduced caregiver participation in a child's school work due to a language barrier (Barac et al., 2014; Kohnert et al., 2005; Moore & Pérez-Méndez, 2006; Schwartz et al., 2010).

The existing evidence for children acquiring two languages, including those with speech and language disorders, demonstrates there are many benefits, and no harm, associated with bilingualism (Barac & Bialystok, 2012; Barac et al., 2014; Carlson & Meltzoff, 2008; Goodrich et al., 2013; Kohnert & Medina, 2009; Kohnert et al., 2005; Mancilla-Martinez & Lesaux, 2011; Miller et al., 2006; Páez & Rinaldi, 2006; Winsler et al., 2014). Furthermore, because a child's skills in one language have been shown to positively influence their skills in their second language, supporting the home language can also lead to better academic outcomes for children who receive instruction in English (Goodrich et al., 2013; Mancilla-Martinez & Lesaux, 2011; Miller et al., 2006; Páez & Rinaldi, 2006; Winsler et al., 2014). Additionally, supporting a child's home language and developing dual-language learners can result in multiple cognitive benefits for the child. A comprehensive review of studies of early childhood bilingualism found that children who are bilingual have many cognitive advantages compared to their monolingual peers (Barac et al., 2014). Bilingual children demonstrate advantages in executive functioning skills and tend to present with stronger metalinguistic abilities, including phonological awareness, and better metacognitive abilities than peers who are monolingual (Barac et al., 2014; McClelland et al., 2007; Raver et al., 2011).

The evidence clearly supports that infants and toddlers with language impairments can learn two languages and benefit significantly from becoming dual-language learners. As EI SLPs, we must be knowledgeable about the evidence supporting bilingualism in the young children we serve, and we should be prepared to share this information with families. By doing so, we can address and support their cultural and linguistic diversity as often as the opportunity presents itself in our practice.

Evaluation and Assessment Considerations When Working With Culturally and Linguistically Diverse Families

When we engage with children and their families who speak a language other than English in the home, we need to gather detailed information about their use of their native or home language, as well as their use of English. Evaluation and assessment of children whose first language is not English, or who are learning more than one language, can be complex; however, these issues are often mitigated by the fact that the infants and toddlers with whom we work in EI have limited linguistic development in any language. These young children typically present prelinguistic or emerging stages of language development. Some English-based, norm-referenced measures provide opportunities for us to examine the children's use of gaze, gesture, and vocal forms of communication. Parent report forms can also be used to assess the emergence of play, gestures, words, and word combinations without engaging in direct or formal assessment by a monolingual SLP (Crais, 2011).

Use of Standardized Evaluation and Assessment Tools

When standardized tests are used, we must ensure they are culturally and linguistically appropriate. Standard scores should not be determined if the norming sample does not adequately represent the individual being assessed (ASHA, n.d.). It is essential to consider the language spoken and even the dialect used by the child before selecting a standardized assessment. We cannot use an assessment tool that has been normed in U.S. English and translate the results; translation of a standardized assessment automatically invalidates the results (Crais, 2011). Standard scores cannot be reported when the assessment has been translated. In such cases, we can use available standardized language assessments for children who speak languages other than English (ASHA, n.d.).

Authentic and Dynamic Assessment Considerations

A comprehensive assessment of young children and their families must involve our identification of the environmental, maturational, and social factors that could affect the child's development and learning (Greenspan & Wieder, 2006). Rich observation through authentic assessment in the child's natural environment, or multiple environments, is another critical source of assessment information. Observing a child engage with family members in familiar tasks provides culturally valid information about how a child functions on a daily basis (Jackson et al., 2009; Westby et al., 1996). Observing children over time and monitoring their acquisition of skills and responsiveness to culturally appropriate and relevant tasks also provides us with important information that will assist in determining the strengths and needs of the child and their family and develop routines-based outcomes and intervention strategies.

Criterion-referenced play-based assessment methods that are developmentally based and take into consideration the child's experiences and cultural background can also be especially useful when assessing infants and toddlers in their natural environments (Casby, 2003; Linder, 2008). When these types of tools are used, the EI team also has the opportunity to observe natural parent–child interactions and the developmental priorities presented by the parents and caregivers, including information that will be useful when we work together to make recommendations and develop the IFSP with the family (Banerjee & Guiberson, 2012).

An additional alternative to standardized testing methods is dynamic assessment. When we conduct a dynamic assessment, we test the child for a particular behavior, provide cues or models to facilitate the child's use of the behavior, and then test the child again. Dynamic assessment is also an evaluation method we can use to identify a child's learning potential. This type of assessment emphasizes the learning process and accounts for the amount and nature of examiner investment. Dynamically assessing a young child also helps us differentiate speech-language differences and disorders when working with children who speak a language other than English. Dynamic assessment focuses on the child's ability to acquire the skills after being tested and after being exposed to instruction. Those who demonstrate significant development of skills over a short window of time or within a small number of EI sessions are more likely to have language differences, whereas those who do not demonstrate change are more likely to have a language disorder (Crais, 2011).

Intervention Considerations When Working with Culturally and Linguistically Diverse Families

As SLPs in EI, we need to be prepared to deliver interventions that are not only evidence-based, but also honor and are responsive to the cultural and linguistic diversity of the children and families we serve. These interventions must incorporate the families' beliefs, values, practices, and context; they should support the development of their home language and the varieties of languages, in addition to English, used by the family.

Intervention strategies that are culturally and linguistically responsive to the needs of children and families can enhance engagement, family satisfaction, and retention in EI programs and services (Bailey et al., 1999; Garcia Coll et al., 2002; Holden et al., 1990; Kumpfer et al., 2002). Additionally, our inclusion of responsive practices is supported by research, which indicates early language and literacy interventions that are culturally and linguistically responsive result in more promising outcomes for both children and family members than interventions that do not address their diversity (Duran et al., 2016; Larson et al., 2020). Dunst et al. (2016) determined that families' perceptions of the appropriateness of early language interventions resulted in greater fidelity and more consistent use of strategies by parents and caregivers between sessions, resulting in enhanced language skills for the children. When we honor, consider, and adapt our intervention strategies and processes to the cultures and languages of the children and families with whom we work, EI will be more enjoyable, engaging, and effective for everyone.

Teaching Families How to Implement Strategies in the Home Language

We first discussed evidence-based practices in EI in Chapter 3. We introduced the family-centered and strengths-based approaches and shared information that supported the RBI and practice-based coaching models. When used in EI, each of these approaches and models supports our ability to implement culturally and linguistically responsive services and ultimately leads to inclusive practice on behalf of the children and families we serve.

The family-centered model guides us to meet families where they are, collaborate with them, and build on and support their capacity to make informed decisions and act on them. As EI providers, we engage with family members to understand their lives, goals, strengths, and challenges and develop a relationship between family and practitioner. We work with them to set goals, strengthen capacity, and implement individualized, culturally responsive, and evidence-based interventions for each family. We also learned about RBI in EI to ensure families are considering and incorporating the strategies we have discussed within their everyday routines and activities to maximize the child's development and learning (Dunst et al., 2012). The evidence supports the approach of embedding skills and strategies within everyday activities and daily routines as an effective way to help parents and caregivers give their children the support to encourage development, engage with, and increase their participation in culturally relevant activities with their families, address their needs within the linguistic structures of their home language, and facilitate carryover of skills between EI sessions (Crawford & Weber, 2014).

The strengths-based model also emphasizes the capacity of families to take ownership of their priorities, needs, and preferences and to identify, value, and mobilize their strengths, capacities, and resources. Rather than focusing on their deficits and their child's delays or disorder, the approach guides us to work with families to identify their social, personal, cultural, and structural constraints and empower them to take control of their goals (McCashen, 2005). The nature of the strengths-based approach in EI also acknowledges and supports the family's language(s) and culture(s) as positive contributors to a child's development (McCashen, 2017). Particularly because of our unique role in regard to a child's communication and language development, this practice encourages us to view multilingualism as an asset and to support children in maintaining their first language while learning English as a second or additional language (Fenton et al., 2015). By using the family-centered and strengths-based approaches as we support RBI, we can effectively provide culturally and linguistically responsive services to our families.

Using the Coaching Model With Culturally and Linguistically Diverse Families

With the shift to family-centered services in EI, we have also learned that best practice includes our use of a coaching model. As EI providers, we can support families during our visits by coaching them as they practice using intervention strategies with their children within their everyday activities and routines (Roberts et al., 2019; Roberts & Kaiser, 2014; Rush & Shelden, 2020). Our understanding of how different cultural beliefs affect parenting practices is essential for us to provide appropriate coaching with families who are culturally or linguistically diverse. The coaching model will only be successful if and when families are actively involved in developing outcomes and intervention strategies for and with their children. Using a one-size-fits-all approach to caregiver training might not be culturally acceptable for many families (van Kleeck, 1994). Calzada et al. (2013) examined how Latina mothers viewed caregiver training programs in the United States. They found that many strategies commonly taught in EI programs by SLPs to families to promote language development and positive behavior of young children were unfamiliar to the mothers and did not align with their perspectives of parenting. Although they understood that play was important for the development of their children, it was not common practice in their culture for parents and caregivers to play with their children. They were also not in support of material reinforcers for good behavior and did not believe in intentionally ignoring or waiting as a strategy to encourage their children to initiate or respond to an action or request. This strategy was considered neglectful, or the parent was judged as disrespectful. This study reminds us that we must connect with our families and value their differences. On the other hand, when coaching has been adapted to align with the cultural values of families, intervention is often considered successful (Agazzi et al., 2010; Domenech Rodríguez et al., 2009; Xu, 2007).

Summary

When we intentionally and proactively incorporate cultural and linguistic responsiveness into our practice with children and families who are from diverse cultures or speak another language, we pave the way for meaningful family engagement and better outcomes for the children we serve. We build stronger relationships with the children, parents, and caregivers in our care; we address their unique needs by recognizing that each family is a whole unit with its own unique set of values. By respecting the choices families make regarding child-rearing and decision-making, serving the family's functional needs, and viewing their culture and home language as the strengths that they are, we can effectively implement the principles of family-centered practice. In this chapter, we discussed statistics, definitions, and concepts that increase our awareness of the importance of inclusion, cultural and linguistic diversity, and family developmental expectations. We spent some time focusing on bilingualism and thoroughly examined language and communication skills and expectations of dual-language learners. We were presented with evidence-based strategies and considerations regarding responsive practices in the areas of collaboration, evaluation and assessment, and intervention when working with diverse children and families. This knowledge and these skills set the foundation from which we will appropriately and successfully respond to and provide inclusive services to the diverse population of families we serve in EI.

Critical Thinking Questions

1. Why is it not surprising that current data indicates families from diverse ethnic/racial backgrounds and families at lower income levels who have participated in EI services are less satisfied with services than Caucasian families and those families at higher income levels?

2. Describe at least 2 policies presented within IDEA that specifically focus on and emphasize culturally and linguistically responsive services.

3. What are the definitions of inclusion, cultural and linguistic diversity, and culturally and linguistically responsive practices as they relate to EI?

4. Describe best practices when working with an interpreter to support EI services.

5. How might you explain the current evidence related to young children acquiring two languages, including those with speech and language disorders, to parents, caregivers, and colleagues?

6. Present at least 3 evaluation and assessment considerations we need to incorporate when working with culturally and linguistically diverse families. What impact might these have on the child's and family's creation of IFSP outcomes and progress?

7. Present at least 3 intervention strategies we can implement to effectively work with children and families who are culturally and linguistically diverse.

8. What strategies might we use to build a relationship with a family when collaborating with a language interpreter?

9. What are some examples of different cultural perspectives from our own background and culture that may influence EI services (e.g. medical treatment and healing, familial roles, children/child rearing)?

10. How might our own cultural and/or linguistic perspectives influence the ways in which we connect with the young children and families we serve?

11. As an SLP engaging in EI, we are likely to go into homes that present a variety of cultural and linguistic differences in addition to varying child-rearing practices. What are some considerations and strategies we might consider as we prepare for this experience?

References

Agazzi, H., Salinas, A., Williams, J., Chiriboga, D., Ortiz, C., & Armstrong, K. (2010). Adaptation of a behavioral parent-training curriculum for Hispanic caregivers: HOT DOCS Español. *Infant Mental Health Journal, 31*(2), 182–200. http://doi.org/10.1002/imhj.20251

Agner, J. (2020). Moving from cultural competence to cultural humility in occupational therapy: A paradigm shift. *The American Journal of Occupational Therapy, 74*(4), 7404347010p1–7404347010p7. https://doi.org/10.5014/ajot.2020.038067

American Speech-Language-Hearing Association. (n.d.). *Late language emergence [Practice Portal]*. https://www.asha.org/practice-portal/clinical-topics/late-language-emergence/

American Speech-Language-Hearing Association. (2021). *Demographic profile of ASHA members providing bilingual services, year-end 2020*. https://www.asha.org/siteassets/surveys/demographic-profile-bilingual-spanish-service-members.pdf

American Speech-Language-Hearing Association. (2023). *Early intervention* [Practice portal]. https://www.asha.org/practice-portal/professional-issues/early-intervention/

Bailey, D. B., Jr., Skinner, D., Rodriguez, P., Gut, D., & Correa, V. (1999). Awareness, use, and satisfaction with services for Latino parents of young children with disabilities. *Exceptional Children, 65*(3), 367–381. https://doi.org/10.1177/001440299906500307

Banerjee, R., & Guiberson, M. (2012). Evaluating young children from culturally and linguistically diverse backgrounds for special education services. *Young Exceptional Children, 15*(1), 33–45.

Barac, R., & Bialystok, E. (2012). Bilingual effects on cognitive and linguistic development: Role of language, cultural background, and education. *Child Development, 83*(2), 413–422. https://doi.org/10.1111/j.1467-8624.2011.01707.x

Barac, R., Bialystok, E., Castro, D. C., & Sanchez, M. (2014). The cognitive development of young dual language learners: A critical review. *Early Childhood Research Quarterly, 29*(4), 699–714. https://doi.org/10.1016/j.ecresq.2014.02.003

Bialystok, E., & Peets, K. F. (2010). Bilingualism and cognitive linkages: Learning to read in different languages. In M. Shatz & L. C. Wilkinson (Eds.), *The education of English language learners: Research to practice* (pp. 234-273). Guilford.

Bosch, L., & Ramon-Casas, M. (2014). First translation equivalents in bilingual toddlers' expressive vocabulary: Does form similarity matter? *International Journal of Behavioral Development, 38*(4), 317–322. https://doi.org/10.1177/0165025414532559

Bradshaw, W. (2013). A framework for providing culturally responsive early intervention services. *Young Exceptional Children, 16*(1), 3–15. https://doi.org/10.1177/1096250612451757

Caesar, L. G. (2013). Providing early intervention services to diverse populations: Are speech-language pathologists prepared? *Infants and Young Children, 26*(2), 126–146. https://doi.org/10.1097/IYC.0b013e3182848340

Calzada, E. J., Basil, S., & Fernandez, Y. (2013). What Latina mothers think of evidence-based parenting practices: A qualitative study of treatment acceptability. *Cognitive and Behavioral Practice, 20*(3), 362–374. http://doi.org/10.1016/j.cbpra.2012.08.004

Camilli, G., Vargas, S., Ryan, S., & Barnett, W. S. (2010). Meta-analysis of the effect of early education interventions on cognitive and social development. *Teachers College Record, 112*(3), 579–620.

Carlson, S. M., & Meltzoff, A. N. (2008). Bilingual experience and executive functioning in young children. *Developmental Science, 11*(2), 282–298. https://doi.org/10.1111/j.1467-7687.2008.00675.x

Casby, M. (2003). The development of play in infants, toddlers, and young children. *Communication Disorders Quarterly, 24*, 163–174.

Casto, G., & Mastropieri, M. A. (1986). The efficacy of early intervention programs: A meta-analysis. *Exceptional Children, 52*(5), 417–424. https://doi.org/10.1177/001440298605200503

Core, C., Hoff, E., Rumiche, R., & Señor, M. (2013). Total and conceptual vocabulary in Spanish-English bilinguals from 22 to 30 months: Implications for assessment. *Journal of Speech, Language, and Hearing Research: JSLHR, 56*(5), 1637–1649. https://doi.org/10.1044/1092-4388(2013/11-0044)

Crais, E. (2011). Testing and beyond: Strategies and tools for evaluating and assessing infants and toddlers. *Language, Speech, and Hearing Services in Schools, 42*, 341–364.

Crawford, M. J., & Weber, B. (2014). *Early intervention every day! Embedding activities in daily routines for young children and their families*. Brookes.

DeNavas-Walt, C., & Proctor, B. D. (2015). In U.S. Census Bureau Current Population Reports (Eds.). *Income and poverty in the United States: 2014* (pp. 60-252). U.S. Government Printing Office.

Division of Early Childhood and the National Association for the Education of Young Children. (2009). *Early childhood inclusion: A joint position statement of the Division for Early Childhood (DEC) and the National Association for the Education of Young Children (NAEYC)*. http://www.decsped.org/uploads/docs/about_dec/position_concept_papers/PositionStatement_Inclusion_Joint_u pdated_May2009.pdf

Domenech Rodríguez, M. M., Donovick, M. R., & Crowley, S. L. (2009). Parenting styles in a cultural context: Observations of "protective parenting" in first-generation Latinos. *Family Process, 48*(2), 195–210.

Dunst, C. J., Raab, M., & Hamby, D. W. (2016). Interest-based everyday child language learning. *Revista de Logopedia, Foniatria y Audiologia, 36*(4), 153–161. https://doi.org/10.1016/j.rlfa.2016.07.003

Dunst, C. J., Raab, M., & Trivette, C. M. (2012). Characteristics of naturalistic language intervention strategies. *Journal of Speech-Language Pathology & Applied Behavior Analysis, 5*, 8–16. https://www.thefreelibrary.com/Characteristics+of+naturalistic+language+intervention+strategies.-a0299887454

Duran, L. K., Hartzheim, D., Lund, E. M., Simonsmeier, V., & Kohlmeier, T. L. (2016). Bilingual and home language interventions with young dual language learners: A research synthesis. *Language, Speech, and Hearing in the Schools, 47*(4), 347–371. https://doi.org/10.1044/2016_LSHSS-15-0030

Early Childhood Technical Assistance Center. (2023). *Fact Sheet: Advancing racial equity in early intervention and preschool special education*. https://ectacenter.org/topics/racialequity/factsheet-racialequity-2023.asp

Fadiman, A. (1998). *The spirit catches you and you fall down: A Hmong child, her American doctors, and the collision of two cultures*. Macmillan.

Fenton, A., Walsh, K., Wong, S., & Cumming, T. (2015). Using strengths-based approaches in early years practice and research. *International Journal of Early Childhood, 47*(1), 27–52.

Garcia Coll, C., Akiba, D., Palacios, N., Bailey, B., Silver, R., DiMartino, L., & Chin, C. (2002). Parental involvement in children's education: Lessons from three immigrant groups. *Parenting: Science and Practice, 2*(3), 303–324. https://doi.org/10.1207/S15327922PAR0203_05

Genesee, Fred. (2006). Chapter 4. Bilingual First Language Acquisition in Perspective. In P. McCardle & E. Hoff (Eds.), *Childhood Bilingualism: Research on Infancy through School Age* (pp. 45-67). Multilingual Matters. https://doi.org/10.21832/9781853598715-005

Goodrich, J. M., Lonigan, C. J., & Farver, J. M. (2013). Do early literacy skills in children's first language promote development of skills in their second language? An experimental evaluation of transfer. *Journal of Educational Psychology, 105*(2), 414–426. https://doi.org/10.1037/a0031780

Greenspan, S. I., & Wieder, S. (2006). *Infant and early childhood mental health: A comprehensive developmental approach to assessment and intervention.* American Psychiatric Publishing.

Hanson, M. J., & Lynch, E. W. (1990). Honoring the cultural diversity of families when gathering data. *Topics in Early Childhood Special Education, 10*(1), 112–132. https://doi.org/10.1177/027112149001000109

Hoff, E. (2006). How social contexts support and shape language development. *Developmental Review, 26*, 55–88. http://dx.doi.org/10.1016/j.dr.2005.11.002

Hoff, E., & Core, C. (2015). What clinicians need to know about bilingual development. *Seminar in Speech and Language, 36*(2), 89–99. https://doi.org.10.1055/2-0035-1549104

Hoff, E., Core, C., Place, S., Rumiche, R., Señor, M., & Parra, M. (2012). Dual language exposure and early bilingual development. *Journal of Child Language, 39*(1), 1–27. https://doi.org/10.1017/S0305000910000759

Hoff, E., Rumiche, R., Ribot, K., & Welsh, S. (2013, April). English language acquisition without heritage language loss: who succeeds. In *Poster presented at: The Meetings of the Society for Research in Child Development.*

Holden, G. W., Lavigne, V. V., & Cameron, A. M. (1990). Probing the continuum of effectiveness in parent training: Characteristics of parents and preschoolers. *Journal of Clinical Child Psychology, 19*(1), 2–8. https://doi.org/10.1016/j.ecresq.2018.12.006

Hopf, S. C., Crowe, K., Verdon, S., Blake, H. L., & McLeod, S. (2021). Advancing workplace diversity through the culturally responsive teamwork framework. *American Journal of Speech-Language Pathology, 30*(5), 1949–1961. https://doi.org/10.1044/2021_AJSLP-20-00380

Huttenlocher, J., Haight, W., Bryk, A., Seltzer, M., & Lyons, T. (1991). Early vocabulary growth: Relation to language input and gender. *Developmental Psychology, 27*(2), 236–248. https://doi.org/10.1037/0012-1649.27.2.236

Individuals With Disabilities Education Improvement Act of 2004, Pub. L. No. 108-446, §

632, 118 Stat. 2744 (2004). http://idea.ed.gov/

Individuals With Disabilities Education Improvement Act. (2011). Part C Final Regulations. 34 C.F.R. §§ 303 (2011). https://www.gpo.gov/fdsys/pkg/FR-2011-09-28/pdf/2011-22783.pdf

Jackson, S., Pretti-Frontczak, K., Harjusola-Webb, S., Grisham-Brown, J., & Romani, J. M. (2009). Response to intervention: Implications for early childhood professionals. *Language, Speech, and Hearing Services in Schools, 40*, 424–434. http://doi:10.1044/0161-1461

Karoly, L. A., Kilburn, M. R., & Cannon, J. S. (2005). *Proven benefits of early childhood interventions*. RAND Corporation. https://www.rand.org/pubs/research_briefs/RB9145.html

Keating, K., Cole, P., Scheider, A., & Schaffner, M. (2021). *State of babies yearbook 2021*. Zero to Three. https://stateofbabies.org/national/

Khetani, M. A., Richardson, Z., & McManus, B. M. (2017). Social disparities in early intervention service use and provider-reported outcomes. *Journal of Developmental and Behavioral Pediatrics, 38*(7), 501–509. https://doi.org/10.1097/DBP.0000000000000474

Kids Count Data Center. (2018). *Children in poverty in United States*. https://datacenter.aecf.org/data#USA/1

Kohnert, K., & Medina, A. (2009). Bilingual children and communication disorders: A 30-year research retrospective. *Seminars in Speech And Language, 30*(4), 219–233. https://doi.org/10.1055/s-0029-1241721

Kohnert, K., Yim, D., Nett, K., Kan, P. F., & Duran, L. (2005). Intervention with linguistically diverse preschool children: A focus on developing home language(s). *Language, Speech, and Hearing Services in Schools, 36*(3), 251–263. https://doi.org/10.1044/0161-1461(2005/025)

Kumpfer, K. L., Alvarado, R., Smith, P., & Bellamy, N. (2002). Cultural sensitivity and adaptation in family-based prevention interventions. *Prevention Sciences, 3*(3), 241–246. https://doi.org/10.1023/A:1019902902119

Larson, A. L., Cycyk, L. M., Carta, J., Hammer, C. S., Baralt, M., Uchikoshi, Y., … Wood, C. (2020). A systematic review of language-focused interventions for children from culturally and linguistically diverse backgrounds. *Early Childhood Research Quarterly, 50*(1), 157–178. https://doi.org/10.1016/j.ecresq.2019.06.001

Linder, T. (2008). *Transdisciplinary play-based assessment*. Brookes.

Mancilla-Martinez, J., & Lesaux, N. K. (2011). Early home language use and later vocabulary development. *Journal of Educational Psychology, 103*(3), 535–546. https://doi.org/10.1037/a0023655

Mancilla-Martinez, J., & Vagh, S. B. (2013). Growth in toddlers' Spanish, English, and conceptual vocabulary knowledge. *Early Childhood Research Quarterly, 28*(3), 555–567. https://doi.org/10.1016/j.ecresq.2013.03.004

McCashen, W. (2005). *The strengths approach*. St. Luke's Innovative Resources.

McCashen, W. (2017). *The strengths approach: Sharing power, building hope, creating change* (2nd ed.). Innovative Resources.

McClelland, M. M., Cameron, C. E., Connor, C. M., Farris, C. L., Jewkes, A. M., & Morrison, F. J. (2007). Links between behavioral regulation and preschoolers' literacy, vocabulary, and math skills. *Developmental Psychology, 43*(4), 947–959.

McManus, B. M., Richardson, Z., Schenkman, M., Murphy, N. J., Everhart, R. M., Hambidge, S., & Morrato, E. (2020). Child characteristics and early intervention referral and receipt of services: A retrospective cohort study. *BMC Pediatrics, 20*(1), 84. https://doi.org/10.1186/s12887-020-1965-x

McWilliam, R.A. (2010). *Routines-based early intervention: Supporting young children and their families*. Brookes.

Meisel, J. M. (1989). Early differentiation of languages in bilingual children. In K. Hyltenstam & L. K. Obler (Eds.), *Bilingualism across the lifespan: Aspects of acquisition, maturity, and loss* (pp. 245-254). Cambridge University Press.

Miller, J. F., Heilmann, J., Nockerts, A., Iglesias, A., Fabiano, L., & Francis, D. J. (2006). Oral language and reading in bilingual children. *Learning Disabilities Research & Practice, 21*(1), 30–43. https://doi.org/10.1111/j.1540-5826.2006.00205.x

Montgomery, W. (2001). Creating culturally responsive, inclusion classrooms. *Teaching Exceptional Children*, 4-9. https://www.smithwlac.com/uploads/2/6/1/1/26117566/culturally_responsive_teaching.pdf

Moore, S., & Pérez-Méndez, C. (2006). Working with linguistically diverse families in early intervention: Misconceptions and missed opportunities. *Seminars in Speech and Language, 27*(3), 187–198. https://doi.org/10.1055/s-2006-948229

Oh, J. S., & Fuligni, A. J. (2010). The role of heritage language development in the ethnic identity and family relationships of adolescents from immigrant backgrounds. *Social Development, 19*(1), 202–220. https://doi.org/10.1111/j.1467-9507.2008.00530.x

O'Hara, N., & Bollmer, J. (2021, July). *Equity requirements in IDEA (Version 2.0)*. IDEA Data Center. https://ideadata.org/sites/default/files/media/documents/2021-07/EquityInIDEA.pdf

Oller, D. K., Pearson, B. Z., & Cobo-Lewis, A. B. (2007). Profile effects in early bilingual language and literacy. *Applied Psycholinguistics, 28*(2), 191–230. https://doi.org/10.1017/S0142716407070117

Páez, M., & Rinaldi, C. (2006). Predicting English word reading skills for Spanish-speaking students in first grade. *Topics in Language Disorders, 26*(4), 338–350.

Paradis, J., & Kirova, A. (2014). English second-language learners in preschool. *International Journal of Behavioral Development, 38*, 342–349.

Patterson, J., & Pearson, B. (2004). Bilingual lexical development: Influences, contexts, and processes. In B. Goldstein (Ed.), *Bilingual language development and disorders in Spanish-English speakers* (pp. 113-129). Brookes.

Pearson, B., Fernandez, S., Lewedeg, V., & Oller, D. (1997). The relation of input factors to lexical learning by bilingual infants. *Applied Psycholinguistics, 18*(1), 41–58. https://doi:10.1017/S0142716400009863

Pearson, B. Z., Fernandez, S. C., & Oller, D. K. (1993). Lexical development in bilingual infants and toddlers: Comparison to monolingual norms. *Language Learning, 43*, 93–120.

Peña, E. D., & Fiestas, C. (2009). Talking across cultures in early intervention: Finding common ground to meet children's communication needs. *Perspectives on Communication Disorders and Sciences in Culturally and Linguistically Diverse Populations, 16*(3), 79. https://doi.org/10.1044/cds16.3.79

Peredo, T. N. (2016). Supporting culturally and linguistically diverse families in early intervention. *Perspectives of the ASHA Special Interest Groups, 1*(1), 154–167. https://doi.org/10.1044/persp1.SIG1.154

Place, S., & Hoff, E. (2011). Properties of dual language exposure that influence 2-year-olds' bilingual proficiency. *Child Development, 82*(6), 1834–1849. https://doi.org/10.1111/j.1467-8624.2011.01660.x

Raver, S. A., & Childress, D. C. (2015). *Family-centered early intervention: Supporting infants and toddlers in natural environments.* Brookes.

Raver, C. C., Jones, S. M., Li-Grining, C., Zhai, F., Bub, K., & Pressler, E. (2011). CSRP's impact on low-income preschoolers' preacademic skills: Self-regulation as a mediating mechanism: CSRP's impact on low-income preschoolers' preacademic skills. *Child Development, 82*(1), 362–378. https://doi.org/10.1111/j.1467-8624.2010.01561.x

Ribot, K. M., & Hoff, E. (2014). "¿Cómo estas?" "I'm good." Conversational code-switching is related to profiles of expressive and receptive proficiency in Spanish-English bilingual toddlers. *International Journal of Behavioral Development, 38*(4), 333–341. https://doi.org/10.1177/0165025414533225

Roberts, M. Y., Curtis, P. R., Sone, B. J., & Hampton, L. H. (2019). Association of parent training with child language development: A systematic review and meta-analysis.

Journal of the American Medical Association Pediatrics, 173(7), 671–680. https://doi.org/10.1001/jamapediatrics.2019.1197

Roberts, M. Y., & Kaiser, A. P. (2011). The effectiveness of parent-implemented language interventions: A meta-analysis. *American Journal of Speech-Language Pathology, 20,* 180–199.

Rogoff, B. (2003). *The cultural nature of human development.* Oxford University Press.

Rowe, M. (2012). A longitudinal investigation of the role of quantity and quality of child directed speech in vocabulary development. *Child Development, 83,* 1762–1774. http://dx.doi.org/10.1111/j.1467-8624.2012.01805.x

Rush, D., & Shelden, M. L. (2020). *The early childhood coaching handbook* (2nd ed.). Paul H. Brookes.

Schwartz, S. J., Unger, J. B., Zamboanga, B. L., & Szapocznik, J. (2010). Rethinking the concept of acculturation: Implications for theory and research. *American Psychologist, 65*(4), 237–251. https://doi.org/10.1037/a0019330

Segal, R., & Beyer, C. (2006). Integration and application of a home treatment program: A study of parents and occupational therapists. *American Journal of Occupational Therapy, 60,* 500–510. https://doi.org/10.5014/ajot.60.5.500

Song, L., Tamis-Lemonda, C. S., Yoshikawa, H., Kahana-Kalman, R., & Wu, I. (2012). Language experiences and vocabulary development in Dominican and Mexican infants across the first 2 years. *Developmental Psychology, 48*(4), 1106–1123. https://doi.org/10.1037/a0026401

Tseng, V., & Fuligni, A. J. (2000). Parent-adolescent language use and relationships among immigrant families with East Asian, Filipino, and Latin American backgrounds. *Journal of Marriage and Family, 62*(2), 465–476. http://www.jstor.org/stable/1566752

U.S. Department of Education, Office of Special Education Programs (2020). *OSEP fast facts: Infants and toddlers with disabilities.* https://sites.ed.gov/idea/osep-fast-facts-infants-and-toddlers-with-disabilities-20/

van Kleeck, A. (1994). Potential cultural bias in training parents as conversational partners with their children who have delays in language development. *American Journal of Speech-Language Pathology, 3*(1), 67–78. http://dx.doi.org/ 10.1044/1058-0360.0301.67

Wayman, K., & Lynch, E. W. (1991). Home-based early childhood services: Cultural sensitivity in a family systems approach. *Topics in Early Childhood Special Education, 10*(4), 56–76. https://doi.org/ 10.1177/027112149101000406

Werker J. (2012). Perceptual foundations of bilingual acquisition in infancy. *Annals of the New York Academy of Sciences, 1251,* 50–61.

Westby, C. (2009). Considerations in working successfully with culturally/linguistically diverse families in assessment and intervention of communication disorders. *Seminars in Speech and Language, 30*(4), 279–289. http://doi.org/10.1055/s-0029-1241725

Westby, C. E., Stevens Dominguez, M., & Oetter, P. (1996). A performance/competence model of observational assessment. *Language, Speech, and Hearing Services in the Schools, 27,* 144–156.

Winsler, A., Burchinal, M. R., Tien, H.-C., Peisner-Feinberg, E., Espinosa, L., Castro, D. C., & De Feyter, J. (2014). Early development among dual language learners: The roles of language use at home, maternal immigration, country of origin, and sociodemographic variables. *Early Childhood Research Quarterly, 29,* 750–764.

Xu, Y. (2007). Empowering culturally diverse families of young children with disabilities: The double ABCX model. *Early Childhood Education Journal, 34*(6), 431–437. doi.org/10.1007/s10643-006-0149-0

Chapter 9
Treatment in the Natural Environment

Learning Outcomes

When we have completed this chapter, we will be able to:

- Present a brief review of evidence-based practices in EI, including practice-based coaching, family-centered services, and RBI, as applied to treatment.

- Describe strategies that focus on the facilitation of prelinguistic communication, including engagement, play, and gestures, of an infant or toddler.

- Recount responsive and directive treatment strategies to address the expansion of a young child's receptive and expressive language development.

- Define milieu teaching and the techniques implemented to model and prompt language in everyday contexts.

- Discuss the basic principles of augmentative and alternative communication to address the needs of young children and their families in EI.

- Share common challenges and possible solutions associated with remote service delivery in EI treatment.

What Will We Learn and How Can We Apply It?

As providers working in EI, we now know how important it is to think and work beyond our traditional speech-language pathology knowledge and skill set. We connect with and teach each individual family we serve by using effective and relationship-enhancing instruction in an environment specifically tailored to meet their needs, priorities, and goals. We offer consultation to both families and colleagues in our areas of expertise as they relate to those areas connected to speech, language, communication, and feeding. We know how to teach adults, coach caregivers, collaborate with colleagues, and furnish consultative services. While engaging in these evidence-based practices, we must also be knowledgeable about and provide treatment that addresses the developmental needs and outcomes of the young children we serve.

In this chapter, we review the best practices and approaches in EI and focus on the arsenal of evidence-based speech-language pathology strategies we can use to support children's language acquisition and enable the expansion of their linguistic repertoire. We take a closer look at how some of these intervention strategies can be used to address the development of specific communication and language skills and the important role AAC plays in our work with young children and their families. We learn about remote service delivery and consider the challenges and opportunities this modality presents. As we look further into treatment in EI, keep in mind the purpose of this chapter is to present the information we need to get us started; not every approach or every strategy is included. Instead, our goal is to learn about and be prepared to implement and coach families to use accessible treatment strategies and approaches that address their children's needs within their own natural environments.

Brief Review of Evidence-Based and Best Practices in Treatment

The research is clear that young children learn best and tend to generalize the skills they acquire when engaged in everyday, natural learning opportunities in familiar places and with familiar people (Chiarello, 2017; Dunst et al., 2001; Hwang et al., 2013; Rush & Shelden, 2020; Trivette et al., 2004). To be effective in our role as service providers in EI, therefore, we must meet families where they are, share our knowledge, skills, and strategies, and build their capacity to support, engage, and teach their children every day and within their own activities and routines.

Coaching parents and caregivers to use early language strategies that support their child's language and communication skills is a highly effective therapy approach (Finestack & Fey, 2013). Therefore, we also need to coach families on how to help their children. Through effective coaching, parents and caregivers learn and implement new strategies with their children, they become empowered and feel more prepared to support their child and their needs, and they are capable of carrying out EI goals when we are not present or available (Douglas et al., 2017, 2018; Meadan et al., 2013; Meadan et al., 2016; Rush & Shelden, 2011, 2020). We use both general and specific coaching strategies in EI to ensure services are family-centered and implemented within everyday activities and routines. General strategies include information sharing and observation and specific strategies include direct teaching, demonstration with narration, guided practice, caregiver practice, general and specific feedback, problem solving, reflection, and review (Friedman et al., 2012; Woods et al., 2011). Be sure to go back to Chapter 4 to review details about each of the strategies involved in our coaching practices.

One of the most challenging parts of coaching can be finding effective ways to invite parents and caregivers to participate and join in interactions with their child. Although Chapter 4 presents the variables we need to support a family's awareness and involvement in collaborative coaching, it is also helpful to explain to families how their engagement with the intervention strategies we use is integral to both support and enable their child's development of language and communication skills. We can begin to empower them by sharing the following information with parents and caregivers. The two critical components that need to be in place during intervention include the quality of interactions and the quality of language input between parents or caregivers and the child. This means that the family members and child need to participate in interactions that make the child *want* to communicate; at the same time, the parent or caregiver needs to model new language that the child can eventually understand and express. Both of these components need to be embedded and established. If there is a breakdown in one, there will likely be a breakdown in the other; ultimately, this leads to a breakdown in the child's ability to learn. Our responsibility is to coach parents and caregivers to recognize, learn, and use intervention strategies that work for them, and to explain how they can seamlessly embed these strategies within the everyday routines and activities important to each family. When we are successful as SLPs in EI, our intervention is focused on helping parents and caregivers learn and use the knowledge and skills they need to help their child.

Supporting Language Acquisition

The strategies we use to support language acquisition tend to focus on the development of a child's prelinguistic communication skills, including joint attention, use of gestures, and both nonverbal and verbal imitation. When we coach parents and caregivers to respond to a child's engagement in an attempt to communicate, we contribute to their knowledge and those skills that serve as a foundation for future language development (Roberts et al., 2016). The techniques we use and share to support, develop, and coach families in EI include engagement-based strategies, (e.g., following their lead, child-directed play, shared reading), multimodal strategies (e.g., touching the child to initiate interaction, combining gestures with words), and quantity-based strategies, including those techniques in which we vary the amount and complexity of language directed toward the child based on their communication skills and needs. We also tend to incorporate milieu teaching, which is a conversation-based approach in which we use a child's interests and initiations as opportunities to model and prompt language in everyday contexts. Regardless of the type or name of the technique we incorporate into our intervention with young children and their families, our first consideration is often the infant or toddler's current level of communication, language development, or both. Recognizing and acknowledging the foundation from which we are addressing the child's needs and priorities is an important step in choosing an appropriate treatment strategy.

Prelinguistic Communication Skills

Prelinguistic communication describes the intentional and unintentional behaviors children display to communicate their wants and needs. Some behaviors are natural reactions, whereas others are more purposeful to access or refuse items, participate in a social interaction, and give or receive more information. The prelinguistic stage is considered the time period between birth and when a child begins to use words, signs, or both to interact with others. During this time, young children begin to use eye gaze, attend to sounds and words, and use facial expressions and affective vocalizations to communicate. Their use of gestures and other nonverbal means begins to emerge. The development of prelinguistic communication builds the foundation for later developing skills, including the use of words (or signs) and the ability to combine these into sentences to communicate. As children engage in intentional attempts to receive and send messages, they begin to demonstrate an understanding and emerging appreciation of the details related to successful communication (Crais & Ogletree, 2016).

Joint Attention

Joint attention occurs when two people share a common interest or shared focus on the same stimulus and there is an understanding between them that they are both interested in the same object, person, sound, or event. Joint attention is achieved when one person alerts the other to the stimulus by using verbal or nonverbal means. This still requires the child's ability to gain, maintain, and shift attention; it is important that a child is able to initiate joint attention and respond to other people when they initiate the child's attention.

We learned in Chapter 5 that joint attention is expected to emerge around 9 months of age and be well-established by 18 months of age. This form of attention is indicative of early social and communicative behavior and requires a young child to gain, maintain, and shift attention. Joint attention (also sometimes called shared attention) might include the use of eye contact, gestures, vocalizations, or verbalizations and provides a critical foundation for social, cognitive, and language development (Levey, 2014). A young child who has difficulty engaging in joint attention might inconsistently respond to our words, gestures, and actions; they might appear to avoid others or to ignore what is said to them; and they might appear to ignore their own names and verbal instructions.

Research suggests the amount of time infants and toddlers and their caregivers spend interacting with each other jointly predicts the frequency with which they use gestures. Families who promote joint attention with their children and who are responsive to their child's focus of attention might also be more likely to respond to their children within interactions that facilitate later gesture and language use (Law et al., 2017). When we coach parents and caregivers to address shared, or joint, attention with their children, we are also focusing on how they recognize and respond to their children's attempts to communicate during play, routines, and everyday activities. Embedding our coaching of joint attention within the family's natural environments and everyday activities supports their awareness as well as the implementation of strategies to facilitate this skill.

Gestures

Recognizing and supporting the development of gestures with the young children we serve is important. The milestones related to infant and toddler gestural development provide us with an index of developing cognitive abilities and help us predict when certain language milestones might emerge. Gestures are the intentional use of actions, including hand and body movements, as well as facial expressions, to communicate. They include acts such as waving, shaking or nodding of the head, showing and giving objects to other people, and pointing. When children use gestures, they are able to communicate effectively even before their first words emerge. This is exciting because it means we can use a young child's gestures as a gauge to anticipate and encourage the emergence and development of language (Goldin-Meadow, 2015).

The use of gestures is an important prelinguistic skill because it supports a child's ability to talk about their experiences, needs, and wants even before they have the words to do so; the use of gestures also offers us cues that the child understands that communication is a social act and supports the message they are trying to convey (Crawford & Weber, 2014). Early gesture use is a strong predictor of later language ability and should be included in our treatment activities (Cameron-Faulkner et al., 2015; Law et al., 2017; O'Neill et al., 2019.)

We should support a child's development and use of gestures through parent and caregiver coaching. The use of gestures by a young child encourages families to model language and to interact with their child in more meaningful ways. Law and colleagues (2017) suggested that children use more gestures, and more frequently, when they spend more time with their parents and caregivers interacting together with objects and activities of interest. When we coach families within a session, we can focus on supporting their recognition and response to their child's attempts at communication and use strategies that encourage their use of gestures during play, routines, and everyday activities.

Imitation

As SLPs, we know how powerful imitation can be when we are attempting to teach and learn a new skill. Imitation involves the intentional copying of a gesture, action, or behavior of another person. It is a prelinguistic skill that begins to develop in infancy and is maintained and used frequently by children to expand their verbal communication skills. A direct correlation has been found between imitation and language skills in young children (Laakso et al., 1999; Zambrana et al., 2013). Additionally, imitation serves as both a learning function, as infants learn new skills and knowledge, and a social function, as infants engage in games with parents and caregivers for social and emotional fulfillment and enjoyment (Ingersoll, 2008; Uzgiris, 1981).

We should not expect young children to imitate words or phrases until they are first demonstrating other prelinguistic skills, including appropriate play with objects, joint attention, and imitation of actions (see Chapter 5 for the milestones expected for each of these skills). Young children also tend to develop imitation skills according to the hierarchy presented in Table 9–1.

Table 9–1. Developmental Hierarchy of Imitation Skills

Imitation of ...	Examples
Actions with an object	• Banging on a drum • Rolling a ball
Big body movements	• Stomping feet • Clapping hands
Communicative gestures	• Waving • Using the sign for "more"
Smaller body movements and facial expressions	• Smiling • Sticking out the tongue

When addressing a child's development of imitation, we should coach the family to support and encourage their imitation skills at their current level, and work with them on progressing from there. It is also important to honor the routines-based approach when we focus on the development of imitation with children. By embedding opportunities for children to imitate actions, and eventually language, into play, routines, or everyday activities with their parents and caregivers, we are often able to follow the children's lead and include their interests to maintain their motivation. We are also able to support further social-emotional, play, and language development by promoting the social role of imitation (Ingersoll, 2008).

Treatment Strategies to Address Prelinguistic Communication

When we work with prelinguistic infants and toddlers, treatment often focuses on engagement, meaningful play, and gestures (Roberts et al., 2016). There are multiple strategies we can employ and coach families to use to support a young child's prelinguistic skills and ensure we have established a strong foundation for language development and learning.

Sit Face-to-Face

The first step is for the parent or caregiver to engage face-to-face with their child. This proximity is essential to creating a connection between the parent and child and encouraging the child to take the lead (Weitzman, 2017). Playing at the child's level and engaging with them face-to-face helps a child develop early social, prelinguistic, and linguistic skills, including joint attention, turn-taking, and conversation skills. We want to encourage the child to look at the adult's face and mouth while they talk and play together; this level of engagement supports their imitation of both oral motor movements and sounds. Coach the parents and caregivers to sit on the floor, or at a small table, at the same level as their child. Their child should be able to easily see their face, including how their mouth moves to form words, their facial expressions, and their gestures. When reading a book, playing with a toy, or eating a snack or meal, encourage the family to directly face their child.

Follow Their Lead

Responding to a child's interests and following their lead has been demonstrated to be an effective, evidence-based strategy to facilitate language development (Venker et al., 2012). Implementation of this strategy involves watching what the child is doing in play, then copying and commenting on the child's actions, sounds, or words. It is important to coach parents and caregivers to follow their child's lead within their chosen activity, rather than attempting to direct the actions or play. This is important because we want the child to hear language related to something they are doing and in which they are interested. We can also coach parents and caregivers to follow their child's lead within their typical routines. By providing the opportunity for the child to guide the activity, we give them space to engage in a way that is meaningful to them. When we are eating a snack and the child looks at their food or drink, we can coach the parents to use words to label and talk about the snack itself. Coach them to keep it simple and in the present moment. Encourage families to create lots of opportunities for their children to participate and stay engaged; by following their lead, we limit the time they might zone out or shut down. We can encourage parents to observe the activities in which their child is interested, watch what they are involved in, and use simple, one- or two-word utterances to provide them with opportunities to hear the words, experience the words, and process the words that relate to their interests and current experiences.

Keep It Simple

While engaged in daily routines within a child's natural environment, we need to pay attention to how we are talking to the child. Toddlers with receptive and expressive language difficulties often need specific and focused models to begin to link words with objects, people, and events. They need help making the connection between the symbol (i.e., vocabulary word), and the referent (i.e., object, action, or concept being labeled or described). Children who have difficulty understanding and processing language need adults who are there to interpret the world for them. They benefit from involved and engaged parents, teachers, and providers who can support them to better understand words and associate them with their environments.

Researchers have determined that labeling, which involves simply stating an object or an event name, is more effective than any other kind of talking to help children maintain attention to what they are doing (Finestack and Fey, 2013; Hadley, Rispoli, & Holt, 2017; Hadley, Rispoli, Holt, et al., 2017). Ultimately, we need to break it down for a child who is struggling to understand by using single words and simple, short phrases when we are talking to them. When we coach parents and caregivers, we need to present clear instructions to talk simply to and with their child. Encourage them to use single words and short phrases and to avoid long explanations or questions. When we are asking a child with a language disorder if they want a cookie, instead of asking, "Do you want one of these yummy chocolate chip cookies that I just bought at the grocery store?" prompt the parent or caregiver to hold up a cookie and ask, "Want a cookie?" Using simple language and repeating the target word gives the child a greater chance to make the connection between the object and the word. We often overwhelm late-talking toddlers by using too many words. They walk away looking disinterested or bored, when they are really trying to tell us they do not understand what we are saying.

Commenting

When we *comment*, we offer children the opportunity to hear language related to the objects they have or the actions in which they are engaged. When coaching parents or caregivers to use this strategy, we want to encourage them to talk about what they and their children are doing, looking at, playing with, touching, or eating. It is important to encourage them to use short, grammatical phrases and repeat key words. They should not expect the child to respond to or imitate them; instead, the intention is for the child to hear lots of language to accompany their routines, activities, and play. There are several forms of comments we can coach families to incorporate into their activities and routines, including self-talk, parallel talk, and toy talk.

Self-Talk. *Self-talk* is describing our own actions with the toy or within the routine (e.g., "This is a ball! I am rolling the ball"). We are modeling language for the child as we verbalize the words and phrases. Initially, parents and caregivers might feel silly talking out loud all day without a response. We need to assure them this practice exposes their child to more words every day and, even though they might not think the child is listening, their brain is processing and learning from the models their family is providing them. The use of self-talk serves as an excellent way to expose children to new and functional vocabulary, speech sounds, and patterns in both words and phrases.

Parallel Talk. *Parallel talk* occurs when an adult describes or narrates the child's actions with a toy or when engaged in a routine (e.g., "You have a ball! You're kicking the ball"). We need to encourage the parents or caregivers to use simple phrases and sentences, as opposed to longer, more complex language, to ensure the child has a greater opportunity to comprehend the words and phrases they are using to describe their actions. Parallel talk is another simple way for families to expose children to vocabulary, and we can encourage them to incorporate this strategy as much as possible throughout the day. Repetition provides a critical component of learning and eliciting language because children must understand what a word means, as well as its context, before they use it. This strategy also makes it easier for children to remember new vocabulary and sentence structures because they are actively participating in the activity and therefore have context for the words or phrases they are hearing.

Toy Talk. This strategy shifts the focus of attention to the toy or object itself; we might describe what the object looks like, where it is located, or its action (e.g., "The ball rolled away").

Wait and Provide Time to Process

We can encourage a child to initiate an interaction by waiting expectantly and using a slow pace to allow time for their initiation. We must remember to grant the child enough time to process the information we are presenting. Often, we need to coach parents and caregivers to purposefully (but silently) count to five before moving on to their next point or before repeating themselves. This might seem like a long time, but we can assure family members this is time their children need in order to create connections between what they are hearing and their meaning.

As the parents and caregivers wait for their children to launch an interaction, we can observe them as well, noting what they say and do, as well as what types of interactions they initiate. We can then coach the parent to wait and give the child time to do or say something. We can also remind the parents to listen intently to the child; they are showing their child that their message is important by responding to what they do or say (Weitzman, 2017).

Match the Child's Turn

Another strategy to share with parents and caregivers is one in which they match their child's turn. This means we coach them to ensure each turn they take in the conversation is about the same length as the child's turn. In many interactions between adults and children, the adult takes at least three turns to every one of the child's turns (Weitzman, 2017). At that pace, a child tends to lose interest in the conversation and shifts attention away from the parents. We can also encourage family members to be sure their turn matches what the child is interested in at that moment to encourage the child to take more turns and stay in the interaction longer. If the child is reluctant to take a turn, the parent or caregiver might need to cue the child to take a turn by giving signals that let the child know it is time to take a turn (e.g., touching their hand; Weitzman, 2017).

Hand-Over-Hand Guidance

Once we have given a child a verbal direction and repeated it once, or twice if they were not initially attending, we can help them follow by first modeling the expected response or action. If we repeat the direction again and the child does not imitate our response, we can coach the parent or caregiver to offer *hand-over-hand guidance*. We should encourage the parent to move closer to the child, get down on their child's level, and gently touch and guide them to redirect their attention to the intended task. This provides the child with a physical connection between the words we have said along with the actions that go along with them. We need to remember to keep our language simple and repeat the direction as we engage the child to ensure they are linking their action to our words.

Hand-Under-Hand Prompting

Hand-under-hand prompting is physical prompting during which an adult guides a child's hands from underneath (rather than over the top of) the child's hands. With hand-under-hand prompting, children are not forced to comply but can move their hands at will. This process is less intrusive than manipulating the child's hands and is particularly beneficial for young children who are tactilely defensive, including those who are deaf and blind (National Center on Deaf-Blindness, 2021).

As an EI provider using or coaching the parent or caregiver to use the hand-under-hand technique, our hands perform the activity while the child's hands rest on top of ours; the infant or toddler can feel what our hands are doing by guiding them in this noninvasive way. If the activity is new to the child and they are at all hesitant to engage, they might feel more secure touching our hands rather than the unknown object or activity. Therefore, we need to remember to introduce the object or activity gradually. Additionally, this strategy provides children with the opportunity to focus their energy on feeling the movements of our hands, rather than on an object or action, because their palms are on our hands. With hand-under-hand prompting, it is common for young children to feel more comfortable and in control; they can move their hands freely with this placement. Finally, we need to remember that it is always important to connect the hand-under-hand prompting with a verbal description of the activity or task in which we are engaging with the child (Miles, 2003; National Center on Deaf-Blindness, 2021).

We revisit the use of this form of prompting in Chapter 12 in the context of services for children who are experiencing sensory and perceptual disorders.

Serve and Return

Responsive, attentive relationships between adults and children build a strong foundation in a child's brain to support ongoing growth and development. Ideally, this engagement allows lots of opportunity for back-and-forth interactions between the child and the adult. A simple, effective strategy to support the development of this foundation is called *serve and return* (Center on the Developing Child, n.d.). We can encourage families to take small moments throughout their day and within their routines to serve and return with their children. As SLPs who want to encourage future conversational turns between children and their families, the following steps guide our coaching when we share this strategy with parents and caregivers.

1. Pay attention to what the child is "serving." Look for opportunities within everyday routines and share the child's focus of attention (e.g., waiting in line at a store, taking a bath, getting them dressed).

2. Support and encourage the child's interest. Return the serve with a sound, word, facial expression, or gesture. Let the child know we have noticed the same thing; pick up the object a child is pointing to or bring the child closer to an object of interest.

3. Name whatever it is the child is seeing, doing, or feeling. Even if the child is not yet demonstrating understanding or verbalizing the words, label and comment on the person, object, action, or feeling.

4. Give the child a chance to "return" by giving them the time they need to respond. Waiting for them is critical and helps maintain and continue the turn-taking.

5. Practice ending and beginning activities. Watch for the child's signals that indicate they are done or ready to move on to a new activity (Center on the Developing Child, n.d.).

Enabling Expansion of the Linguistic Repertoire

When we focus our treatment on expanding a child's receptive and expressive language development, we typically use a combination of responsive strategies and directive strategies. Responsive strategies model target communication behavior, but do not require a response (ASHA, 2008). These include self-talk, parallel talk, modeling, and expansion or recasting of the child's verbalizations. Directive strategies include adult-directed teaching approaches through which we assist or help the child facilitate an adult-desired response (ASHA, 2008; Owens, 2019). The most common and effective directive strategies in EI include prompting and cueing, use of questions and choices, and communication temptations or environmental sabotage.

Receptive and Expressive Language Skills

Receptive language refers to our ability to understand and comprehend spoken language. Young children typically understand language before can produce it. Until a child is age 3 or older, it is often difficult to separate receptive language and cognition. Although it is true that some children demonstrate cognitive strengths, such as a good memory or exceptional visual skills, we often discover that poor language comprehension is linked to underlying cognitive deficits. Therefore, when we address the cognitive skills of an infant or toddler, we are often supporting the development of their receptive language skills as well. Likewise, by targeting receptive language development, we are accessing and focusing on their cognitive development.

Expressive language is the ability to express wants and needs through verbal or nonverbal communication. Infants typically have the ability to express themselves at birth via their cries or their facial expressions. We know to expect the emergence of first words around a child's first birthday and exponential expansion of their expressive language, including the development of semantics, morphology, syntax, phonology, and pragmatic skills, over the next several years. If and as needed, return to Chapter 5 for a detailed review of both receptive and expressive language development milestones.

Treatment Strategies to Address Receptive and Expressive Language

As EI SLPs, we are often faced with addressing the needs of infants and toddlers who present with either expressive language disorder in isolation, or with delays in both receptive and expressive language. When addressing the needs of young children with delays in both comprehension and expression, we need to consider how we develop and focus their IFSP outcomes as well as what treatment strategies result in the most effective outcomes.

As discussed in Chapter 7, IFSP outcomes are statements about what the family wants their child to learn or do. Each statement should include emergent literacy and language skills developmentally appropriate for the child and should include the criteria, procedures, and timelines we will use to determine progress toward achieving the outcome. Outcomes should be individualized for each child and family and each one should be contextualized, functional, and discipline-free. Outcomes should also be relevant to the family and focused on the whole child and their participation in activities and within settings important to the family (IDEA, 2004, 2011). With regard to language development, does it make sense to develop IFSP outcomes that directly target receptive language skills? Or should we focus on the child's abilities to effectively connect and communicate with the people in their lives and to learn the skills they need to get their needs and wants met?

Empirical evidence supports the fact that receptive language skills serve as the predecessor to many expressive language abilities (Chapman et al., 2000; Owens, 2012, 2019; Paul, 2000). Additionally, among children with delayed language development, comprehension skills at 12 to 24 months are a significant predictor of later receptive and expressive language (Lyytinen et al., 2001; Wetherby et al., 2002; Wetherby et al., 2003). We have also learned that children with typical comprehension skills and delayed expressive language skills are more likely to catch up in their language production than children with delayed comprehension skills. This explains why we do not often diagnose or work with young children in EI who present with a receptive language disorder in the absence of an expressive language delay. With this knowledge, we again need to consider whether to address the receptive language skills of a young child in isolation from expressive language skills. Based on evidence-based and best practices and approaches in EI, knowledge and research regarding language development, and the consideration of functional goals for the children and families we serve, we recommend addressing receptive language as a step or objective toward reaching the goal of effective expression. With this in mind, many of the strategies presented in the sections that follow focus on addressing receptive language development; we can implement and coach families to use these stepping stones as we lean into their children's development and include them in our repertoire of techniques to address expressive language as well.

Visual Cues

Children who have language delays and disorders, particularly those with delays in comprehension, rely heavily on visual cues because they do not consistently understand, or process words presented to them verbally. It is important that we give them additional information, using cues they can see, if we want them to develop their language skills. Coach the parents and caregivers to point to an object or activity to direct their child's attention. When practical, show them the actual object. When sharing a book, encourage the family to point directly to a picture, label it, and add a short comment about it. Other visual cues include leading the child toward or moving objects within their line of vision to be sure they are attending to the same object or activity as adults. Because they need visual cues, children with language disorders might depend on our facial expressions to add meaning to our comments. We need to coach parents to use expressions that match their words.

Some children need picture schedules to help them know what to expect. We can help families brainstorm and create a visual system that will work for them to further support their children; these can be used to facilitate choices, prepare children for and help them anticipate routines, and adjust to new or novel activities throughout the day.

Simple Commands

Until a child is following directions consistently, we can coach parents and caregivers to limit themselves to simple commands with a single concept and concrete vocabulary (e.g., "Get your cup," rather than "Take your cup to the sink"; "Look at my eyes," rather than "Please look at me"). When providing children with basic directions, we should model and coach them to use grammatically correct language, regardless of the level of simplicity (i.e., "Pick up your cup," vs. "Pick up cup"). These simple commands should be embedded within every day, repeated activities and daily routines to ensure the child has lots of opportunities to make the connection between the word(s) and the objects, action words, and expectations. As the child demonstrates an increased understanding of the words within these simple commands, we can work with the family to appropriately expand the directions to include two or more components (e.g., "Get your shoes and bring them to Mommy").

Repetition

Toddlers with receptive language delays need lots of extra repetition to be able to process the words and the information that has been presented. Resist the urge to say, "I've already told you once (or twice)." Repetition helps a child create connections in the brain to solidify and store information. The more repetition, the more likely it is that the child will be able to process and recall information that has been presented earlier. If we feel like we have repeated a word too many times and are tired of hearing ourselves say something repeatedly, we probably have not yet said it enough.

Verbal routines involve a description of each specific task in which the child engages on a consistent basis. We can encourage parents and caregivers to use the same phrase every time to describe each routine (e.g., "lights on," "arms up"). This practice exposes the child repeatedly to specific language, supporting their eventual ability to anticipate our words, and fill in the blanks, accordingly.

A parent or caregiver can also be coached to consistently prompt a child within everyday activities or family routines to: "Show me [person or object]," or ask, "Where's [person or object]?" If the child is not yet pointing, we can encourage them to look around to find the person or object we have asked them to locate. Other activities or daily routines in which repetition can be embedded by the family are presented in Table 9–2.

Table 9–2. Everyday Activities and Routines in Which Repetition Can Be Embedded

• Point to pictures in books. Focus on the names of objects and actions (e.g., "Where's the dog?" "Show me who is sleeping.").
• Once the child has mastered basic names for objects and common actions, move on to other types of words. Target object use and function (e.g., "Which one is for riding?" "Which one goes on your feet?" "Which one do we use to drink?" "Which one says moo?"). • Help the child identify parts of an object rather than the whole picture (e.g., "Show me the door on the car, the window in the kitchen, the cat's tail").
• Provide instructions for the child to retrieve objects. Ask them to get items or put away specific toys upon request (e.g., "Get your ball"; "Bring me the puzzle").
• Have the child perform tasks with which they are familiar, and that are related to daily routines. Toddlers can get their own diapers or wipes, throw things in the trash, put their own cups in the sink, take off their own shoes and socks, close doors, wipe off the tray on their high-chair, and help clean up toys by putting them in baskets. Involving young children in their everyday activities and expecting them to follow through expands their opportunities to comprehend and follow directions.

- When engaged in play, give short directions and help the child perform the action (e.g., "Put the ball in" [and then help them do it!]).

- When playing with puzzles, hold up each piece and label it with a single word. When the child is finished, ask them to retrieve the puzzle pieces one at a time by prompting: "Give me the _____."

- When dressing, instruct the child to put one arm in their sleeve or one leg in their pants. Hold up a sock and shoe and prompt them to "get the sock."
- When engaged in the bathtub or during a diaper change, ask the child to point to their body parts; help them follow through by pointing or providing hand-over-hand support.

Choices

Offering choices rather than asking yes–no questions encourages a child to respond, interact, and even use words. Choices can also be embedded into any activity, including play, and every family's daily routines. When coaching parents and caregivers to use choices, we want to coach them to make the choices visual. Showing the child two options by presenting them as they name each one helps the child connect the words with the objects and process the choices more easily. The adult can clearly and simply label the options and encourage the child to repeat the name of the option they choose. Parents can visually highlight each item by lifting it up, holding it closer to the child, or holding one object at a time while repeating its name. We can encourage the family to accept the child's response in the form of eye gaze, pointing, gestures, sounds, or words. We also need to coach parents and caregivers to accept any of these responses and to name the item the child chooses before giving it to them.

Offering a choice between objects or options gives the child a sense of control. Many young children with whom we work are unable to do many things for themselves and do not have many choices presented to them. This strategy often helps eliminate some frustrations among both the child and their family members.

Communication Temptations

This is a strategy in which we structure or manipulate the environment in such a way that the child must use some form of communication to obtain a desired item or outcome. The use of this technique encourages a child's communication by tempting them with something they might want but cannot get independently. *Communication temptations* are useful to encourage and facilitate early language skills for the following reasons:

- They offer the child a reason and an opportunity to communicate with another person.

- They provide the child with an opportunity to initiate communication or interaction in some form.

- This is particularly helpful for young children who have difficulty using language to request and/or make their needs known. If the child is already capable of consistently initiating interactions, communication temptations offer opportunities for the child to practice their skills.

The communication temptation should fit within the family's routines. Within a session, we can first observe the parents or caregivers and child in a play activity or daily routine. We should look for opportunities where they can use temptations to encourage more communication from their child. Coaching the family to start with just one or two communication temptations, we can encourage them to gradually build up the opportunities until they are using a wide range within multiple routines as well as throughout their day. These could include the following examples:

Within play

- Use toys that are difficult for the child to operate independently (e.g., wind-up toys).
- Put desired items in the child's view and out of their reach.
- Place toys inside a clear, hard-to-open box (e.g., with clip-locks on the lid or a screw top).

Within daily routines

- At snack time, coach the parent or caregiver to begin eating the child's snack in front of them.
- Give the child their toothbrush but "forget" to wet it or put toothpaste on the brush.
- Give the child a cup of yogurt but "forget" to give them a spoon.

Table 9–3 offers additional suggestions for using communication temptations to support and encourage a young child's use of communication.

Table 9–3. Suggestions to Support Implementation of Communication Temptations

Brainstorm with the family and determine what motivates the child.   What are desirable objects or materials we can use that will encourage the child to initiate communication?
Reflect on the skills the child is already using, and what skills we are targeting.   How will the communication temptation we use help us work with the child to use these skills?

> **Consider how the child communicates.**
> What is their current level of communication?
> Are our expectations realistic?

> **Remember to model the target behavior.**
> Does the child know what we expect from them within the routine or activity?

Linguistic Mapping

Linguistic mapping is a responsive behavior in which we interpret a child's interest in something they do not have the vocabulary to verbalize, based on either a nonverbal act or their attempt to communicate, and we use a word or phrase to describe it. The following is an example of this form of mapping.

- The child reaches for a ball.
- The parent or caregiver immediately exclaims, "You want the ball!"

This is a powerful strategy because it provides the family with easily accessible opportunities to respond to their child's interests; the child is consistently exposed to vocabulary to communicate something in which they have already shown an interest. When parents or caregivers embrace the strategy, they demonstrate how much they value their role as their child's first and most important teacher. We can coach them to watch for their child's communication acts, and to respond with language that will eventually empower them.

Linguistic mapping is a form of modeling language. When modeling language in this way, however, we want to keep it free of expectation. We should confirm with the family that their child does not have to imitate their words to receive the benefit of this strategy. Over time and with repetition and practice, parents and caregivers might report their children do begin to imitate them, and this is where the next strategy comes into play.

Modeling and Prompting

Although these strategies might seem obvious for us as SLPs, *modeling* and *prompting* words does not come naturally to many adults (Owens, 2012). We will often need to support parents and caregivers to identify when and how to speak to their children to encourage and facilitate their language development.

A child's use of expressive language often begins with imitation; the more often they hear a word used in a meaningful context, especially those used consistently within their everyday activities and routines, the more likely a young child is to begin to verbalize that word themselves. Earlier in this chapter, we discussed the importance of repetition, particularly for those children who have receptive and expressive language delays or disorders. When parents and caregivers model words repeatedly, within activities and across routines, they provide their children with the opportunity to process the language they are hearing in their natural environments and with the people who are most familiar to them. It could take several hundred exposures before a child attempts to produce a word (Owens, 2012). We should coach families to be realistic and consistent in their use of modeling.

In addition to modeling, we might need to support a child to recognize and then repeat, or imitate, the words we are using. One strategy we can coach parents to use to convey this expectation is prompting their child. The following are several ways in which we might prompt the child:

- We can choose to simply wait patiently until the child responds. The longer we wait, the more likely the child will react to our pause.

- We can use facial expressions or body language to cue the child. We can give them an expectant look, raise our eyebrows, tilt our head, or lean in to indicate that it is their turn in the conversation.

- We can tap our finger to the corner of our lower lip. This action serves as a cue for the child to say something.

- Adding a contextual question to the modeled word indicates that a response is expected. For example, the parent models the word "cookie." We can coach the parent to then expand their model with the prompt as follows: "Cookie. What do you want?"

- Instruct the child to "Tell me [model word or phrase]." We want to keep the verbal exchange as conversational as possible. Therefore, instead of prompting the child to "repeat" or "say" the word or phrase that has been modeled, we should coach the parents or caregivers to use a more natural prompt. Requesting their child to "tell me milk" is conversational in nature; instructing the child to "say milk" prompts them to repeat rather than request an object.

- This prompt can also be added to the question-based prompt: "Cookie. What do you want? Tell me cookie."

Expansions and Extensions

We have learned and coached parents and caregivers to watch and wait to see what the child wants to do and what they have to say. We have commented, through both self-talk and parallel talk, and have modeled and prompted them to elicit their verbalizations. Next, we need to coach the parents to imitate any words or phrases their child produces. If the child is just beginning to vocalize and verbalize and they use any sounds or word approximations, we want to encourage them to imitate those as well. Once we have the child's attention, we continue to imitate their actions, gestures, sounds, and words.

What's next? If the child gestures for an object, we coach the family to imitate the gesture and expand on it with the word before giving the child the desired object or performing the desired action. If the child produces a sound, we can imitate it and then expand it with either a reduplication or an expansion of it into a word (e.g., turn blowing into a repetitive sound with a silly expression on our face; imitate the car sound multiple times and then say "Go!"). If they simply engage in a play action, we should imitate it and expand on the play sequence (e.g., if the child stirs a pot, we should stir a pot, pretend to smell it, and say "Mmmmm").

This strategy is known as *language expansion,* and it involves the adult adding one or two more gestures or words to a child's action or utterance. We model how to expand their action, word, or phrase by using additional sounds, word combinations, or sentences in response to their own verbalizations. When coaching parents or caregivers, we need to be sure they understand the importance of first repeating the word or words as the child said them, before adding more words to make the message complete (Weitzman, 2017). We do not want to add too much new information, but we can also use this strategy to coach parents and caregivers to teach different types of words to expand their child's lexicon. We can encourage them to expand a child's verbalization by adding a color word, size description, or even carrier phrase (e.g., "I want"; "I see") to their language. When a child is already talking and using two- to three-word combinations, our expansions add semantic and syntactic details to incomplete phrases. For example, if the child puts a figure of a dog in the house and says "dog house," we can expand their utterance and model additional semantic and syntactic structures by verbalizing "The dog is in the house."

The use of *extensions* takes expansions a step further by adding even more information to the child's utterance. To extend a child's comments, we acknowledge and respond to what they have said and add additional information to support both language and communication intent. For example, the child is pointing to a baby and saying, "baby cry." We can coach the parent or caregiver to extend the child's utterance by responding, "Yes, the baby is sad," or "Oh no! The baby has a boo-boo." The extension, in this case, presented additional information and an explanation as to why the baby was crying. Children tend to respond positively when their parents or caregivers extend their words and phrases. They appear to recognize that the adult has listened to them and enjoys engaging in verbal turn-taking with them (Paul & Elwood, 1991).

Milieu Teaching

Milieu teaching is an evidence-based approach in which the provider, parent, or caregiver manipulates or arranges stimuli in a young child's natural environment to create a situation or setting that encourages the child to engage in a targeted behavior (Akamoglu & Meadan, 2019; Akemoglu et al., 2020; Whalon et al., 2015). Using a child's interests and initiations as opportunities to model and prompt language use in everyday contexts, we can arrange the environment to increase the probability that the child will initiate communication; respond to the child's initiations with prompts, expansions, or recasts to support their targeted goals; and naturally and functionally reinforce the child's communicative attempts (Owens, 2012). In milieu teaching, the responsive strategies we learned about in the earlier sections of this chapter are combined in natural, play-based, or routines-based intervention. More directive strategies can also be used in enhanced milieu teaching, through which we can effectively coach families to embed treatment approaches into their everyday activities, routines, and play to facilitate the child's language development (Lang et al., 2009; Mobayed et al., 2000; Patterson et al., 2012; Roberts & Kaiser, 2015). These include the mand-model, expectant delays, and incidental teaching. We might notice an overlap between these, and the strategies presented earlier in this chapter.

Mand-Model

The *mand-model approach* involves the arrangement of the environment in a way that will gain or earn the child's interest. We wait for children to show interest; as soon as they express their interest, we verbally request (mand) a response from them. We might provide a choice related to the materials we have arranged or ask an open-ended question (e.g., "Do you want the apple or the cheese? What do you want?"). If the child responds with the desired communicative behavior, such as a gesture or a word, we reinforce them via praise and an appropriate response (e.g., handing them want they want). If the child does not respond, or responds inappropriately, we model the desired communicative behavior. Once we present a model, we wait a short amount of time for the desired behavior. As needed, we should coach the parents and caregivers to repeat the models or add a prompt to support the child.

Expectant Delays

This milieu teaching strategy has been used to successfully cue young children to communicate in response to environmental stimuli (Owens, 2012). When we set up an *expectant delay*, we arrange the environment in a way in which the child will require assistance by communicating in some way. Expectant delays work best in predictable routines between parents and their child. We can coach parents and caregivers to break established patterns within appropriate routines or activities in which they tend to naturally support and meet their child's needs. For example, if a parent typically opens the container of bubbles after taking them out of the cabinet, the child will expect them to do so during subsequent encounters with the bubbles. When implementing expectant delays, however, the routine is broken: The parent simply sets the bubbles on the table within reach of the child and sits quietly nearby for a predetermined time. If, by the end of the time interval, the child has not communicated a need for the bottle to be opened, we coach the parent to look toward their child with an expectant facial expression. If the child responds with an appropriate communicative behavior, the parent responds by opening the bubbles. If the child does not make a request, the parent is encouraged to model, and subsequently prompt, the child to initiate a behavior to indicate their desire.

Incidental Teaching

When we engage in *incidental teaching*, we include many of the strategies we have already learned about in this chapter. Everyday activities and routines are used as the foundation on which the intervention is supported. With the family, we can brainstorm the best situations in which communication occurs naturally or has the potential to occur. We can then determine the best strategies to elicit and prompt the child to communicate within these situations.

Augmentative and Alternative Communication

As SLPs in EI, we are well aware that during the first years of life, communication serves as the foundation of a child's overall development and connection with family. When infants and toddlers face significant challenges learning to communicate via speech, they are often unable to convey basic needs, wants, knowledge, and emotions with their families, caregivers, and communities. Some children might also experience delays in other modes of communication such as gesture use or eye contact. Regardless of the cause or onset of this delay or disability, all children should have access to some form of AAC. AAC manifests in many modes ranging from gestures, sign language, low-tech pictures, and symbols to high-tech voice output devices. At one time, it was believed that AAC was a last resort reserved for older children who exhibited certain foundational skills (Romski & Sevcik, 2005). We now know this is not the case; secondary to increased availability of technology, all young children with communication deficits are able to access AAC (Cress & Marvin, 2003; Romski et al., 2015; Wilkinson & Hennig, 2007). As EI providers, it is within our scope of practice to encourage access to any young child who will benefit from AAC (ASHA, 2008). Therefore, although we do not dive deeply into AAC in this text, we address the basic principles of AAC intervention to effectively address the needs of the young children and families who we serve within the context of EI.

In alignment with the evidence-based practices we have discussed throughout this textbook, using a family-centered approach to intervention is also necessary for successful AAC system consideration and implementation with a young child in EI (Wright & Quinn, 2016). As always in EI, we need to recognize each family's unique strengths, needs, and priorities for their child and as a unit; build a strong relationship with the family to ensure they engage as an integral member of the EI team; provide them with choices regarding AAC resources; and address their needs as a family through individualized services (Epley et al., 2010; Wright & Quinn, 2016).

In EI, involving family members in intervention is integral to their success in using AAC with their children (Granlund et al., 2008; Light & McNaughton, 2012). Providing family-centered services is especially difficult for children with severe to profound communication impairments. Frequently, parents and caregivers will prioritize those activities that meet their child's basic needs (feeding, dressing, medicating); by doing so, they leave less time to address strategies that focus on their child's communication development. We can observe, collaborate with, and coach family members to embed communication strategies into their everyday activities and routines. Additionally, we can support the family's choices for communication functions (e.g., protesting, requesting, commenting, and sharing information) to ensure we are addressing those areas that result in the most functional interactions between parents, caregivers, and their children. Although many communication interventions address the need to meet basic wants and needs initially, other important functions can and should be addressed including refusing, communicating for social closeness, and gaining attention (Light et al., 2002). We also need to ensure we implement the child's AAC as well as strategies for them to communicate with the families across different settings both in and beyond their home (IDEA, 2004). We can work with families to determine which strategies will be most effective for them to support their child's use of AAC within a variety of communication functions across all of their natural environments (Wright & Quinn, 2016).

Finally, we are negligent if we do not consider and understand how a family's cultural, ethnic, and socioeconomic background could affect their decisions about the use of assistive technology (AT) and AAC with their children. Culturally and linguistically based values might influence family perceptions of AT and the successful implementation of AT solutions agreed on by team members. Multiple studies have found differences in family reactions to AT across cultures (Family Center on Technology and Disability, 2005a, 2005b; Hourcade et al., 1997; Huer & Wyatt, 1999; Judge & Parette, 1998; Parette & McMahan, 2002; Parette & Petch-Hogan, 2000). It is our responsibility as SLPs in EI to do our research, maintain our cultural humility, and be prepared to engage in these conversations with families.

Providing Remote Services

As we noted in Chapter 4, we have been able to offer EI services via remote delivery and telehealth for more than a decade through the use of advanced tools; remote training programs for families, caregivers, and service providers; and protocols for direct clinical services (Buzhardt & Meadan, 2022). Until the spring of 2020, when the COVID-19 pandemic forced EI programs to limit or stop providing face-to-face interactions, these protocols and processes were viewed as an option through which to expand access to evidence-based practices, regardless of location. Remote services in EI were typically used in special circumstances and with specific populations, including families who lived in remote areas or those who were restricted from participating in home visits. Over the past 4 years, however, the demand for remote services and telehealth in EI has resulted in swift, widespread changes in how infants, toddlers, and their families receive services. These changes have included the way in which technology is used to afford access across diverse populations, practical considerations that providers need to consider, and the evidence that has emerged to support the approaches through which we should engage and connect with children, parents, and caregivers when providing remote services in EI.

In regard to best practices in EI when engaging in remote service delivery, recent research supports our use of telehealth as an effective alternative or supplement to face-to-face methods to offer both diagnostic and assessment services, as well as to offer treatment via our coaching approach (Ferguson et al., 2019; Greenwood et al., 2022; Wallisch et al., 2019). According to the literature, EI providers most effectively use coaching when providing remote services by working with parents, caregivers, and siblings to embed strategies into their everyday routines and activities that promote the child's engagement, development, and learning. Current evidence indicates that our use of coaching or direct intervention in the EI arena is effective, and the strategies we have shared throughout this chapter can and should also be implemented via remote services (Akemoglu et al., 2022; McCarthy et al., 2019; Poole et al., 2020).

Table 9–4 presents common challenges and possible solutions associated with providing EI via remote service delivery.

Table 9–4. Engaging Families During Remote Service Delivery

Prior to the visit
Prepare with the parent or caregiver.
• Connect with the parent or caregiver by phone before the virtual visit to discuss their technological needs, and also answer any questions they might have.

- Plan for how we will connect, what device the parent will use, and how it will be positioned so the parent can see us and we can observe the parent–child interaction.
- Determine how the parent will access the link we will send to the virtual meeting platform.
- Chat with the parents about ideas for what we will do during the visit. We need to be prepared to follow the parents' lead, which means they need to know we will engage with whatever they do during the visit. We can also plan activities and should discuss which routines and activities will be happening and who else might be present at the time of the visit.

Prepare for our session.
- Before the virtual visit, we need to collect our own thoughts.
- Remember we will not need toys because our focus will be on coaching the parent or caregiver; we are not trying to engage the child! We might, however, need a prop to model ways in which to engage (e.g., using a doll to show the parent what we are asking them to do with their child).

During the visit

- **Take time to check in with the parent or caregiver.** Just as we would during any visit, we should begin the session by asking the family how they are doing, and check in on their child's progress.

- **Use our voice to join** the activity either we or the parent has planned, or search for opportunities based on what we see. Observe parent–child interaction, watch the siblings play, and use coaching tools to share our observations, ask questions with opportunities for the parent to reflect, and provide guidance on how to use intervention strategies.

- When we provide guidance, share observations, or give feedback, we need to be specific and describe what we see and strategies we suggest. It may be difficult for some parents, especially those who are used to watching us, to follow verbal directions; be sure to take the necessary time, and to check in frequently.

- **Be flexible!** If the visit is a little shorter than usual, that is okay. If what was planned with the parent does not work out, try something else. If we end up discussing development more than observing it, especially on the first remote visit, this is acceptable. Use the "show me …" prompt to move from discussion to observation and support; this is a simple yet effective tool in any visit.

- **Remember our focus should be on the parents, as they are the ones facilitating the child's learning.** Use coaching tools to keep the focus on the parents; the child will ultimately benefit from the intervention provided by their parents.

• **Write down the joint plan.** Plan with the parent as we would in an in-person visit, but also write down the joint plan at the end or after the visit. Email or text the plan to the parent shortly after the session. Be sure to follow up on the plan at the start of the next visit.
After the visit
• Share the plan with the parent via email or text shortly after the session has wrapped up. Offer the parent an opportunity to ask questions or to voice concerns about the session and the plan. • Be sure to address and follow up, with a focus on the plan, at the start of the next visit.

Note. Adapted from "10 strategies for engaging parents (not children?) during tele-intervention," by the Partnership for People with Disabilities, 2020 (https://www.veipd.org/earlyintervention/2020/04/14/10-strategies-for-engaging-parents-not-children-during-tele-intervention/); "Inside the virtual visit: Using tele-intervention to support families in early intervention," by M. Poole, A. Fettig, R. McKee, & A. Gauvreau, 2020.

Summary

In this chapter, we briefly reviewed best practices and approaches in EI before turning our attention toward a set of evidence-based speech-language pathology strategies to support language acquisition, and the expansion of a young child's linguistic repertoire. We discussed how to work with families to choose and coach them in the use of these intervention strategies to address the development of the communication and language skills needed by their child. We touched on the importance of considering and including families in the utilization of AAC for those children who might need AT to engage with others. We also shared challenges, opportunities, and strategies to effectively use remote service delivery to provide accessible services to the children and families in EI.

As we move forward, we discuss considerations related to speech sound development and expectations to address articulation, phonology, and intelligibility with infants and toddlers in EI in Chapter 10. An examination of our roles and responsibilities as SLPs in EI when addressing feeding and swallowing development and disorders are presented in Chapter 11. Finally, information related to assessment and intervention practices with infants and toddlers in the neonatal intensive care unit (NICU), as well as several other special populations with whom we tend to work in EI, is shared in Chapter 12.

Critical Thinking Questions

1. Present a brief review of evidence-based practices related to practice-based coaching, family-centered services, and routines-based intervention, as applied to treatment.

2. Describe the treatment strategies we can incorporate to focus on the facilitation of prelinguistic communication, including engagement, play, and gestures, with an

infant or toddler.

3. What is the difference between hand-over-hand guidance and hand-under-hand prompting? When and why might we choose to use one of these strategies to support the communication development of a young child?

4. What is serve and return? Describe the instructional steps we might provide within our coaching when sharing this strategy with parents or caregivers.

5. Describe at least 5 treatment strategies we might incorporate and/or coach when addressing the receptive and/or expressive language development of an infant or toddler.

6. What is the difference between expansion and extension? Provide a scenario in which we might incorporate each of these strategies.

7. Define milieu teaching; what are the techniques we can implement to model and prompt a young child's language within everyday routines and contexts?

8. What are the basic principles of AAC as they relate to the intervention needs of young children and their families in EI?

9. What are the common challenges associated with remote service delivery in EI treatment? Provide at least 3 possible solutions to the challenges we may face when engaged in remote services.

References

Akemoglu, Y., Hinton, V., Laroue, D., & Jefferson, V. (2022). A parent-implemented shared reading intervention via telepractice. *Journal of Early Intervention, 44*(2), 190–210.

Akamoglu, Y., & Meadan, H. (2019). Parent implemented communication strategies during storybook reading. *Journal of Early Intervention, 41*(4), 300–320.

Akemoglu, Y., Muharib, R., & Meadan, H. (2020). A systematic and quality review of parent-implemented language and communication interventions conducted via telepractice. *Journal of Behavioral Education, 29,* 282–316.

American Speech-Language-Hearing Association. (2008). *Core knowledge and skills in early intervention speech-language pathology practice.* https://doi.org/10.1044/policy.KS2008-00292

Buzhardt, J., & Meadan, H. (2022). Introduction to the special issue: A new era for remote early intervention and assessment. *Journal of Early Intervention, 44*(2), 104–109.

Cameron-Faulkner, T., Theakston, A., Lieven, E., & Tomasello, M. (2015). The relationship between infant holdout and gives, and pointing. *Infancy, 20,* 576–586. https://doi.org/10.1111/infa.12085

Center on the Developing Child. (n.d.). *5 steps for brain-building serve and return.* Harvard

University. https://developingchild.harvard.edu/resources/5-steps-for-brain-building-serve-and-return/

Chapman, R., Seung, H., Schwartz, S., & Bird, E. (2000). Predicting language production in children and adolescents with Down syndrome: The role of comprehension. *Journal of Speech, Language, and Hearing Research, 43*, 340–350.

Chiarello, L. (2017). Excellence in promoting participation: Striving for the 10 Cs—Client-centered care, consideration of complexity, collaboration, coaching, capacity building, contextualization, creativity, community, curricular changes, and curiosity. *Pediatric Physical Therapy, 29*, 16–22. https://doi.10.1097/PEP.0000000000000382

Crais, E., & Ogletree, B. (2016). Prelinguistic communication development. In D. Keen, H. Meadan, N. Brady, & J. Halle (Eds.), *Prelinguistic and minimally verbal communicators on the autism spectrum* (pp. 9–32). Springer. https://doi.org/10.1007/978-981-10-0713-2_2

Crawford, M. J., & Weber, B. (2014). *Early intervention every day! Embedding activities in daily routines for young children and their families*. Brookes.

Cress, C. J., & Marvin, C. A. (2003). Common questions about AAC services in early intervention. *Augmentative and Alternative Communication, 19*(4), 254–272.

Douglas, S. N., Nordquist, E., Kammes, R., & Gerde, H. (2017). Online parent communication training for young children with complex communication needs. *Infants and Young Children, 30*(4), 288–303. https://doi.org/10.1097/IYC.0000000000000101

Douglas, S. N., Kammes, R., Nordquist, E., & D'Agostino, S. (2018). A pilot study to teach siblings to support children with complex communication needs. *Communication Disorders Quarterly, 39*(2), 346–355. https://doi.org/10.1177/1525740117703366

Dunst, C. J., Bruder, M. B., Trivette, C. M., Hamby, D., Raab, M., & McLean, M. (2001). Characteristics and consequences of everyday natural learning opportunities. *Topics in Early Childhood Special Education, 21*(2), 68–91. https://doi.org/10.1177/027112140102100202

Epley, P., Summers, J. A., & Turnbull, A. (2010). Characteristics and trends in family-centered conceptualizations. *Journal of Family Social Work, 13*(3), 269–285. doi:10.1080/10522150903514017

Family Center on Technology and Disability. (2005a). *Family and cultural issues in assistive technology*. http://www.fctd.info/reviews/reports/webboardTranscript.php?id=484

Family Center on Technology and Disability. (2005b). *Family and cultural issues in AT service delivery*. http://www.fctd.info/reviews/reports/webboardTranscript.php?id=474

Ferguson, J., Craig, E. A., & Dounavi, K. (2019). Telehealth as a model for providing behaviour analytic interventions to individuals with autism spectrum disorder: A systematic review. *Journal of Autism and Developmental Disorders, 49*(2), 582–616. https://doi.org/10.1007/s10803-018-3724-5

Finestack, L. H., & Fey, M. E. (2013). *Evidence-based language intervention approaches for young talkers.* In L. A. Rescorla & P. S. Dale (Eds.), *Late talkers: Language development, interventions, and outcomes.* Brookes.

Friedman, M., Woods, J., & Salisbury, C. (2012). Caregiver coaching strategies for early intervention providers: Moving toward operational definitions. *Infants & Young Children, 25*(1), 62–82. https://doi.org/10.1097/IYC.0b013e31823d8f12

Goldin-Meadow, S. (2015). Gesture as a window onto communicative abilities: Implications for diagnosis and intervention. *Perspectives on Language Learning and Education, 22*, 50–60.

Granlund, M., Björck-Åkesson, E., Wilder, J., & Ylvén, R. (2008). AAC interventions for children in a family environment: Implementing evidence in practice. *Augmentative and Alternative Communication, 24*(3), 207–219.

Greenwood, C., Higgins, S., McKenna, M., Buzhardt, J., Walker, D., Ai, J., ... Grasley-Boy, N. (2022). Remote use of individual growth and development indicators (IGDIs) for infants and toddlers. *Journal of Early Intervention, 44*(2), 168–189.

Hadley, P. A., Rispoli, M., & Holt, J. K. (2017). Input subject diversity accelerates the growth of tense and agreement: Indirect benefits from a parent-implemented intervention. *Journal of Speech, Language, and Hearing Research, 60*(9), 2619–2635. https://doi.org/10.1044/2017_JSLHR-L-17-0008

Hadley, P. A., Rispoli, M., Holt, J. K., Papastratakos, T., Hsu, N., Kubalanza, M., & McKenna, M. M. (2017). Input subject diversity enhances early grammatical growth: Evidence from a parent-implemented intervention. *Language Learning and Development: The Official Journal of the Society for Language Development, 13*(1), 54–79. https://doi.org/10.1080/15475441.2016.1193020

Huer, M. B., & Wyatt, T. (1999). *Cultural factors in the delivery of AAC services to the African-American community.* http:// www.asha.ucf.edu/huer.wyatt.html

Hourcade, J. J., Parette, H. P., & Huer, M. B. (1997). Family and cultural alert! Considerations in assistive technology assessment. *Exceptional Children, 30*(1), 40–44.

Hwang, A. W., Chao, M. Y., & Liu, S. W. (2013). A randomized controlled trial of routines-based early intervention for children with or at risk for developmental delays. *Research in Developmental Disabilities, 34*(10), 3112–3123. https://doi.org/10.1016/j.ridd.2013.06.037

Individuals With Disabilities Education Improvement Act of 2004, Pub. L. No. 108-446, § 632, 118 Stat. 2744 (2004). http://idea.ed.gov/

Individuals With Disabilities Education Improvement Act. (2011). Part C Final Regulations. 34 C.F.R. §§ 303 (2011). https://www.gpo.gov/fdsys/pkg/FR-2011-09-28/pdf/2011-22783.pdf

Ingersoll, B. (2008). The social role of imitation in autism: Implications for treatment of imitation deficits. *Infants & Young Children*, *21*(2), 107–119.

Judge, S. L., & Parette, H. P. (1998). Family-centered assistive technology decision making. Infant–toddler intervention. *The Transdisciplinary Journal*, *8*(2), 185–206.

Laakso, M.-L., Poikkeus, A.-M., Katajamäki, J., & Lyytinen, P. (1999). Early intentional communication as a predictor of language development in young toddlers. *First Language*, *19*(56), 207–231. https://doi.org/10.1177/014272379901905604

Lang, R., Machaliecek, W., Rispoli, M., & Regester, A. (2009). Training parents to implement communication interventions for children with autism spectrum disorders (ASD): A systematic review. *Evidence-Based Communication Assessment and Intervention*, *3*, 174–190.

Law, J., Charlton, J., Dockrell, J., Gascoigne, M., McKean, C., & Theakston, A. (2017). *Early language development: Needs, provision, and intervention for preschool children from socioeconomically disadvantaged backgrounds: A report for the Education Endowment Foundation.* Education Endowment Foundation and Public Health England. https://educationendowmentfoundation.org.uk/public/files/Law_et_al_Early_Language_Development_final.pdf

Levey, S. (2014). *Introduction to language development.* Plural Publishing.

Light, J., & McNaughton, D. (2012). Supporting the communication, language, and literacy development of children with complex communication needs: State of the science and future research priorities. *Assistive Technology*, *24*, 34–44.

Light, J., Parsons, A., & Drager, K. (2002). "There's more to life than cookies": Developing interactions for social closeness with beginning communicators who require augmentative and alternative communication. In J. Reichle, D. Beukelman, & J. Light (Eds.), *Exemplary practices for beginning communicators: Implications for AAC* (pp. 187–218). Brookes.

Lyytinen, P., Poikkeus, A., Laakso, M., Eklund, K., & Lyytinen, H. (2001). Language development and symbolic play in children with and without familial risk of dyslexia. *Journal of Speech, Language, and Hearing Research*, *44*, 873–885.

McCarthy, M., Leigh, G., & Arthur-Kelly, M. (2019). Telepractice delivery of family-centered early intervention for children who are deaf or hard of hearing: A scoping review. *Journal of Telemedicine and Telecare, 25*(4), 249–260.

Meadan, H., Ostrosky, M. M., Santos, R. M., & Snodgrass, M. R. (2013). How can I help? Prompting procedures to support children's learning. *Young Exceptional Children, 16*(4), 31–39. https://doi.org/10.1177/1096250613505099

Meadan, H., Snodgrass, M. R., Meyer, L. E., Fisher, K. W., Chung, M. Y., & Halle, J. W. (2016). Internet-based parent-implemented intervention for young children with autism: A pilot study. *Journal of Early Intervention, 38*(1), 3–23. https://doi.org/10.1177/1053815116630327

Miles, B. (2003). *Talking the language of the hands to the hands*. The National Information Clearinghouse on Children Who Are Deaf-Blind. file:///C:/Users/cherd/Downloads/hands-to-hands-english.pdf

Mobayed, K. L., Collins, B. C., Strangis, D. E., Schuster, J. W., & Hemmeter, M. L. (2000). Teaching parents to employ mand-model procedures to teach their children requesting. *Journal of Early Intervention, 23*, 165–179.

National Center on Deaf-Blindness. (2021). *Hand-under-hand technique: NCDB practice guide*. https://www.nationaldb.org/media/doc/HandUnderHandTechnique_a.pdf

O'Neill, H., Murphy, C. A., & Chiat, S. (2019). What our hands tell us: A two-year follow-up investigating outcomes in subgroups of children with language delay. *Journal of Speech, Language, and Hearing Research, 62*(2), 356–366. https://doi.org/10.1044/2018_JSLHR-L-17-0261

Owens, R. (2012). *Language development: An introduction* (8th ed.). Pearson Education.

Owens, R. (2019). *Language development: An introduction* (10th ed.). Pearson Education.

Parette, H. P., & McMahan, G. A. (2002). What should we expect of assistive technology: Being sensitive to family goals. *Teaching Exceptional Children, 23*(1), 56–61.

Parette, H. P., & Petch-Hogan, B. (2000). Approaching families: Facilitating culturally/linguistically diverse family involvement. *Exceptional Children, 33*(2), 4–10.

Partnership for People With Disabilities. (2020). *10 strategies for engaging parents (not children?) during tele-intervention*. https://www.veipd.org/earlyintervention/2020/04/14/10-strategies-for-engaging-parents-not-children-during-tele-intervention/

Patterson, S. Y., Smith, V., & Mirenda, P. (2012). A systematic review of training programs for parents of children with autism spectrum disorders: Single subject contributions. *Autism, 16*, 498–522.

Paul, R. (2007). *Language disorders from infancy through adolescence: Assessment and intervention* (3rd ed.). Mosby.

Paul, R., & Elwood, T. J. (1991). Maternal linguistic input to toddlers with slow expressive language development. *Journal of speech and hearing research, 34*(5), 982–988. https://doi.org/10.1044/jshr.3405.982

Poole, M., Fettig, A., McKee, R., & Gauvreau, A. (2020). Inside the virtual visit: Using tele-intervention to support families in early intervention. *Young Exceptional Children, 25*(1), 3–14. https://doi.org/10.1177/109625620948061

Roberts, M. Y., Hensle, T., & Brooks, M. K. (2016). More than "Try this at home"—Including parents in early intervention. *Perspectives of the ASHA Special Interest Groups, 1*(1), 130–143. https://doi.org/10.1044/persp1.SIG1.130

Roberts, M. Y., & Kaiser, A. P. (2015). Early intervention for toddlers with language delays: A randomized controlled trial. *Pediatrics, 135*(4), 686–693. https://doi.org/10.1542/peds.2014-2134

Romski, M., & Sevcik, R. A. (2005). Augmentative communication and early intervention: Myths and realities. *Infants & Young Children, 18*(3), 174–185.

Romski, M., Sevcik, R. A., Barton-Hulsey, A., & Whitmore, A. S. (2015). Early intervention and AAC: What a difference 30 years makes. *Augmentative and Alternative Communication, 31*(3), 181–202.

Rush, D. D., & Shelden, M. L. (2011). *The early childhood coaching handbook*. Brookes.

Rush, D. D., & Shelden, M. L. (2020). *The early childhood coaching handbook* (2nd ed.). Brookes.

Trivette, C. M., Dunst, C. J., & Hamby, D. (2004). Sources of variation in consequences of everyday activity settings on child and parenting functioning. *Perspectives in Education, 22*(2), 17–36. https://eric.ed.gov/?id=EJ687912

Uzgiris, I. C. (1981). Two functions of imitation during infancy. *International Journal of Behavioral Development, 4*, 1–12.

Venker, C. E., McDuffie, A., Ellis Weismer, S., & Abbeduto, L. (2012). Increasing verbal responsiveness in parents of children with autism: A pilot study. *Autism: The International Journal of Research and Practice, 16*(6), 568–585. https://doi.org/10.1177/1362361311413396

Wallisch, A., Little, L., Pope, E., & Dunn, W. (2019). Parent perspectives of an occupational therapy telehealth intervention. *International Journal of Telerehabilitation, 11*(1), 15–22. https://doi.org/10.5195/ijt.2019.6274

Weitzman, E. (2017). *It takes two to talk: A practical guide for parents of children with language delays*. The Hanen Centre.

Whalon, K., Martinez, J. R., Shannon, D., Butcher, C., & Hanline, M. F. (2015). The impact of reading to engage children with autism in language and learning (RECALL). *Topics in Early Childhood Special Education, 35*, 102–115.

Wetherby, A., Allen, L., Cleary, J., Kublin, K., & Goldstein, H. (2002). Validity and reliability of the Communication and Symbolic Behavior Scales Developmental Profile with very young children. *Journal of Speech, Language, and Hearing Research, 45*, 1202–1218.

Wetherby, A., Goldstein, H., Cleary, J., Allen, L., & Kublin, K. (2003). Early identification of children with communication disorders: Concurrent and predictive validity of the CSBS Developmental Profile. *Infants & Young Children, 16*, 161–174.

Wilkinson, K. M., & Hennig, S. (2007). The state of research and practice in augmentative and alternative communication for children with developmental/intellectual disabilities. *Mental Retardation and Developmental Disabilities, 13*, 58–69.

Woods, J. J., Wilcox, M. J., Friedman, M., & Murch, T. (2011). Collaborative consultation in natural environments: Strategies to enhance family-centered supports and services. *Language, Speech, and Hearing Services in Schools, 42*(3), 379–392.

Wright, C. A., & Quinn, E. D. (2016). Family-centered implementation of augmentative and alternative communication systems in early intervention. *Perspectives of the ASHA Special Interest Groups, 1*(1), 168–174.

Zambrana, I. M., Ystrom, E., Schjølberg, S., & Pons, F. (2013). Action imitation at 1½ years is better than pointing gesture in predicting late development of language production at 3 years of age. *Child Development, 84*(2), 560–573. https://doi.org/10.1111/j.1467-8624.2012.01872.x

Chapter 10

Best Practices for Assessment and Treatment of Speech Sound Development

Learning Outcomes

When we have completed this chapter, we will be able to:

- Define articulation, phonology, and intelligibility.

- Differentiate between speech sound disorders, articulation disorders, and phonological disorders.

- Share evidence-based developmental expectations of articulation, phonology, and intelligibility of young children.

- Present data related to referral and diagnosis of speech sound development and disorders in EI.

- Describe what and how to assess speech sound development of infants and toddlers.

- List the patterns (i.e., red flags) that indicate speech sound production difficulties in early childhood.

- Discuss best practices for differential diagnosis of speech sound disorders, including childhood apraxia of speech, in EI.

- Explain the speech-related needs of young children with cerebral palsy or cleft lip and cleft palate.

- Provide evidence to support and strategies to implement embedding of speech sound development in EI treatment.

What Will We Learn and How Can We Apply It?

In previous chapters, we discussed evaluation and assessment strategies and considerations, as well as how to work with families to implement intervention strategies that address the development of their children's communication and language skills. We did not, however, address or include speech sound development or disorders in these discussions. Although many parents and caregivers will come to us, as SLPs in EI, with specific concerns about their children's pronunciation and their ability to understand them, there is a dearth of literature to guide us regarding the treatment of speech sound development and disorders in very young children. In fact, most of the literature that addresses intervention for speech sound disorders (specifically articulation and phonology) is focused on children over 3 years of age (e.g., Brumbaugh & Smit, 2013). There is an important reason for the lack of information related to speech sound development and disorders in EI.

What does this mean for the services we provide to families who are concerned about their child's "speech," and how do we address their concerns, needs, and priorities when they are struggling to communicate with their children? We rarely assess and treat speech sound production as the primary concern in EI; to support the children and families we serve, however, our knowledge and skills about expectations and best practices related to assessment and treatment regarding development and disorders in this area are integral to our work. This chapter presents a review of the typical development of speech sounds, phonological patterns, and expectations related to intelligibility with infants and toddlers. We consider the differences between articulation and phonological delays or disorders, developmental apraxia of speech, and organic speech disorders, as well as what to expect in the differential diagnosis of these disorders with children under the age of 3 years. We also consider the evidence regarding speech sound use by young children, considerations for embedding speech sounds in the development of IFSP outcomes, and within the family-centered RBI, we coach and implement with parents and caregivers to address their children's needs.

What Is a Speech Sound Disorder?

As we discussed in Chapter 5, speech sound disorders refer to any difficulty or combination of difficulties a child might have with perception, motor production, or phonological representation of speech sounds or speech segments. Speech sound disorders can be organic and result from an underlying motor, neurological, structural, sensory, or perceptual cause. These disorders can also be functional and have no known cause. In the past, we have referred to functional speech sound disorders as either articulation disorders or phonological disorders. *Articulation disorders* focus on errors made in the production of individual speech sounds. *Phonological disorders* focus on predictable, rule-based errors that affect more than one sound. As SLPs, we know it is often difficult to clearly differentiate between articulation and phonological disorders, especially in the early years; therefore, in more recent years, we have turned to the broader term *speech sound disorder* when referring to speech errors of unknown cause (ASHA, 2023b).

Referral and Diagnosis of Speech Sound Disorders in Early Intervention

According to Broomfield and Dodd (2004), speech sound referrals (including phonological and articulatory-related concerns) represent approximately 60% of all speech-language pathology referrals for children between the ages of 3 and 4 years; for children 2 years old and younger, referrals to address concerns with speech sound development constitute less than 9%. This distinction is most likely due to limited speech sound use by most infants and toddlers in the early stages of language development (Broomfield & Dodd, 2004). Additionally, young children with limited expressive language might not be able or willing to name pictures associated with standardized testing or to imitate an adult model on command.

Multiple sources recommend waiting until after the age of 3 to differentially diagnose a child with a developmental speech sound disorder (Bowen, 2014; DeVeney & Peterkin, 2022; Sosa, 2011). With the evidence to support us, it makes sense to question the appropriateness of a speech-related referral in EI (DeVeney & Peterkin, 2022; Sosa, 2011). When an infant or toddler is referred to us for an evaluation and assessment, and the primary concern is speech production, we must consider early milestones and development expectations, as well as empirical data, to make evidence-based decisions regarding our role in providing intervention that directly targets speech sound disorders for infants and toddlers in EI. Let's review these considerations.

Speech Sound Development

To support family concerns regarding a child's speech-sound development by providing preventive services for children who are at risk of continuing difficulty with speech production and possible long-term difficulty with speech, language, and literacy development, EI practitioners first need evidence-based information that specifically addresses speech development in children under the age of 3. This information includes relationships between speech and language skills in early development, how to assess speech sound development in children with delays and disorders in language and communication, how to identify which children are at special risk for continuing to have difficulty with speech sound production, and functional approaches to support the development of speech skills within the EI framework.

Articulation

The first signs of communication occur when an infant learns that crying leads to the acquisition of food, comfort, and attention. Newborns also begin to recognize important sounds in their environment, including the voice of their mother or primary caregiver. As they grow, infants begin to sort out the speech sounds that make up the words of their language. By 6 to 9 months of age, most babies recognize the basic sounds of their native language (Rossetti, 2005). This does not mean that they are producing the sounds at this age; however, it simply means that they have learned the sounds by hearing them, and they are beginning to process and organize the speech sounds in their environment in preparation for producing them. Between the ages of 6 and 12 months, an infant begins babbling sounds in different vowel and consonant combinations. First words tend to emerge just around the time a young child turns 1 year old (Rossetti, 2005). When young children do begin to produce words, we do not expect the sounds to be clear and distinct. They need time to coordinate the movement of their lips, tongue, teeth, palate, and respiratory system to develop effective *articulation* skills.

When we begin to consider whether a young child is producing speech as expected, we tend to use consonant acquisition or developmental norms as a benchmark for evaluation, assessment, and diagnosis. Once we have diagnosed a child with a speech sound disorder, we also use these norms to consider eligibility and select intervention targets (Ireland & Conrad, 2016; Ireland et al., 2020; McLeod & Baker, 2014; Porter & Hodson, 2001; Storkel, 2019). Even though the ability to speak encompasses a broad range of skills, as SLPs, we have traditionally and continue to focus on the acquisition of consonant sounds and combinations of sounds in words to guide our clinical decisions regarding speech development and disorders (McLeod et al., 2013). Table 10–1 presents a review of the expected acquisition of speech sounds. Because we are taking a closer look at these expectations as they relate to the assessment and treatment of speech sound production in this chapter, it is important we review the data here.

Table 10–1. Age of Acquisition of English Language Consonants

Average Age of Acquisition	**English Consonants**
2 years	p, b, d, m, n, h, w
3 years	t, k, g, ng, f, y
4 years	v, s, z, sh, ch, j, l
5 years	th (voiced), zh, r
6 years	th (voiceless)

Note. Adapted from "Children's English Consonant Acquisition in the United States: A Review," by K. Crowe & S. McLeod, 2020.

It is worth noting that the data presented in Table 10–1 are a result of a comprehensive review of studies that met strict inclusion and exclusion criteria that described English consonant acquisition by 18,907 children living in the United States (Crowe & McLeod, 2020). Based on this review, the evidence indicates that 13 consonants (including all plosives, nasals, and glides) are typically acquired between 2;0, and 3;11 years of age; seven additional consonants are typically acquired between 4;0, and 4;11 years of age; and the remaining four consonants are typically acquired between 5;0 and 6;11 years of age (Crowe & McLeod, 2020). These findings echo the crosslinguistic findings of McLeod and Crowe (2018) across 27 languages that most consonants are acquired by 5;0 years of age. These data are comprehensive and current; they should inform our clinical decision-making and consideration of eligibility for services and determination of appropriate and functional IFSP outcomes.

Phonology

We are reminded that phonology includes the study of the individual sounds of a language (the phonemes), their patterns, how they are learned (which is called phonological development), and how they work together (ASHA, 2023b). When we consider phonological processes, we are referring to the typical patterns children use to simplify their phonology as they learn to speak. A child is not born with the ability to immediately produce every sound pattern in our language. As children learn to speak English, they will simplify sounds and sound patterns. For example, a young child might simplify the word "bottle" to sound more like "baba." A toddler might say "goggie" for "doggie" and "nail" for "snail." We might observe a 2-year-old deleting the final consonants of their words as they work through new vocabulary; as such, "please" becomes "pee," and "ball" might be produced as "baw."

All the sounds in the English language are organized into different classes based on their place, voice, and manner (ASHA, 2023b).

- *Place* refers to the location in the oral cavity where the sound is actually produced (e.g., /b/ is produced between the lips; /d/ is produced in the front of the oral cavity with the tongue pushed up against the hard palate; /g/ is produced in the back of the oral cavity with the back of the tongue pushed up against the soft palate).

- *Voice* refers to whether the sound requires voice (e.g., /b/ or /g/) or is voiceless (e.g., /p/ or /k/).

- *Manner* indicates the way in which the air is pushed through the vocal tract and the degree or type of closure of the vocal tract when a sound is produced (e.g., when we produce an /s/ sound, we push the air between our teeth and our lips; in contrast, when we produce a /p/ sound, we pop the air out between closed lips).

Therefore, when we refer to phonological processes, we are talking about the typical patterns children use while taking into consideration their use of place, manner, and voice to simplify their speech as they learn to speak. Just as typically developing children develop their articulation skills within expected age ranges, there are ages when children are also expected to stop using different phonological processes; interestingly, the deletion of these processes, or patterns, do not emerge until after a child is 3 years old. Table 10–2 presents the phonological processes we observe in children in EI, as well as the age by which children are expected to eliminate the process.

Table 10–2. Elimination of Phonological Processes

Phonological Process	Example	Age by Which 90% of Children Eliminate Process
Context-sensitive voicing	pig = big	3 years
Word-final devoicing	pig = pick	3 years
Stopping of /f/	fish = tish	3 years
Stopping of /s/	soap = dope	3 years
Final consonant deletion	comb = coe	3.3 years
Fronting	car = tar	3.6 years
Stopping of /v/	very = berry	3.6 years
Stopping of /z/	zoo = doo	3.6 years
Consonant harmony	mine = mime	3.9 years
Weak syllable deletion	elephant = efant	4 years

Cluster reduction	spoon = poon	4 years
Stopping of "sh"	shop = dop	4.6 years
Stopping of /j/	jump = dump	4.6 years
Stopping of "ch"	chair = tare	4.6 years
Gliding of liquids	run = won	5 years
Stopping of voiceless "th"	thing = ting	5 years
Stopping of voiced "th"	them = dem	5 years

Note. Adapted from *"Children's speech sound disorders 2nd edition,"* by E. Bowen, 2014; *"The new phonologies: Developments in clinical linguistics,"* by M. Ball & R. Kent, 2007.

Intelligibility

Now that we have reviewed articulation and phonological development, we need to consider how this information relates to intelligibility. As SLPs, we often hear from parents that their children are difficult to understand. Because we have established a clear understanding of the time and expectations involved in speech sound development, we recognize why we very well might have difficulty understanding the young children with whom we work. It is also within our scope of practice in EI to share with our families why and how their child's lack of intelligibility could be developmentally appropriate. Throughout infancy, toddlerhood, and the preschool years, children are continuously improving the clarity and accuracy of their speech sound productions.

The term *intelligibility* refers to speech clarity or the percentage of a speaker's output that a listener can readily understand. For those demonstrating typical development, as children learn to talk, their intelligibility, or how clear their speech is to others, steadily increases. In young children, there is often a marked difference between the intelligibility of single-word productions and conversational speech, as well as in their intelligibility to close family members and caregivers and those who are unfamiliar listeners. There also might be a difference in intelligibility when a child is talking about or within a known context versus talking about unknown or novel topics. Within families, siblings are often more adept than parents or other caregivers at understanding or comprehending what their younger brothers or sisters are saying (Bowen, 2014). The most recent empirical data suggest that young children are expected to be difficult for adults, including those who are both familiar and unfamiliar with the child, to understand. According to Hustad et al. (2021), children between the ages of 31 and 47 months are only expected to be 50% intelligible at the single-word level; at the multiword level, children between the ages of 34 and 46 months are expected to reach 50% intelligibility.

Table 10–3 presents a breakdown of the current intelligibility criteria; we can share this information with families when answering their questions and working together to determine functional IFSP outcomes and treatment strategies for their young children.

Table 10–3. Single-Word and Multiword Utterance Intelligibility Expectations

Percentage of Expected Intelligibility	Single-Word Utterances: Age Range for (Average) Children Demonstrating Expressive Language in the 50th Percentile	Multiword Utterances: Age Range for (Average) Children Demonstrating Expressive Language in the 50th Percentile
25%	18 months	
50%	31 months (2 years, 7 months)	34 months (2 years, 10 months)
75%	49 months (4 years, 1 month)	46 months (3 years, 10 months)
90%	83 months (6 years, 11 months)	62 months (5 years, 2 months)
Percentage of Expected Intelligibility	Single-Word Utterances: Age Range for (Delayed) Children Demonstrating Expressive Language in the 5th Percentile	Multiword Utterances: Age Range for (Delayed) Children Demonstrating Expressive Language in the 5th Percentile
50%	46 months (3 years, 10 months)	46 months (3 years, 10 months)
75%	87 months (4 years, 1 month)	61 months (5 years, 1 month)
90%	120 months (6 years, 11 months)	87 months (7 years, 3 months)

Note. Adapted "Children's speech sound disorders 2nd edition," by E. Bowen, 2014; "Speech development between 30 and 119 months in typical children I: Intelligibility growth curves for single-word and multiword productions," by K. C. Hustad, T. J. Mahr, P. Natzke, & P. J. Rathouz, 2021.

Assessment of Speech Sound Development in Early Intervention

Now that we have reviewed the developmental expectations of articulation, phonology, and intelligibility in young children, we need to consider how we should assess infants and toddlers regarding their speech-sound development. As part of any evaluation or assessment in EI, we are familiar with the comprehensive set of activities in which we engage to identify a child's strengths and challenges, address the family's concerns and priorities, and develop a plan for the next steps and opportunities for the child and family (Crais, 2011; Raver & Childress, 2015). Evaluating a child's speech sound development is simply one component of this comprehensive process.

Our interview with the parents and caregivers includes the child's developmental history and family background, environmental stressors affecting the family and child, and language history and proficiency of the child and family. Based on our family interview and by engaging in both observation and play-based activities with the child, we listen for the sounds and the patterns they are currently using, and we assess their current articulation and phonological development. We also consider the report by the parents or caregivers regarding their ability to understand their child. We could ask families the following questions to determine the rating of their child's intelligibility:

- Do you have difficulty understanding your child when they speak?

- How much of your child's speech do you understand? More than half? Less than [%]?

Basing our observations on the development milestones and the potential red flags presented in the next section, we listen for atypical phonological patterns and consider the child's speech sound development to date to determine whether their speech production is an area of concern. If we have significant concerns during an initial evaluation or at any time within the EI pathway, we can assess early speech skills by collecting a phonetic inventory of the child's home language. We do this by simply counting the different consonant sounds produced in a sample of spontaneous interaction, without regard to the adult target, or evaluating their syllable complexity by counting the number of closed syllables or syllables that contain two or more different consonants (Crais, 2011; Olswang et al., 1987; Paul, 2007).

Above and beyond our observations and assessment of the child's speech productions, we also need to determine whether this child is using the language skills developmentally expected for their age. Toddlers who are extremely difficult to understand often embed a significant percentage of jargon in their vocalizations secondary to a lack of vocabulary, a delay in their use of grammatical markers, or the inability to combine words into phrases. We know all these skills are expected by 2 years of age. We typically expect that jargon (which can be considered "babbling with intent") will begin to fade at about 18 months and completely disappear by 24 months (Levey, 2014; Owens, 2019). If a toddler has an expressive language delay or disorder, however, their intelligibility will also be affected as they might continue to use jargon in lieu of words. Instead of recognizing that jargon is a substitute for real words or grammar that should have developed, we often misinterpret the jargon to be speech sound production errors (Levey, 2014; Owens, 2019).

Red Flags Related to Speech Sound Development

As we consider young children's speech sound production and the patterns they demonstrate in regard to their articulation and phonology, there are several patterns we might observe that we should not ignore. Each of these red flags could be an indication that the child, under the age of 3 years, might be experiencing difficulty with speech sound production beyond developmental expectations. When we are conducting a comprehensive intake and evaluation of an infant or toddler, there are several speech-related behaviors we should take into consideration. A child who presents with any of the following on a pervasive, consistent basis (i.e., not an isolated word or observed by the parents or caregivers on occasion) could be at greater risk for later or long-term difficulty with their speech sound development.

- Difficulty with inclusion of syllables (e.g., one syllable instead of two: /ah/ for apple).

- Difficulty with or deletion of initial sounds (e.g., /ama/ for /mama/).

- Extremely restricted consonant inventory.

- Babbling remains simple (i.e., reduplicated); no emergence of variegated babbling.

- Reduced vowel inventory or distorted vowels.
- Low intelligibility as rated by parents and caregivers.
- Poor stimulability of errors (i.e., ability to correct errors with modeling and curing).

In a recent study, To et al. (2022) reviewed the relationship between risk factors presented in toddlers and the normalization of speech sound development over time. They found that children who were more likely to normalize their speech sound development or normalize their speech sound development in a shorter window of time were stimulable to all errors and were more intelligible, as rated by their caregivers. Additionally, children who demonstrated atypical errors did not necessarily take longer to normalize. To et al. (2022) also determined that delays in expressive language ability were not significantly associated with speech sound development. Therefore, we could choose to include speech sound development and production more intentionally in our IFSP outcomes and treatment strategies for these children, as their speech errors could be less likely to resolve naturally.

Diagnosis of Speech Sound Disorders

As SLPs, we will typically diagnose a speech sound disorder if a child demonstrates a delay of at least 6 to 12 months in the production of certain sounds or deletion of patterns in phonology, based on the ages at which mastery of the sounds and patterns are expected. Because the earliest developing sounds, including /p, m, h, n, and w/, are not expected to be mastered until the age of 3, a child between the ages of birth and 3 years is not expected to produce any sounds correctly (Cane & McLeod, 2020). Therefore, when we consider the empirical evidence supporting these expectations of speech sounds and the elimination of phonological processes, we recognize a child should not be differentially diagnosed with a speech sound disorder before the age of 3 years old. Unless we see some major red flags, we should not diagnose an infant or toddler with a speech sound disorder. Young children are still developing their speech production skills; there are no sounds or phonological processes that should be mastered prior to or by the age of 3 years (Bowen, 2014; Cane & McLeod, 2020).

Childhood Apraxia of Speech

What about *childhood apraxia of speech* (CAS)? CAS is a neurological, pediatric speech sound disorder in which the precision and consistency of movements underlying speech are impaired in the absence of neuromuscular deficits (e.g., abnormal reflexes, abnormal tone) (Shriberg et al., 2019). CAS could occur because of neurological impairment, in association with complex neurobehavioral disorders of known and unknown origin, or as an idiopathic (i.e., unknown origin) neurogenic speech sound disorder (ASHA, 2023a). The core difficulties with planning and programming parameters of movement sequences result in errors in speech sound production and prosody (ASHA, 2007, 2023a). CAS is an uncommon speech disorder that accounts for less than 3% of speech sound disorders in preschool-aged children (Shriberg et al., 2019).

For a child to speak correctly, the child's brain must learn how to make plans that tell the speech muscles how to move the lips, jaw, and tongue in ways that result in accurate sounds and words (Tshering Pema, 2016). The child's brain also plans these movements so that they speak with normal speed and rhythm. When a child has CAS, the brain struggles to develop plans for speech movement. As a result, children with CAS do not learn accurate movements for speech with normal ease. The speech muscles are not weak but do not perform normally because the brain has difficulty directing or coordinating the movements. Some characteristics help distinguish apraxia from other speech sound disorders. The characteristics associated specifically with CAS include (ASHA, 2023a; Tshering Pema, 2016) the following.

- Difficulty moving smoothly from one sound, syllable, or word to another.
- Groping movements with the jaw, lips, or tongue to make the correct movement for speech sounds.
- Vowel distortions (e.g., attempting to use the correct vowel but saying it incorrectly).
- Using the wrong stress in a word (e.g., producing "syllable" as "syll-OBle").
- Separation of syllables (e.g., including a pause or gap between syllables: "syll … a … ble").
- Inconsistency in errors (i.e., presenting a different error in speech when repeating the same word).
- Difficulty imitating simple words.

There are several characteristics presented by most children with language delays or disorders that are not specific to CAS (ASHA, 2023a):

- Reduced amount of babbling or vocal sounds from the ages of 7 to 12 months old.
- Speaking first words late (after ages 12–18 months old).
- Using a limited number of consonants and vowels.
- Frequently leaving out (i.e., omitting) sounds.
- Difficult to understand a child's speech productions.

According to ASHA (2023a), there are multiple challenges to diagnosing CAS in the birth-to-3 population. These include the following:

- The potential presence of developmental disabilities, comorbid conditions, or both.
- The lack of a single validated list of diagnostic features differentiates CAS from other types of childhood speech sound disorders (e.g., those due to phonological-level deficits or neuromuscular disorder).
- The fact that some primary characteristics of CAS (e.g., word inconsistency, a predominant error pattern of omission, etc.) are characteristic of emerging speech in typically developing children under the age of 3.

- The lack of a sufficient speech sample size for making a more definitive diagnosis.
- The challenge of sorting out inability versus unwillingness to provide a speech sample or to attempt a speech target.
- The possibility that changes occurring prior to age 3 (e.g., developmental maturation, social and linguistic peer exposure, and beneficial effects of therapy) might alter the diagnostic label.

Overby and Caspari (2012, 2013) also reported that rather than a definitive diagnosis of CAS before the age of 3 years, we should instead categorize difficulties an infant or toddler presents with motor planning with a provisional diagnostic classification such as "CAS cannot be ruled out," "signs are consistent with problems in planning the movements required for speech," or "suspected to have CAS." This is the same terminology used in the 2007 ASHA Position Statement on Childhood Apraxia of Speech. Furthermore, the three assessment tools considered most valid and reliable for diagnosis of CAS, including the Verbal Motor Production Assessment for Children, the Kaufman Speech Praxis Test, and the Screening Test for Developmental Apraxia of Speech, provide a minimum appropriate age range for administration of 3 years, 4 years, and 5 years, respectively. Therefore, although it is our responsibility to assess and monitor a child's motor planning and to determine any difficulties they might have in this area, a differential diagnosis of CAS in EI is not appropriate.

Special Populations

Who else should we keep in mind when considering the diagnosis of speech sound disorders in young children? Most children continue to develop their speech production abilities through the preschool and early school-age years, but some children are diagnosed with organic disorders that affect their speech development; their communication skills are often also characterized by comorbid delays or disorders in language development (Bashina et al., 2002; Chenausky et al., 2017).

Young children could demonstrate delays with the development of speech sounds related to cleft lip or palate or dysarthria related to cerebral palsy (CP). These are legitimate concerns that relate to the coordination of muscle movement (as in the case of dysarthria) and weakness of or damage to the oral structure (related to cleft lip or palate). We might need to address these issues in EI and discuss them further in the following sections.

Cerebral Palsy

Cerebral Palsy (CP) is the most common childhood physical disability (Rosenbaum et al., 2007). Although CP is permanent and nonprogressive, the clinical presentation is heterogenous and changes over time (Rosenbaum et al., 2007). Motor speech impairments are neurologically based speech difficulties that arise from interference in the motor planning, motor control, or motor execution of speech (Shriberg & Strand, 2018) and are common in children with CP (Nordberg et al., 2013). The most common motor speech impairment in children with CP is dysarthria; up to 78% of children with CP present with difficulties in speech-motor control or execution of movements (Mahr et al., 2020; Shriberg & Strand,

2018). When this is the case, they experience weakness, spasticity, or the inability to control the muscles in and around the oral cavity that allow them to produce speech. For a child with dysarthria secondary to CP, producing speech sounds is difficult because their muscles do not move as far, as quickly, or as strongly. Children with dysarthria might also have a hoarse, soft, or even strained voice or slurred or slow speech (Shriberg & Strand, 2018).

Children with dysarthria secondary to CP have difficulty producing speech sounds, poor speech intelligibility, and, subsequently, low communicative participation (Korkalainen et al., 2023). It is important to consider these issues and address them with the child and their family. We need to be aware of the weakness or the spasticity with which the child is dealing and consider the possible inability of the child to control the muscles they need to produce speech. We should discuss and consider AAC options for children with CP who struggle to produce speech sounds and have difficulty communicating their needs and wants.

We can support families by providing them with information and facilitating the children's communication through any possible means and modalities. We continue our discussion regarding children with CP in Chapter 12, where we discuss additional opportunities to ensure we are engaging in best practices in EI with this population.

Cleft Lip and Cleft Palate

Infants and toddlers with a *cleft lip* or *cleft palate* often present specific challenges in speech sound development and production (Scherer, 1999). A recent study by Lane and colleagues (2022), in which the researchers systematically reviewed the efficacy of IE speech-specific interventions for children with cleft palate, resulted in mixed findings. They determined naturalistic and routines-based approaches, including milieu strategies, led to the children's growth in the use of consonants and phonemic inventories. Several studies also reported significant positive outcomes when parents and caregivers were trained by SLPs to use strategies that addressed specific sounds within their everyday activities and routines. Overall, however, the findings were inconclusive regarding specific strategies that focused on speech sound development, either before or after surgery, and their impact on the children's long-term articulation, phonology, and intelligibility (Lane et al., 2022). We should, therefore, engage in and coach families to implement treatment strategies in the natural environment that focus on the overall communication and language development of these children, but there are several additional considerations we need to address with these children.

Prior to a child's lip or palate repair, it is often difficult for a child with a cleft to learn to produce sounds that require air pressure to build up in the mouth (i.e., /p/, /b/, /d/). We need to be sure they hear these sounds frequently, though, as they are still learning them and will begin to use them after their palate surgery. Before a palate repair, we need to work with the families to help their children learn to produce sounds by using their lips and tongue (Scherer, 1999). We do not want to encourage the child to learn to use their throat to make sounds (e.g., grunting); we also want to avoid encouraging or facilitating the infant or young toddler's use of "rough sounds" (e.g., truck noises or gruff animal sounds). Although it is normal for children to use some throat sounds, especially as infants, children with cleft palates could get into a habit of using these sounds too often as they get older; this can then make it more difficult for them to learn new sounds in words (Scherer, 1999). Instead, we want to encourage the infant or young toddler to use sounds that they are producing successfully. These sounds tend to include those that do not require the palate to work yet (e.g., m, n, w, y, and h). If, when we are working with young children with a cleft lip or palate, they are making a lot of grunting or throat sounds, we should reinforce their attempt to vocalize and model a different sound or the true word for the child. For example, if the child says "uh" for "truck," we can respond with "Yes! Truck!" Regardless of their productions, we need to coach families to consistently praise their children for using sounds and words to communicate and to provide models for the words they can functionally use in their everyday play, activities, and routines. In Chapter 12, we revisit children with cleft lip and palate and discuss additional considerations for providing best practices in EI to this special population and their families.

Submucosal Cleft Palate

The *submucosal cleft palate* is a type of cleft palate about which we should be aware. It results from a congenital condition associated with abnormal development in muscle tissue of the soft palate (Gilleard et al., 2014). In comparison to a complete or incomplete cleft palate, a submucosal cleft palate is characterized by the disconnected muscle tissue and unbroken lining only in the middle of the soft palate (Reiter et al., 2011). Young children with a submucosal cleft palate might present hypernasal speech from velopharyngeal insufficiency (VPI), as well as otitis media and hearing loss from the malfunction of the Eustachian tube and a bifid uvula. Hypernasality is the most common symptom of VPI, and it accounts for approximately 50% of individuals with a submucous cleft palate (Reiter et al., 2011). Our nasal and oral cavities are completely separated from one another while speaking, swallowing, blowing, and vomiting by closing off the velopharynx. Velopharyngeal closure is a particularly important part of our physiology in producing pressure-sensitive sounds (Ko, 2018). For those children with a submucosal cleft, abnormal muscle development within the soft palate often leads to abnormal velopharyngeal closure; the result is hypernasality and unintelligible speech, often characterized by substitutions of nasal sounds for all other sound productions.

As SLPs in EI, we are often the first providers to recognize a child who presents the signs and symptoms of a submucosal cleft, VPI, or both. If we observe these characteristics when assessing or working with a young child, our first step is to communicate our concerns with the family and refer them to a medical professional for further evaluation. On diagnosis, surgical intervention will be considered in combination with continued speech therapy. Submucosal cleft palate tends to be diagnosed late; our role in early diagnosis is important as the palate can and should be repaired at an early age to support improved outcomes in speech and hearing (Reiter et al., 2011).

Addressing Speech Sound Development Within Early Intervention Services

Because speech sounds are still developing and phonological processes are still expected in children under the age of 3, we know we should not be addressing speech sound development as a disorder. Despite current clinical practices and the associated rationale regarding limited intervention for speech sound productions prior to the age of 3, there is empirical evidence to support embedding speech sound production when we implement treatment and coach families in EI. Parents and SLPs reported that young children who are unintelligible have difficulty participating in many everyday activities that involve engaging in conversations, relating to others, focusing their attention, handling stress, and learning (McCormack et al., 2010). Additionally, EI has been associated with positive outcomes when speech sound productions are embedded in intervention for toddlers (Girolametto et al., 1997; Munro et al., 2021); therefore, it stands to reason that when a family is concerned about their child's articulation, phonology, or intelligibility, we can engage in evidence-based best practices by strategically embedding speech sounds within their IFSP outcomes and incorporating them within a young child's everyday activities, play, and routines.

Incorporating Speech Sound Development in IFSP Outcomes

When we work with young children who are struggling to communicate, they certainly need to be able to produce sounds to produce words. We can address children's ability to obtain their needs and wants by working with parents and caregivers to determine specific words the children can use to label desired objects or to make verbal choices. To request a drink, ask for more, or label the boots a child wants to wear to play in the snow, the child must be able to produce an approximation of the words: "milk," "more," and "boots." The outcome itself is not to produce the /m/ or /b/ sounds; however, the production of these sounds can be embedded into the child's activities and routines to facilitate their development.

How do we embed speech sound development into our outcomes? How do we effectively incorporate speech sounds into EI in a natural, engaging way that also addresses the child's functional outcomes with our families? By focusing on the strengths, needs, and priorities of the families with whom we work, we can easily provide best practices by coaching families to facilitate speech-sound development within (rather than separate from) outcomes and activities that target functional communication by and with the child.

Embedding Specific Words in Outcomes

Literature addressing intervention for speech sound production in children under 3 years old suggests that by focusing on words with specific characteristics, children can improve their speech sound production skills while directly targeting their language skills (Scherer, 1999; Storkel, 2018). Therefore, an effective strategy is to embed single words from different semantic categories, such as nouns, verbs, prepositions, and adjectives, into the IFSP outcomes to facilitate the child's expression of different ideas. How we select the target words should be based on typical vocabulary development, as well as a child's interests, the family's priorities, and everyday opportunities in which they can use and practice these words. We want to choose vocabulary that can be naturally embedded by the family into their everyday routines and activities.

We tend to begin with nouns. Nouns are considered words of substance because we can choose those that are concrete in nature and represent specific objects or people. These target words could include names of favorite toys, desired foods, family member names, or even pets. Other words we want to consider as targets include *relational* terms; these words express a relationship with a noun and tend to express a variety of meanings. They could include verbs, adjectives, and prepositions (Storkel, 2018). We might also choose several relational terms when addressing an infant's or toddler's communication skills. It is important to include one or two relational words in our outcomes and as targets of intervention when we are trying to expand a child's ability to express a variety of intentions and to help a child eventually prepare for the transition to two- to three-word combinations. Relational words express a variety of meanings and include the following (Storkel, 2018):

- Action words are essentially verbs such as "eat," or "open," or "help."

- Descriptive words include adjectives such as "hot," "wet," and "dirty."

- Common location terms include "up" and "in."

- Recurrence terms, or words that express the reappearance of an object or repetition of an event; "more" is a word that can be used within multiple activities and routines by both children and their parents or caregivers.

- Rejection and denial words might include the word "no" and nonexistence or disappearance words or phrases like "all done" and "all gone."

- We also often think of the word "mine" when considering a relational word of possession.

Although we want to provide children with a variety of options, we also need to limit the number of target words we include within the IFSP outcomes. We should work with parents and caregivers to be intentional about which words we want to target first to ensure children are exposed to fewer words more frequently while reducing the demand on their language processing system. In addition to a handful of nouns embedded in the child's outcomes, we might focus on including two to three action words. As is the case with relational words, action words tend to play an important role in a child's ability to transition from single-word utterances to short phrases and early sentences.

Examples of Embedded Speech Sounds in Outcomes and Intervention

Speech sound development and production can easily be embedded into our services to ensure the development of articulation and phonology are naturally supported within interactions with the family and the child's everyday activities and routines. Table 10–4 offers examples of two children for whom we can support their intelligibility, and overall communication skills, by embedding speech sound development within language-based outcomes.

Table 10–4. Examples of Embedded Speech Sounds in Outcomes and Intervention

Child 1: Olive

Concern

Olive points to pictures in a book and tries to imitate the words sometimes. According to her mother, she is very hard to understand and gets mad when others don't understand her.

Outcome

During evening reading time every night for 1 week, Olive will name 5 to 10 pictures in a book using sounds her parents can understand.

Embedding Speech Sounds
- Her mother will use wait time when asking Olive what something is or when giving her a choice (i.e., "Is this a puppy or a kitty") while reading.
- Her mother will repeat what Olive says, provide her with the correct model, and reinforce her for responding.
- Her mother will make matching sounds as appropriate. She will also look for opportunities to reinforce the same words when playing with toys, eating, or playing outside.

Child 2: August

Concern

August attends his child-care center every day; he is very social and loves playing with his peers. The teachers report that other children have difficulty understanding him and often choose to play with other peers, leaving August to play by himself.

Outcome

August will use words his peers can understand during playtime with blocks at his child-care center each day for 3 consecutive days. We will know he can do this when the children he is playing with understand what he is saying without August having to show them what he wants or means.

> **Embedding Speech Sounds**
> - The SLP will visit the child-care center and talk with the teacher about this goal. The teacher will model the sounds and words August says during block play, including "block," "bang," "build," "more," and "mine," and repeat them several times to provide him with multiple models. She will encourage his peers to participate by providing August with models as well. The teacher will reinforce words by giving August verbal choices during play.

Embedding Speech Sound Development in Treatment

There is no doubt the evidence supports our services in natural environments to ensure authentic learning experiences are provided for the child and promote successful communication with the caregivers. We want to be sure the functional communication skills we are coaching families to address are generalized within their natural, everyday contexts. For a child to process information, it needs to be presented within a normal, naturally occurring event or opportunity in their own environment. Using flashcards to teach sounds or words or creating superficial teaching opportunities like pushing the child to imitate specific sounds in isolation (e.g., "Say /ba/") is not going to work. For most children, when functional language and communication needs are addressed within the natural environment, their speech will develop as well (ASHA, 2008; Edwards et al., 2011; Stoel-Gammon, 2011; Vihman, 2017).

To ensure we are providing best practices in EI, as we have learned about throughout the previous chapters in this textbook, we also need to embed speech sound development into the routines and everyday activities of the families. We can use the evidence-based treatment strategies presented in Chapter 9 to embed speech sound development and production in our sessions with families. We need to consider acknowledging with parents and caregivers that these strategies might feel uncomfortable at first; they might not feel natural or easy when we first encourage a family to use these approaches.

Self-Talk

The strategy of self-talk is all about encouraging parents or caregivers to talk about what they are doing when they are around their child. We can encourage them to pair their words with their actions. This strategy helps build the child's language while targeting specific sounds and can be incorporated into every setting and situation.

For example, we can coach the parents to engage in self-talk when they are making a snack for the children. The grandparents (i.e., Pawpaw and Mawmaw) are coming to visit, and they want to work on the child's use of the /m/ and /p/ sounds; the parent might verbalize: "I am making pancakes. I need to put more milk in the batter." The parent can model, stress, and repeat the /p/, /m/, and /b/ within the context of the words embedded within the activity itself. In this example, we also want to encourage the inclusion of the target words in their self-talk. If they want to encourage the child's use of these sounds in their attempts to say their grandparents' names, we should coach the parents to name Pawpaw and Mawmaw as well: "Pawpaw and Mawmaw are going to love these pancakes when they visit!"

Parallel Talk

As we learned in Chapter 9, parallel talk is similar to self-talk; in this case, however, we provide a running commentary about what the child is doing and saying. Consider yourself a sports announcer, describing each action the child is doing. For example, if the child is playing with toy cars while he is pushing, you might say, "Oh, Caleb is playing with the car. You are pushing the car! P-p-push! Push the red car! Oh, it crashed into the purple truck. Oops!" The concept is to let the child know we are aware of his actions and intentions while intentionally embedding a speech sound (e.g., /p/) to encourage the child's verbalizations.

Self-talk and parallel talk are also complementary approaches. We often find ourselves using both strategies within the same routine or activity. When we coach the caregivers and parents to include multiple strategies when engaged with their child within their routines and activities, we present additional opportunities for repetition and generalization of skills between EI sessions.

Wait…and Then Prompt

This is probably the simplest concept to understand and the most difficult to apply. We all tend to layer question upon question and often forget to give children the time they need to process and respond on their own. When we do not provide a young child with the chance to process information, we limit their opportunities to practice and develop their communication development. This strategy requires us, as adults, to be patient when waiting for a child to respond to our requests or questions. A good rule of thumb is to wait between 5 and 10 seconds after asking a question or making a request.

We can encourage parents and caregivers to implement wait time by reminding them that by pausing and providing additional time, they are letting their children know they care about what they have to say. We are also supporting an opportunity to engage in a more functional turn-taking exchange, which ultimately leads to conversation. For example, we ask a child the question: "Where is your car going?" while playing with race cars. We then wait for at least 5 seconds before repeating our question or adding a comment. By waiting, we have allowed the child time to attend to the actions in which they are involved and to consider what we are contributing to the interaction; we have given the child time to process the information they have heard that they might later use themselves.

Modeling With Natural Prompts

Children learn well through imitation; modeling is all about the demonstration of a behavior or skill and the expectation that someone will imitate the presented model. We can use modeling in a variety of ways. We might demonstrate how to accurately produce a sound in a word that the child is having difficulty saying, or we might model what to say to facilitate a response when a child is attempting to ask for a desired object.

In addition to modeling language or communication skills, we could take the opportunity to add a *natural prompt* to encourage the child to imitate sounds and words as well. Once we have the child's attention, based on the self-talk and parallel talk a parent has been providing, we can begin to prompt the child to imitate us. We will want to prompt a young child in the most natural way possible.

As always, we want to coach the families to embed this strategy within an everyday conversation or turn-taking routine. As such, we should encourage the parents or caregivers to avoid using "You say _____." Instead, coach them to prompt with "Tell me____," or "Show me___," or by providing the model of the sound or word before asking a direct question. For example, if we are spending time with a grandmother who is making cookies with her grandchild, we might coach the grandmother to model, "We are making cookies. ... What are we making?" If the child does not respond, remind the grandmother to wait 5 to 10 s and then prompt with "Cookies! Yum! Tell me cookies!" During a shared snack experience, we can model and prompt the child with "I need a spoon. What do you need?" If the child does not respond after 10 seconds, we can prompt again with "Tell me, spoon," while holding the spoon up in front of them.

Modeling is often a strategy in which parents and caregivers are already engaging; they just might not realize how effectively they are already doing it. When we coach families to incorporate and add natural prompts, we are supporting them to interact with their children in a way that is fun, engaging, and natural.

Expanding and Recasting

We waited to see what the child wants to do and what they might have to say. We have commented, through self-talk and parallel talk, modeled, and prompted. Now, we want to follow the child's lead and imitate their actions, sounds, and words. We want to coach the parents and caregivers to do the same. Once the family has their child's attention, they should continue to imitate the child's actions, gestures, signs, and sounds and then expand on them. If the child uses a gesture (e.g., pointing) to request an object, the parent should imitate the gesture and expand on it with the associated word before giving the child the desired object. If the child makes a sound, we can coach the parent or caregiver to imitate the sound and then expand it with either a reduplication or an extension into a word (e.g., turn the raspberry sound into a funny, repeated speech sound with a silly facial expression; imitate the car sound multiple times and then verbalize "Go!"). If the child simply engages in a play action, imitate the action and expand on the play with a representative sound or word (e.g., as the child stirs a pot, the parent stirs a pot, smells it, and says "Mmmmm" or "Yum").

Recasting is a strategy we use to gently correct a child's speech or language. Young children tend to respond to their parents or caregivers when provided with feedback on how to correctly say a certain sound, word, or even phrase. It is important, however, to coach the family members to present this feedback in a gentle, embedded manner. When we use this strategy, we respond with a correct speech or language model in a way that encourages the child to continue communicating while also learning and developing their speech sound productions or language skills. For example, if a child says, "I want to pay" (instead of "play"), we might respond with, "Oh, you want to play? Yay! Let's play!" The accurate sound productions have been restated (or recast) so the child hears the correct form; although corrected, we have presented the accurate model in a natural and positive way. By directly correcting a child who is still developing speech sounds, we might inadvertently halt the learning process, stop the conversation, or even take the fun out of communicating (ASHA, 2008; Owens, 2019; Weitzman, 2017).

Summary

We have reviewed empirical data regarding the development of speech sounds, phonological processes, and intelligibility for young children. We have also discussed characteristics of speech sound development that merit further consideration, as well as considerations of special populations for whom speech sound development follows a different path. Based on this information, we now have a stronger understanding of our expectations and best practices for evaluation, assessment, and diagnosis when working with infants and toddlers in EI. We also have a better appreciation for and knowledge about how to support families when they come to us with concerns about their child's speech. This chapter presented information and examples of appropriate and functional IFSP outcomes, as well as the most effective ways to incorporate speech sound development within our practice to address these concerns. We also revisited the treatment strategies presented in Chapter 9 and discussed how and when to use these to facilitate and embed natural speech sound development opportunities into the everyday activities and routines of the children and families we serve in EI.

Critical Thinking Questions

1. What are the definitions of articulation, phonology, and intelligibility?

2. Define and differentiate between speech sound disorders, articulation disorders, and phonological disorders.

3. Why is it important we are familiar with the evidence-based developmental expectations of articulation, phonology, and intelligibility of young children?

4. How does the current data related to referral and diagnosis of speech sound development and disorders in infants and toddlers inform our practice in EI?

5. What and how should we assess in regard to speech sound development when working in EI with infants and toddlers?

6. List the patterns (i.e., red flags) indicative of speech sound production difficulties in early childhood. Why is it important we are aware of and monitor for these patterns in EI?

7. Based on the evidence, what are the best practices in regard to differential diagnosis of speech sound disorders, including childhood apraxia of speech, in EI?

8. Describe the speech-related needs of young children with cerebral palsy or cleft lip and cleft palate.

9. How can we effectively embed speech sound development in EI treatment? Why might we incorporate these strategies into our intervention practices?

Case Study and Critical Thinking Questions

Caleb is 25 months old. His parents contacted their local EI intake coordinator when they were concerned about his intelligibility and inability to effectively communicate his needs or wants. They reported that he uses approximately 15 words but "talks in such a garbled manner" that both parents and Caleb's older siblings become frustrated when they do not know what he is saying or requesting. When asked to describe Caleb's speech, his father noted that it sounds like: "babble-babble-babble-mama-babble-babble-babble as if he knows he should be talking in longer sentences, but he doesn't have the vocabulary yet to form the actual sentence". His mother added that he sometimes sounds like he is humming around his words: "mmmmmmm-ball-mmmmm." Caleb loves playing with balls. His family often takes an extra ball with them to Caleb's brother's soccer practice. While his brother practices, Caleb and his Dad kick the ball. According to Caleb's parents, they find his speech particularly frustrating before mealtimes; they shared that he loves to help them choose and prepare food for snack time every day but that they often do not understand which foods and/or drinks he is requesting or suggesting.

1. What other authentic learning opportunities might you use to facilitate Caleb's expressive language development during snack time and ball play during his brother's soccer practice?

2. What are some other ways in which you can help Caleb's family incorporate naturally occurring opportunities to embed speech sound development into these experiences along the way?

References

American Speech-Language-Hearing Association. (2007). *Childhood apraxia of speech* [Technical report]. https://www.asha.org/practice-portal/clinical-topics/childhood-apraxia-of-speech/

American Speech-Language-Hearing Association. (2008). *Core knowledge and skills in early intervention speech-language pathology practice.* https://doi.org/10.1044/policy.KS2008-00292

American Speech-Language and Hearing Association. (2023a). *Childhood apraxia of speech.* https://www.asha.org/practice-portal/clinical-topics/childhood-apraxia-of-speech/

American Speech-Language and Hearing Association. (2023b). *Speech sound disorders—Articulation and phonology.* https://www.asha.org/practice-portal/clinical-topics/articulation-and-phonology/

Ball, M., & Kent, R. (Eds.). (2007). *The new phonologies: Developments in clinical linguistics.* Singular Publishing Group, Inc.

Bashina, V. M., Simashkova, N. V., Grachev, V. V., & Gorbachevskaya, N. L. (2002). Speech and motor disturbances in Rett syndrome. *Neuroscience and Behavioral*

Physiology, 32, 323–327.

Bowen, C. (2014). *Intervention approaches*. In C. Bowen (Ed.), Children's speech sound disorders 2nd ed. (pp. 174–226). Wiley. https://doi.org/10.1002/9781119180418.ch4

Broomfield, J., & Dodd, B. (2004a). Children with speech and language disability: Caseload characteristics. *International Journal of Language & Communication Disorders, 39*(3), 303–324. https://doi.org/10.1080/13682820310001625589

Brumbaugh, K. M., & Smit, A. B. (2013). Treating children ages 3–6 who have speech sound disorder: A survey. *Language, Speech, and Hearing Services in Schools, 44*(3), 306–319. https://doi.org/10.1044/0161-1461(2013/12-0029)

Chenausky, K., Kernbach, J., Norton A., & Schlaug, G. (2017). White matter integrity and treatment-based change in speech performance in minimally verbal children with autism spectrum disorder. *Frontiers in Human Neuroscience, 11*, 1-9. 10.3389/fnhum.2017.00175

Crais, E. (2011). Testing and beyond: Strategies and tools for evaluating and assessing infants and toddlers. *Language, Speech, and Hearing Services in Schools, 42*, 341–364.

Crowe, K., & McLeod, S. (2020). Children's English consonant acquisition in the United States: A review. *American Journal of Speech-Language Pathology, 29*(4), 2155–2169. https://doi.org/10.1044/2020_AJSLP-19-00168

DeVeney, S. L., & Peterkin, K. (2022). Facing a clinical challenge: Limited empirical support for toddler speech sound production intervention approaches. *Language, Speech, and Hearing Services in Schools, 53*(3), 659-674. https://doi.org/10.1044/2022_LSHSS-21-00104

Edwards, J., Munson, B., & Beckman, M. E. (2011). Lexicon-phonology relationships and dynamics of early language development—A commentary on Stoel-Gammon's "Relationships between lexical and phonological development in young children." *Journal of Child Language, 38*(1), 35–40. https://doi.org/10.1017/s0305000910000450

Gilleard, O., Sell, D., Ghanem, A. M., Tavsanoglu, Y., Birch, M., & Sommerlad, B. (2014). Submucous cleft palate: A systematic review of surgical management based on perceptual and instrumental analysis. *Cleft Palate Craniofacial Journal, 51*, 686–695. https://doi:10.1597/13-046

Girolametto, L., Pearce, P. S., & Weitzman, E. (1997). Effects of lexical intervention on the phonology of late talkers. *Journal of Speech, Language, and Hearing Research, 40*(2), 338–348. https://doi.org/10.1044/jslhr.4002.338

Hustad, K. C., Mahr, T. J., Natzke, P., & Rathouz, P. J. (2021). Speech development between 30 and 119 months in typical children I: Intelligibility growth curves for single-word and multiword productions. *Journal of Speech, Language and Hearing Research, 64*(4), 3707–3719. https://doi.org/10.1044/2021_JSLHR-21-00142

Ireland, M., & Conrad, B. J. (2016). Evaluation and eligibility for speech-language services in schools. *Perspectives of the ASHA Special Interest Groups, 1*(16), 78–90. https://doi.org/10.1044/persp1.SIG16.78

Ireland, M., McLeod, S., Farquharson, K., & Crowe, K. (2020). Evaluating children in U.S. public schools with speech sound disorders: Considering federal and state laws, guidance, and research. *Topics in Language Disorders, 40*(4), 326–340. https://doi.org/10.1097/TLD.0000000000000226

Ko, S. O. (2018). Management of velopharyngeal dysfunction: What is the role of oral and maxillofacial surgeons? *Journal of the Korean Association of Oral Maxillofacial Surgery, 44*, 1–2. https://doi.org/10.5125/jkaoms.2018.44.1.1.

Korkalainen, J., McCabe, P., Smidt, A., & Morgan, C. (2023). Motor speech interventions for children with cerebral palsy: A systematic review. *Journal of Speech, Language, and Hearing Research, 66*, 110–125. https://doi.org/10.1044/2022_JSLHR-22-00375

Lane, H., Harding, S. A., & Wren, Y. E. (2022). A systematic review of early speech interventions for children with cleft palate. *International Journal of Language and Communication Disorders, 57*(1), 226–245. https://doi.org/10.1111/1460-6984.12683

Levey, S. (2014). *Introduction to language development.* Plural Publishing.

Mahr, T. J., Rathouz, P. J., & Hustad, K. C. (2020). Longitudinal growth in intelligibility of connected speech from 2 to 8 years in children with cerebral palsy: A novel Bayesian approach. *Journal of Speech, Language, and Hearing Research, 63*(9), 2880–2893. https://doi.org/10.1044/2020_jslhr-20-00181

McCormack, J., McLeod, S., Harrison, L. J., & McAllister, L. (2010). The impact of speech impairment in early childhood: Investigating parents' and speech-language pathologists' perspectives using the ICF-CY. *Journal of Communication Disorders, 43*(5), 378–396. https://doi.org/10.1016/j.jcomdis.2010.04.009

McLeod, S., & Baker, E. (2014). Speech-language pathologists' practices regarding assessment, analysis, target selection, intervention, and service delivery for children with speech sound disorders. *Clinical Linguistics & Phonetics, 28*(7–8), 508–531. https://doi.org/10.3109/02699206.2014.926994

McLeod, S., & Crowe, K. (2018). Children's consonant acquisition in 27 languages: A cross-linguistic review. *American Journal of Speech-Language Pathology, 27*, 1546–1571. https://doi.org/10.1044/2018_AJSLP-17-0100

McLeod, S., Verdon, S., Bowen, C., & International Expert Panel on Multilingual Children's

Speech. (2013). International aspirations for speech-language pathologists' practice with multilingual children with speech sound disorders: Development of a position paper. *Journal of Communication Disorders, 46*(4), 375–387. https://doi.org/10.1016/j.jcomdis.2013.04.003

Munro, N., Baker, E., Masso, S., Carson, L., Lee, T., Wong, A. M.-Y., & Stokes, S. F. (2021). Vocabulary acquisition and usage for late talkers treatment: Effect on expressive vocabulary and phonology. *Journal of Speech, Language, and Hearing Research, 64*(7), 2682–2697. https://doi.org/10.1044/2021_JSLHR-20-00680

Nordberg, A., Miniscalco, C., Lohmander, A., & Himmelmann, K. (2013). Speech problems affect more than one in two children with cerebral palsy: Swedish population-based study. *Acta Paediatrica, 102*(2), 161–166. https://doi.org/10.1111/apa.12076

Olswang, L., Stoel-Gammon, C., Coggins, T., & Carpenter, R. (1987). *Assessing prelinguistic and early linguistic behaviors in developmentally young children.* University of Washington Press.

Overby, M., & Caspari, S. (2012, November). *Early phonetic and phonological characteristics of childhood apraxia of speech* [Paper presentation]. Annual Convention of the American Speech-Language Association, Atlanta, GA.

Overby, M., & Caspari, S. (2013, November). *Phonological development of children with CAS: Birth to 24 months* [Paper presentation]. Annual Convention of the American Speech-Language Association, Chicago, IL.

Owens, R. (2019). *Language development: An introduction* (10th ed.). Pearson Education.

Paul, R. (2007). *Language disorders from infancy through adolescence: Assessment and intervention* (3rd ed.). Mosby.

Porter, J. H., & Hodson, B. W. (2001). Collaborating to obtain phonological acquisition data for local schools. *Language, Speech, and Hearing Services in Schools, 32*(3), 165–171. https://doi.org/10.1044/0161-1461%282001/015%29

Raver, S. A., & Childress, D. C. (2015). *Family-centered EI: Supporting infants and toddlers in natural environments.* Brookes.

Reiter, R., Brosch, S., Wefel, H., Schlömer, G., & Haase, S. (2011). The submucous cleft palate: Diagnosis and therapy. *International Journal of Pediatric Otorhinolaryngology, 75*(1), 85–88. https://doi.org/10.1016/j.ijporl.2010.10.015

Rosenbaum, P., Paneth, N., Leviton, A., Goldstein, M., Bax, M., Damiano, D., … Jacobsson, B. (2007). A report: The definition and classification of cerebral palsy. *Developmental Medicine & Child Neurology, 49*(Suppl. 109), 8–14. https://doi.org/10.1111/j.1469-8749.2007.tb12610.x

Rossetti, L. M. (2005). *The Rossetti Infant Toddler Language Scale: A measure of communication and interaction.* Linguisystems.

Scherer, N. J. (1999). The speech and language status of toddlers with cleft lip and/or palate following early vocabulary intervention. *American Journal of Speech-Language Pathology, 8*, 81–93.

Shriberg, L. D., Kwiatkowski, J., & Mabie, H. (2019). Estimates of the prevalence of motor speech disorders in children with idiopathic speech delay. *Clinical Linguistics & Phonetics, 33*(8), 679–706. https://doi:10.1080/02699206.2019.1595731

Shriberg, L., & Strand, E. A. (2018). *Speech and motor speech characteristics of a consensus group of 28 children with childhood apraxia of speech* (Tech. Rep. No. 25). https://waismanphonology.wiscweb.wisc.edu/wp-content/uploads/sites/532/2018/05/TREP25.pdf

Sosa, A. V. (2011). *Too young to test? Assessing phonology in infants and toddlers* [Oral presentation]. Arizona Speech-Language-Hearing Association Annual Convention, Tempe, AZ.

Stoel-Gammon, C. (2011). Relationships between lexical and phonological development in young children. *Journal of Child Language, 38*(1), 1–34. https://doi.org/10.1017/s0305000910000425

Storkel, H. L. (2018). Implementing evidence-based practice: Selecting treatment words to boost phonological learning. *Language, Speech, and Hearing Services in the Schools, 49*(3), 1–15. https://doi:10.1044/2017_LSHSS-17-0080

Storkel, H. L. (2019). Using developmental norms for speech sounds as a means of determining treatment eligibility in schools. *Perspectives of the ASHA Special Interest Groups, 4*(1), 67–75. https://doi.org/10.1044/2018_PERS-SIG1-2018-0014

Tshering Pema, W. (2016). Childhood apraxia of speech (CAS) – Overview and teaching strategies. *European Journal of Special Education Research, 0*. https://doi.org/10.46827/ejse.voio.15

To, C. K. S., McLeod, S., Sam, K. L., & Law. T. (2022). Predicting which children will normalize without intervention for speech sound disorders. *Journal of Speech, Language, and Hearing Research, 65*, 1724–1741.

Weitzman, E. (2017). *It takes two to talk: A practical guide for parents of children with language delays*. The Hanen Centre.

Vihman, M. M. (2017). Learning words and learning sounds: Advances in language development. *British Journal of Psychology, 108*(1), 1–27. https://doi.org/10.1111/bjop.12207

Chapter 11

Feeding and Swallowing Assessment and Intervention

Learning Outcomes

When we have completed this chapter, we will be able to:

- Describe basic definitions, physiological processes, and development milestones associated with and necessary for safe and engaging feeding and swallowing in infants and toddlers.

- Identify the signs, symptoms, and causes of feeding and swallowing disorders in young children.

- Present our scope of practice as SLPs related to feeding difficulties and dysphagia in EI.

- List our roles and responsibilities, as members of an interprofessional team, in evaluating, assessing, and providing evidence-based intervention in the areas of feeding and swallowing.

- Describe how the evidence-based, guiding practices of EI are embedded into intervention focused on feeding and swallowing.

- Describe specific assessment protocols, goals and outcomes, and treatment strategies to address feeding and swallowing disorders with infants and toddlers.

- Explain how family-centered and routines-based behavioral strategies can be used to support and coach parents and caregivers who are concerned about their child's feeding development and skills.

What Will We Learn and How Can We Apply It?

As SLPs, we play an important role in the assessment, diagnosis, and treatment of infants and toddlers with feeding and swallowing disorders in EI. Our responsibilities in these areas include prevention, evaluation, planning, treatment, and advocacy services as we focus on the children's needs and the needs and priorities of their families. This chapter provides the basic information we need to feel confident in our ability to identify, assess, and treat feeding and swallowing disorders in EI. We begin with a review of basic definitions and processes, then move on to development milestones associated with as well as necessary for safe and engaging feeding and swallowing and the signs, symptoms, and causes of feeding and swallowing disorders in infants and toddlers. We focus our attention on our own scope of practice as SLPs attending to the needs of young children and families faced with feeding difficulties, dysphagia, or both. Next, we walk through our roles and responsibilities, as members of an interprofessional team, in evaluating, assessing, and providing evidence-based intervention in the areas of feeding and swallowing.

The evidence-based approaches we have been discussing throughout this text, which serve as the foundation of our EI services, can and should also be embedded into our practices when addressing the feeding and swallowing needs of young children and their families. We discuss what this looks like within the context of these areas as well, before diving into specific treatment strategies to target feeding and swallowing disorders with infants and toddlers. Finally, family-centered and routines-based behavioral strategies are offered to ensure we have a set of straightforward techniques to share with parents and caregivers who are concerned about their child's feeding development and skills.

Introduction to Feeding and Swallowing

Before diving into our roles and responsibilities related to assessment and treatment of feeding and swallowing disorders in EI, we must first have a clear understanding of the functions themselves. We begin with the basic definitions.

Feeding is the process involving any aspect of eating or drinking and includes the gathering and preparing of food and liquid for intake, sucking and/or chewing, and swallowing (Arvedson & Brodsky, 2002). *Swallowing* is a complex process during which saliva, liquids, and foods are transferred from the mouth to the stomach, all while the airway is protected. Swallowing is typically divided into the following four phases (Arvedson & Brodsky, 2002; ASHA, n.d.; Logemann, 1998):

- *Oral preparatory phase*: This volitional phase occurs when food or liquid is manipulated in the mouth to form a cohesive bolus; this process includes sucking liquids, manipulating soft boluses, and chewing solid food.

- *Oral transit phase*: This voluntary phase begins with the posterior thrust of the bolus by the tongue and ends with the initiation of the pharyngeal swallow.

- *Pharyngeal phase*: This phase begins with a voluntary pharyngeal swallow that pushes the bolus through the pharynx by way of an involuntary contraction of the pharyngeal constrictor muscles.

- *Esophageal phase*: This involuntary phase occurs when the bolus is carried to the stomach through the process of esophageal peristalsis.

Developmental Milestones and Skills Related to Feeding and Swallowing

The most complex sensorimotor process of a newborn is the coordination of sucking, swallowing, and breathing required for oral feeding (Arvedson, 2006). To successfully engage in this process and refine their skills, a young child's anatomy and physiology needed for eating, drinking, and swallowing safely must grow and mature in sequence. We introduced oral motor and feeding development in Chapter 5; here we look deeper into the details needed to assess and treat feeding and possible swallowing difficulties.

As infants and toddlers grow, the size and shape of their oral and pharyngeal structures change (ASHA, n.d.). In infancy, the tongue fills the oral cavity, and the velum hangs lower. The hyoid bone and the larynx are located higher than in adults, and the larynx elevates less than in adults during the pharyngeal phase of the swallow (Logemann, 1998). When the infant is breastfeeding or using a bottle, they use sequential swallowing (i.e., multiple swallows in rapid succession). Once they begin eating pureed food, each swallow is separate, and the oral and pharyngeal phases are similar to those of an adult. As young children mature, their intraoral space increases as the mandible grows down and forward; the oral cavity elongates. The space increases between the tongue and the palate while the larynx and the hyoid bone lower, ultimately elongating and enlarging the pharynx (Logemann, 1998).

In conjunction with the growth and maturation of their anatomy and physiology, infants and toddlers are expected to develop multiple feeding and oral sensorimotor skills in their first few years of life. In follow-up to the developmental expectations presented in Table 5–10, an expansion of the early developmental milestones, from birth to 36 months, necessary for safe and effective eating, drinking, and swallowing are shared in Table 11–1.

Table 11–1. Developmental Milestones That Support Feeding and Swallowing

Age	Oral Motor	Sensory	Motor & Postural Stability
At birth	• Reflexes that support eating are present: • Swallow reflex • Phasic bite reflex • Palmomental reflex • Transverse tongue reflex		• Sucking is automatic
2 months		• Rejects sour flavors	
2.5–3.5 months	• Transitions to volitional sucking instead of relying on reflex	• Detects flavor differences (e.g., increased suckling to new flavors)	• Achieves steady head control • Maintains a semiflexed (curled) posture during feeding

4–6 months	• Integration of rooting, palmomental, phasic bite reflexes (between 2–6 months) • Loss of neural network supporting sucking rhythms • Opens mouth when spoon approaches/ touches the lips • Uses tongue to move purees to back of mouth for swallow • Munching (up-and-down) jaw movements • Lateral (side-to-side) jaw movements • Diagonal jaw movements (beginning of a more mature rotary chew) • Lateral tongue movements (helps with eating efficiency)	• Preference for salty flavors emerges	• Begins hand-to-mouth play (independent oral exploration of objects) • Increased reaching skills • Reaches for bottle or spoon when hungry
6–7 months			• Trunk control is sufficient for independent sitting for more than 3–5 seconds • Stable head control in sitting (no

				head bobbing) • Transfers toys and food from one hand to the other • Holds bottle in both hands
7–8 months	• Brings upper lip down to draw food off of the spoon • Full lip closure emerges • Consistent tongue lateralization when foods are presented to sides of tongue • Active movement of foods from side of mouth to central tongue groove and back • Mature tongue lateralization emerges • Diagonal rotary movements			
8–10 months	• Circular rotary movements emerge • Transitions to slightly more texture (small bumps, fork mash, thicker purees) • With assistance, breaks off pieces of foods that melt in mouth			• Trunk rotation and weight shift • Begins to move in and out of positions • Voluntary release patterns emerge

	• Chews (by munching) softer food		• Uses fingers to rake food toward self • Puts finger in mouth to move food and keep it in • Cup drinking is introduced
10–12 months	• Licks food off of lips • Simple tongue protrusion may occur • More controlled biting; isolated from body movements • Full transfer of foods from side to side in mouth with tongue without difficulty • Rotary movements emerge		• Sits independently in a variety of positions • Pincer grasp is developing • Pokes food with index finger • Uses fingers to self-feed soft, chopped foods
12–14 months	• Chews and swallows firmer foods without choking • Chews foods that produce juice • Keeps most bites in mouth during chewing		• Cofeeds with a parent (i.e., parent feeds bites, child independently takes bites) • Grasps spoon with whole hand • Holds and tips bottle • Holds cup with two hands

Age	Oral/Chewing Skills		Self-Feeding Skills
14–16 months	<ul><li>Uses tongue to gather shattered pieces</li><li>Sweeps pieces into a bolus with the tongue</li><li>Chews bigger pieces of soft table foods</li><li>Working on chewing foods increasing in texture "hardness"</li></ul>		<ul><li>Finger feeding becomes efficient</li><li>Practices utensil use (vs. effective use for volume)</li></ul>
18–24 months	<ul><li>Working on increased speed and efficiency</li><li>Improved chewing strength</li><li>Better able to manage hard-to-chew foods</li></ul>		<ul><li>Picks up, dips, and brings foods to mouth</li><li>Increases utensil use (although not efficient until after 24 months of age)</li><li>Scoops purees with utensil and brings to mouth</li></ul>

24–36 months	<ul><li>Improved circulatory jaw movements</li><li>Chews with lips closed</li><li>Continues working on increased speed, strength, and efficiency with larger pieces of chewy table food</li></ul>		<ul><li>Uses fingers to fill spoon</li><li>Fork skills improve</li><li>Drinks with open cup without spilling</li><li>Holds cup with one hand</li></ul>

Note. Adapted from "Feeding behaviors and other motor development in healthy children (2-24 months)," by B. Caruth & J. Skinner, 2002; "Pediatric swallowing and feeding: Assessment and management," by J. Arvedson, L. Brodsky, & M. Lefton-Greif, 2020; "Swallowing and feeding in infants and young children," by J. Arvedson, 2002.

Feeding and Swallowing Disorders

From birth, infants eat by sucking. As they grow and develop, they learn how to eat solid foods and drink from a cup. This process involves the development and refinement of specific skills over time. Infants and toddlers might spill food and drinks from their mouths. They might push food back out or gag on new tastes and textures. Some of these behaviors are normal and should resolve over time. A young child with a feeding or swallowing disorder, however, will continue having difficulties and might have an especially hard time eating or drinking; they might refuse to eat foods, eat only certain foods, or take a long time to eat. They might continue to gag or choke on their food and drink (ASHA, n.d.).

A *feeding disorder* is the term we use to describe an issue with a range of eating activities that might or might not include difficulty with swallowing. According to Goday et al. (2019), pediatric feeding disorder (PFD) is "impaired oral intake that is not age-appropriate and is associated with medical, nutritional, feeding skill, and/or psychosocial dysfunction" (p. 129). According to Goday et al. (2019), PFD could be associated with oral sensory function and can be characterized by one or more of the following behaviors (Arvedson, 2008):

- Refusal of age-appropriate or developmentally appropriate foods or liquids.

- Acceptance of a restricted variety or quantity of foods or liquids.

- Disruptive or inappropriate behaviors at mealtime, based on developmental levels.

- Failure to master self-feeding skills expected for developmental levels.

- Failure to use developmentally appropriate feeding devices and utensils.

- Decreased growth according to expectations.

According to ASHA (n.d.), a *swallowing disorder*, also known in our field as *dysphagia*, can occur in one or more of the four phases of swallowing and can result in aspiration, in which food, liquid, or saliva passes into the trachea, or the retrograde flow of food into the nasal cavity. A young child can present with dysphagia at any one or more than one of the stages of swallowing. During the oral phase, they might have difficulty sucking, chewing, or moving food or liquid from the mouth into the throat. During the pharyngeal phase, they might have issues starting the swallow and squeezing food down their throat. Because the body needs to close off the airway to keep food or liquid out, food going into the airway typically results in coughing and choking. At the esophageal phase, the esophagus squeezes food down to the stomach; issues could involve food that gets stuck in the esophagus, or a child might throw up frequently during and after eating if there is a problem with the esophagus (ASHA, n.d.).

When infants or toddlers have feeding or swallowing disorders, they could experience multiple long-term consequences, including the following (ASHA, n.d.):

- Aspiration pneumonia or compromised pulmonary status.
- Dehydration.
- Food aversion.
- Gastrointestinal complications, such as motility disorders, constipation, and diarrhea.
- Ongoing need for gastrointestinal or intravenous nutrition.
- Oral aversion.
- Poor weight gain or undernutrition.
- Psychosocial effects on the child and the family.
- Undernutrition or malnutrition.
- Unintentional and reflexive regurgitation of undigested food (may include the rechewing and re-swallowing of food).

Avoidant/Restrictive Food Intake Disorder

According to the *Diagnostic and Statistical Manual of Mental Disorders* (5th ed.; American Psychiatric Association, 2016), Avoidant/Restrictive Food Intake Disorder (ARFID) is "an eating or feeding disturbance manifested by persistent failure to meet appropriate nutritional or energy needs associated with one (or more) of the following":

- Significant weight loss.
- Failure to achieve expected weight gain.
- Significant nutritional deficiency.
- Dependence on feeding or oral nutritional supplements.
- Considerable interference with psychosocial functioning.

ARFID could present as a supposed lack of interest in eating or in food, avoidance based on sensory characteristics of food, or concern about aversive consequences of eating (APA, 2016). As SLPs, we might screen or make referrals for ARFID; we do not, however, diagnose this disorder. ARFID presents differently than a PDF, as the diagnosis does not include children whose primary challenge is a skill deficit (e.g., dysphagia); additionally, the diagnosis requires that the severity of the eating difficulty exceeds the severity typically associated with another diagnosed condition (e.g., Down syndrome). The definition of ARFID also considers nutritional deficiency, whereas the diagnosis and definition of PFD does not take this variable into consideration (Goday et al., 2019). PFD and ARFID can exist separately or concurrently (APA, 2016; ASHA, n.d.).

Signs of Feeding and Swallowing Disorders

Signs of feeding and swallowing disorders in infants and toddlers vary, based on the phase or phases affected, and the child's age and developmental level. As SLPs, we need to be aware of these signs and be prepared to respond effectively. Table 11–2 presents the behaviors we might observe that indicate a child is presenting with a possible feeding or swallowing disorder.

Table 11–2. Signs and Symptoms of Possible Feeding or Swallowing Disorders

- Back arching.
- Change in breathing rate or breathing difficulties during feeding; these may be presented as
    - An increased respiratory rate (tachypnea).
    - Changes in the normal heart rate (bradycardia or tachycardia).
    - Skin color change (e.g., turning blue around the lips, nose, and fingers and toes).
    - Temporary cessation of breathing (apnea).
    - Frequent stopping due to an uncoordinated suck–swallow–breathe pattern.
    - Oxygen desaturation.
- Color change during or after feeding.
- Coughing.
- Choking.
- Congestion during or after feeding; noisy or wet vocal quality during and after eating.
- Crying during mealtimes.
- Decreased responsiveness during feeding.
- Delayed development of a mature swallowing or chewing pattern.
- Difficulty chewing foods that are texturally appropriate for age (might spit out, retain, or swallow partially chewed food).
- Difficulty coordinating sucking, swallowing, and breathing while bottle-feeding or drinking from a cup or straw.

- Difficulty initiating swallowing.
- Difficulty managing secretions (including non-teething-related drooling of saliva).
- Evidence of food or liquid in a tracheotomy tube during or after eating.
- Failure to gain weight.
- Frequent respiratory illnesses or history of pneumonia.
- Gagging.
- Lengthy feeding times (greater than 30 min).
- Limited intake of food or liquids.
- Refusal of foods of certain textures, brands, colors, or other distinguishing characteristics.
- Refusal of previously accepted food or liquids.
- Sensation of food being stuck in the throat.
- Stridor (i.e., noisy breathing, high-pitched sound) or stertor (i.e., noisy breathing, low-pitched sound, sounds like snoring).
- Taking only small amounts of food, overpacking the mouth, or pocketing foods.

Note. Adapted from "Feeding and swallowing," by J. Kisenwether in R. Owens, "Early language intervention for infants, toddlers, and preschoolers," 2018; "Pediatric feeding and swallowing," by the American Speech-Language and Hearing Association, n.d. (https://www.asha.org/practice-portal/clinical-topics/pediatric-feeding-and-swallowing/).

Causes of Feeding and Swallowing Disorders

As SLPs in EI, it is important we recognize and are also aware of the underlying etiologies associated with pediatric feeding and swallowing disorders. These could include complex medical conditions (e.g., heart disease, pulmonary disease, allergies, gastroesophageal reflux disease, delayed gastric emptying), genetic syndromes, developmental disability, neurological disorders, factors affecting neuromuscular coordination (e.g., prematurity, low birth weight, hypotonia, hypertonia), structural abnormalities (e.g., cleft lip or palate and other craniofacial abnormalities, laryngomalacia, tracheoesophageal fistula, esophageal atresia, choanal atresia, restrictive tethered oral tissues), and medication side effects (e.g., lethargy, decreased appetite) (Beckett et al., 2002; Johnson & Dole, 1999). Feeding and swallowing disorders could also be related to behavioral and socioemotional factors or sensory issues as a primary cause, or secondary to limited food availability when children are infants or toddlers (Beckett et al., 2002; Johnson & Dole, 1999).

Atypical eating and drinking behaviors can also develop in association with dysphagia, aspiration, or as a result of a choking event. These behaviors might also be associated with sensory disturbances (e.g., hypersensitivity to textures), stress reactions (e.g., consistent or repetitive gagging), traumatic events increasing anxiety, or undetected pain (e.g., teething, tonsillitis) (ASHA, n.d.).

Tethered Oral Tissues

Tethered oral tissues (TOTs) is a term we use to describe tight, restrictive connective tissue between oral structures. This connective tissue is called *frena*. We all have frena; when this tissue is thick, tight, and restrictive of typical movement, however, we label this as a *tie*. Lip ties, tongue ties, and buccal, or cheek, ties fall under the category of TOTs. These ties can negatively affect a young child's feeding skills, proper facial structure development, breathing, sleeping, and speech and language development (Merkel-Walsh & Overland, 2018; Zimmerman-Pine, 2018).

An infant or toddler with a TOT could face issues with eating, drinking, and swallowing safely. Tongue-ties can significantly affect the lateral, anterior, and posterior movements of the tongue. Infants who have difficulty latching or establishing a fluid suck–swallow–breath pattern, who make clicking sounds during breastfeeding, tongue hump, or cause their mothers significant nipple pain might have tongue-tie. Impeded tongue movement continues to negatively affect feeding skills later in life, as well, and can result in difficulty clearing the molars of residue, moving a bolus from side to side in the mouth during feeding, maintaining correct tongue posture during swallowing, and correct oral tongue posture at rest throughout the day. Lip-ties can also impair an infant's ability to establish a latch during breastfeeding. As children grow and develop, a lip-tie could affect their ability to seal their lips during feeding and swallowing and when their mouth is at rest. Lip-ties can also contribute to habitual mouth breathing. Buccal-ties can significantly impede an infant's ability to establish a solid latch during breastfeeding and clear food from their cheeks (Merkel-Walsh & Overland, 2018; Zimmerman-Pine, 2018).

As SLPs in EI, it is within our scope of practice to diagnose TOTs and evaluate their impact on feeding, swallowing, and even the speech production of the young children we serve. Once we have conducted the evaluation and determined a TOT might be affecting an infant or toddler's development, we need to refer the family to their pediatrician, specialized physician, dentist, or oral surgeon for further evaluation. TOTs are most often remediated with a frenectomy. This surgical procedure involves the cutting of the frenula tissue to increase structural mobility, and is also known as frenuloplasty, tongue-tie release, lip-tie release or buccal-tie release. Frenectomy is most often performed by a specialized physician (e.g., neonatologist; ear, nose, and throat specialist), dentist, or dental surgeon and can be performed with a laser or a scalpel. If we have the appropriate training, which could include specialization in orofacial myofunctional therapy, we can offer our young children and their families pre- and post-surgery intervention. This could include tissue stretches, as well as specific feeding positions and strategies with infants and toddlers (Merkel-Walsh & Overland, 2018; Zimmerman-Pine, 2018).

Incidence and Prevalence of Feeding and Swallowing Disorders With Infants and Toddlers

It is estimated that approximately 116,000 newborn infants are discharged from short hospital stays every year with a diagnosis of feeding difficulties (National Center for Health Statistics, 2010). Prevalence of feeding and swallowing disorders is estimated to be 30 percent to 80 percent for children with developmental disorders (Arvedson, 2008; Brackett et al., 2006; Lefton-Greif, 2008; Manikam & Perman, 2000). Oropharyngeal dysphagia or feeding dysfunction in children with CP is estimated to be 19.2 percent to 99.0 percent, and rates increase with greater severity of cognitive impairment and decline in gross motor function (Benfer et al., 2014, 2017; Calis et al., 2008; Erkin et al., 2010; Speyer et al., 2019). For children with autism spectrum disorders, the odds of having a feeding problem increase by two to five times when compared with children who do not have an autism spectrum disorder (Seiverling et al., 2018; Sharp et al., 2013). Rates of oral dysphagia in children with craniofacial disorders are estimated to be 33 to 83 percent (Caron et al., 2015; de Vries et al., 2014; Reid et al., 2006). Furthermore, silent aspiration is estimated to occur with 41 percent of children who have laryngeal cleft, 41 percent to 49 percent of children with laryngomalacia, and 54 percent of children who present with unilateral vocal fold paralysis (Jaffal et al., 2020; Velayutham et al., 2018).

We assume the incidence of feeding and swallowing disorders in young children continues to increase secondary to improved survival rates of children with complex and medically fragile conditions (Lefton-Greif, 2008; Lefton-Greif et al., 2006; Newman et al., 2001) and the improved longevity of infants and toddlers with dysphagia (Lefton-Greif et al., 2017). We should note these reports, reflecting incidence and prevalence of pediatric feeding and swallowing disorders, tend to vary widely due to multiple factors, including variations in the conditions and populations sampled, how pediatric feeding and swallowing disorders are defined, and the choice of assessment methods and measures used to diagnose them (Arvedson, 2008; Lefton-Greif, 2008).

Roles and Responsibilities of SLPs Regarding Feeding and Swallowing Disorders

According to ASHA (2016b), as SLPs serving young children with feeding and swallowing difficulties and disorders and their families, our roles vary and could include the following responsibilities:

- Sharing information and educating families of children at risk for pediatric feeding and swallowing disorders.

- Educating and collaborating with other professionals regarding the needs of children with feeding and swallowing disorders and our own role in diagnosis and management.

- Conducting comprehensive assessments, including clinical and instrumental evaluations as appropriate.

- Considering each family's culture, routines, and systems as they pertain to food choices, habits, perception of disabilities, and beliefs about intervention.

- Diagnosing pediatric oral and pharyngeal swallowing disorders (dysphagia).

- Referring the child to other professionals, as needed, to rule out other conditions, determine etiology, and facilitate child and family access to comprehensive services.

- Recommending and participating in the development of safe swallowing and feeding outcomes and plans for the IFSP.

- Educating children and families about how to prevent complications related to feeding and swallowing disorders.

- Serving as an essential member of an interprofessional feeding and swallowing team.

- Consulting and collaborating with colleagues, family members, caregivers, and others to facilitate the development of an intervention program and provide supervision, evaluation, or expert testimony, as appropriate.

- Staying abreast of current research in the area of pediatric feeding and swallowing disorders while helping to advance the knowledge base related to the nature and treatment of these disorders.

- Advocating for families and individuals with feeding and swallowing disorders at the local, state, and national levels.

In addition to our knowledge, skills, and experience specific to pediatric feeding and swallowing disorders, the ASHA Code of Ethics (ASHA, 2016a) clearly notes that those of us who serve the pediatric population should be specifically educated and appropriately trained to work with infants, toddlers, and their families. As such, we must have extensive knowledge of embryology, prenatal and perinatal development, medical issues common to preterm and medically fragile newborns, typical early infant development, neuroprotection, neonatal care, respiratory support, medical comorbidities common in the NICU, and the role of providers in the NICU (ASHA, 2016a). Although we do not cover these areas in depth, we touch on several throughout the remainder of this chapter.

Interprofessional Team Approach

We have learned how important collaboration within and among the interprofessional team is to providing effective, evidence-based EI services. The causes and consequences of feeding disorders and dysphagia with infants and toddlers tend to cross traditional boundaries between professional disciplines, and management of these issues could require the input of multiple specialists. As EI providers, we are not alone when providing services to young children with feeding and swallowing difficulties; it is often, however, our responsibility to coordinate the efforts of, and collaborate with our colleagues within an interprofessional team to ensure exceptional services are offered to families.

Because the severity and complexity of feeding and swallowing disorders vary widely with infants and toddlers, the team approach is necessary for appropriately diagnosing and managing these disorders (Goday et al., 2019; Henton, 2018; McComish et al., 2016). As SLPs, we play an integral role on the interprofessional team. We often serve as team coordinators when addressing the needs of a child with a feeding disorder or dysphagia. In many regions of the United States, however, OTs might also be recognized as having primary expertise in pediatric feeding disorders (Cohen & Dilfer, 2022); we tend to work closely with OTs when addressing this population and they could also serve as the team's coordinator in these cases.

In addition to the SLP and dependent on the etiology, nature, and needs of the child, an EI team that supports an infant or toddler with a feeding or swallowing disorder might include the following members:

- Developmental therapist.
- Family and caregivers.
- Hearing and vision specialists.
- Lactation consultant (when working with an infant).
- Mental health professional.
- Nurse.
- Occupational therapist.
- Physicians (i.e., pediatrician, neonatologist, otolaryngologist, gastroenterologist, dentist, psychologist, or psychiatrist).
- Physical therapist.
- Registered dietician.
- Service coordinator.
- Social worker.

As is the case with any interprofessional team in EI, open communication and strong collaboration among all members are imperative to ensure the child's and family's outcomes are met and their services are successful.

Impact of Feeding and Swallowing Disorders

Feeding and swallowing challenges in infants and toddlers tend to be complex and can significantly impact their nutrition, growth, health, development, psychosocial function, and overall well-being (Goday, Huh, & Silverman, 2019; Grantham-McGregor & Ani, 2001; Manikan & Perman, 2000). According to Cohen and Dilfer (2022), feeding and swallowing difficulties in early childhood might also lead to negative or even traumatic experiences associated with eating and drinking secondary to invasive medical testing or interventions and avoidance of or decreased engagement in food-related activities that support the development of a child's feeding skills or expansion of their diet. While decreased intake of specific nutrients might have an impact on long-term health outcomes (Sharp et al., 2013), nutritional deficits may contribute to gastrointestinal distress, irritability, poor regulation, and poor growth (Robea et al., 2020). Ultimately, these disorders might lead to:

- dehydration
- malnutrition
- poor weight gain
- respiratory problems

- aspiration
- food aversions

As SLPs working with young children with issues related to feeding and swallowing, we need to recognize these disorders have an impact on parents and caregivers as well and may also negatively affect relationships within the family (Cohen & Dilfer, 2022). Simione and colleagues (2020) conducted a study in which the perspectives of caregivers of children with feeding disorders were examined. Results indicated feeding and swallowing difficulties impacted the daily lives and social participation of both the children and their caregivers. Families shared their children's feeding difficulties impacted their everyday activities and routines, particularly as they related to meal and snack times. They noted that meals tended to take longer than developmentally appropriate, their children had difficulty sitting at the table for the duration of the meal, they were messier when eating than developmentally expected, and they often required special assistance or support when eating. Parents and caregivers also noted their children ate better for other people than the primary caregiver, whereas for some families, the child would only eat for the primary caregiver. In addition to the impact on their daily activities, they shared their children's participation at school and social outings, including play dates, birthday parties, and family functions, were also affected by their feeding challenges (Simione et al., 2020; Simione et al., 2023).

When a feeding disorder affects a family's everyday activities and routines, we must also recognize the influence of these changes on parents and/or caregivers. Parents tend to experience higher levels of stress and often face challenges balancing the needs of their child with other family, personal, and work-related responsibilities (Cohen & Dilfer, 2022; Simione et al., 2020; Simione et al., 2023). Caregivers with children with feeding and swallowing challenges reported that they are often worried about their child's health, nutrition, and weight; they felt pressure for their children to eat and gain weight secondary to societal and cultural expectations (Simione et al., 2020). Cohen and Dilfer (2022) confirm the connection between feeding and swallowing difficulties in early childhood and challenges by both children and parents during mealtimes (Cohen & Dilfer, 2022).

In addition to the issues related to a child's nutrition, growth, health, and overall development, it is important that we consider the impact a feeding and swallowing disorder may have on the family's routines and relationships. As such, assessment and treatment approaches should be family-centered and focus on functional and meaningful outcomes to improve the health and quality of life of the young children and families we serve (Cohen & Dilfer, 2022; Simione et al., 2020; Simione et al., 2023). As we dive deeper into both assessment and treatment, these considerations must be prioritized within our practices.

Assessment of Feeding and Swallowing Disorders

An effective feeding assessment in EI is a comprehensive process (ASHA, n.d.). We must use our knowledge of a child's history and the development of their skills to ensure we are integrating all domains within our assessment (Cohen & Dilfer, 2022). In our role as an SLP, we ask the family about the concerns they have regarding their child's feeding and swallowing.

We gather information regarding their medical, developmental, and feeding history. During the assessment itself, we will consider and try strategies and techniques to support the development and use of the child's feeding and/or swallowing skills. We will review the results and recommendations with parents and caregivers on the day of the appointment and may recommend intervention, if and as appropriate.

A clinical evaluation of oral-motor skills and swallow function, including the use of a feeding-specific assessment tool, if necessary, must be completed. We need to consider possible referrals for instrumental assessment of swallowing or medical consultations. We also need to consider the relationship between the child and their caregivers, the perspectives of as well as the actions in which the family engages when feeding their child, the natural environment in which the child and family engage in feeding activities, the everyday routines of each family, socioeconomic variables, and cultural practices related to feeding (Cohen & Dilfer, 2022).

Components of a Comprehensive Assessment

In accordance with the World Health Organization's (WHO) International Classification of Functioning, Disability and Health framework (WHO, 2001), a comprehensive assessment of a young child's feeding and swallowing development, skills, and needs involves the identification and description of the following variables (ASHA, 2016b):

- Impairments in structure and function, including which swallowing phases are affected.

- Comorbid deficits or conditions, including developmental disabilities or syndromes.

- Limitations in activity and ability to participate, including the impact on overall health and the child's participation in routine and everyday activities.

- Contextual factors, including those that are environmental and personal, that serve to support or impede successful nutritional intake (e.g., child's food preferences and the family support in implementing strategies for safe eating and drinking).

- Quality of life related to feeding and swallowing issues for both the child and their family.

There are also multiple factors we need to consider that could specifically affect the feeding and swallowing of infants and toddlers. According to ASHA (n.d.), these include the following considerations with this population:

- Congenital abnormalities and chronic conditions could affect feeding and swallowing function.

- Feeding skills of premature infants will be consistent with neurodevelopmental level rather than chronological age or adjusted age.

- Positioning limitations and abilities could affect intake and respiration (e.g., a child who is unable to sit upright, a child who uses a wheelchair).

- Infants are unable to verbally describe their symptoms or even when they are in pain; toddlers with delayed or disordered communication skills might also have significant difficulty verbalizing their feeding and swallowing difficulties. We must, therefore, rely on secondary sources of information to determine the characteristics of the issues they are facing. These sources include a thorough case history, parent interviews, the child's weight gain and growth trajectory, data from monitoring devices (e.g., for infants in the NICU), nonverbal forms of communication (e.g., behavioral cues), and observations of the parents' or caregivers' behaviors and ability to read their child's cues as they feed them.

A clinical evaluation is the first step in determining the presence or absence of a feeding or swallowing disorder. The clinical evaluation typically begins with our collection of the child's case history, based on a comprehensive review of medical and clinical records and interviews with the family and other health-care professionals. Our evaluation might address eating, drinking, secretion management, oral hygiene, sensory status, the ability of the child to accept food, the amount of diversity in the child's diet, management of oral medications, and the parents' or caregivers' behaviors while feeding their child.

Before we observe the infant or toddler drinking or eating anything, we must also consider and assess the following variables (ASHA, n.d.):

- Overall physical, social, behavioral, and communicative development.

- Structures of the face, jaw, lips, tongue, hard and soft palate, oropharynx, and oral mucosa.

- Cranial nerve function.

- Functional use of muscles and structures used in swallowing; these include their symmetry, sensation, strength, tone, range and rate of motion, and coordination of movement.

- Head–neck control, posture, oral and pharyngeal reflexes, and involuntary movements and responses based on the child's expected developmental level.

- Observation of the child eating or being fed by a family member or caregiver using foods from the home.

- Observation of the child's oral abilities (e.g., lip closure and rounding) related to utensils that are typically used or utensils that the child might reject or find challenging.

- Functional swallowing ability, including but not limited to, typical developmental skills and tasks, such as suckling and sucking in infants, mastication (i.e., chewing), oral containment, manipulation and transfer of the bolus, and the amount of time it takes the infant or toddler to drink or eat.

- Behavioral factors, including acceptance of the pacifier, nipple, spoon, and cup; the range and texture of developmentally appropriate foods and liquids tolerated; and the willingness of the child to participate in mealtime experiences with caregivers.

- Level and/or impact of fatigue on feeding and swallowing safety.

- Coordination of respiration and swallowing.

- Secretion management, as deemed appropriate for developmental level.

- Referrals to and interventions provided by medical or surgical specialists, dentists, registered dietitians, psychologists or social workers, occupational therapists, and/or physical therapists.

Assessment Considerations Related to Family

When we assess a young child's feeding and swallowing development and skills, we must consider the dynamics between the infant or toddler and the parents, caregivers, and family members. Each of these individuals plays an important and unique role in the child's feeding experiences. Each one has their own beliefs, concerns, and motivations that affect how they interact with the child about feeding. When parents or caregivers experience stress around the child's eating or drinking, they could have difficulty problem solving during mealtimes; secondary to their stress, they might also use strategies that involve greater control and less flexibility to support their child's feeding (Adamson & Morawska, 2017; Martin et al., 2013).

Because they choose when, what, and how food and drink are offered, parents and caregivers also have a significant influence on both the tasks and the environment in which the child is eating or drinking. We need to ask questions that relate to these variables and observe the impact feeding has on the family for insight into how the family is managing mealtimes and supporting their child's feeding and swallowing difficulties and needs. This information helps us determine where, when, and how best to offer our support to the child and their parents or caregivers (Thompson et al., 2023).

Evaluation of Feeding and Swallowing for Infants

A feeding and swallowing evaluation of an infant, between birth and 1 year of age, includes the assessment of the child's pre-feeding skills, readiness for oral feeding, breastfeeding and bottle-feeding ability, and observations of the parents and caregivers feeding the child. According to ASHA (n.d.), the clinical evaluation of an infant typically involves the following components:

- Case history, including gestational and birth history and pertinent medical history.

- Physical examination, including developmental assessment, respiratory status assessment, assessment of sucking and swallowing problems, and determination of abnormal anatomy and physiology that might be associated with these findings (Francis et al., 2015; Webb et al., 2013).

- Determination of oral feeding readiness.

- Assessment of the infant's ability to engage in nonnutritive sucking.
- Developmentally appropriate clinical assessments of feeding and swallowing behavior (nutritive sucking), as appropriate.
- Identification of additional disorders that could affect feeding and swallowing.
- Determination of the optimal feeding method.
- Assessment of the duration of mealtime experience, including potential effects on oxygenation.
- Assessment of issues related to fatigue and volume limitations.
- Assessment of the effectiveness of parent/caregiver and infant interactions for feeding and communication.
- Consideration of the infant's ability to obtain sufficient nutrition and hydration across settings.

Infant Evaluation Criteria

When we conduct a comprehensive assessment of an infant's feeding skills, we must engage in multiple layers of observation and evaluation. These include consideration of variables related to infants' readiness for oral feeding and their abilities related to nonnutritive sucking, nutritive sucking, breastfeeding, bottle feeding, and spoon feeding. To determine readiness for oral feeding, we must consider infants' physiological stability, including their digestive, respiratory, heart rate, and oxygenation parameters; motoric stability, which includes their muscle tone, flexion, and midline movements; and behavioral state, including their ability to become and remain alert to a stimulus (ASHA, n.d.). According to ASHA (n.d.), nonnutritive sucking involves the infant's ability to suck for comfort without the release of fluid (e.g., with a pacifier, finger, or recently emptied breast), and nutritive sucking skills are evaluated during either or both breastfeeding and bottle feeding, depending on which method(s) of feeding parents have chosen for their infant. When we assess breastfeeding, we need to first communicate and collaborate with the mother, nurses, and lactation consultants, as this process requires a working knowledge of breastfeeding strategies (ASHA, n.d.). For our consideration, Table 11–3 presents additional criteria to ensure we conduct comprehensive evaluations of an infant's readiness for oral feeding, nonnutritive sucking, nutritive sucking, breastfeeding, bottle feeding, and spoon feeding.

Table 11–3. Non-instrumental Evaluation Considerations for an Infant

Behavior	Evaluation Includes	Notes
Non-nutritive sucking	- Oral structures and functions, including palatal integrity, jaw movement, and tongue movements for cupping and compression.	Any loss of stability in physiologic, motoric, or behavioral state from baseline should be taken into consideration in regard

	• Ability to turn the head and open the mouth (rooting) when stimulated on the lips or cheeks and to accept a pacifier into the mouth. • Ability to use and strength of both compression (positive pressure of the jaw and tongue on the pacifier) and suction (negative pressure created with tongue cupping and jaw movement). • Ability to maintain a stable physiological state (e.g., oxygen saturation, heart rate, respiratory rate).	to the infant's readiness for nutritive sucking.
Nutritive sucking	• Ability to coordinate the sucking, swallowing, and breathing pattern. • Volume of intake per minute. • Ability to remain engaged throughout the feeding while sustaining appropriate feeding patterns. • Interaction between the infant and the individual conducting the feeding.	Nutritive skills should be assessed during both breastfeeding and bottle feeding if the family intends to use both modalities. The infant's communication behaviors during feeding might communicate their ability to tolerate bolus size, the need for more postural support, and if and when swallowing and breathing are no longer synchronized.
Breastfeeding	• General health. • Medical comorbidities. • Current respiratory rate and heart rate. • Behavior (e.g., positive rooting, willingness to suckle at the breast).	This assessment requires a working knowledge of breastfeeding strategies to facilitate safe and efficient swallowing and optimal nutrition. SLPs should collaborate with the mother, nurse, and lactation consultant prior to

		<ul><li>Position (e.g., well supported, tucked against the mother's body).</li><li>Ability to latch onto the breast.</li><li>Efficiency and coordination of the suck-swallow-breathe pattern.</li><li>Health of the mother's breast.</li><li>Mother's behavior (e.g., comfort with breastfeeding, confidence in handling the infant, awareness of the infant's cues during feeding).</li></ul>	assessing breastfeeding skills.
Bottle feeding		<ul><li>General health.</li><li>Medical comorbidities.</li><li>Respiratory rate and heart rate.</li><li>Behavior (willingness to accept nipple).</li><li>Caregiver's behavior while feeding the infant.</li><li>Efficiency and coordination of the suck-swallow-breathe pattern.</li><li>Nipple type and form of nutrition (breast milk or formula).</li><li>Position.</li><li>Quantity of intake.</li><li>Length of time for one feeding.</li><li>Response to attempted interventions, including:<ul><li>Different nipple for flow control.</li><li>External pacing.</li><li>A different bottle to control air intake.</li></ul></li></ul>	

	○ Different positions (e.g., side feeding).	
Spoon feeding	Infant's ability to: • Move their head toward the spoon and then open their mouth. • Turn their head away from the spoon to show that they have had enough. • Close their lips around the spoon. • Clear food from the spoon with their top lip. • Move food from the spoon to the back of their mouth. • Attempt to spoon-feed independently.	This assessment should also include an evaluation of type of spoon to determine optimal choice.

Note. Adapted from "Pediatric feeding and swallowing," by the American Speech-Language and Hearing Association, n.d. (https://www.asha.org/practice-portal/clinical-topics/pediatric-feeding-and-swallowing/); "Reading the feeding," by C. S. Shaker, 2013b.

Evaluation of Feeding and Swallowing for Toddlers

In addition to the areas of assessment already presented, when we evaluate the feeding and swallowing of a toddler between the ages of 1 and 3 years, we could choose to include the following components (ASHA, n.d.):

- Review of any past diagnostic test results.
- Review of current treatment strategies and their outcomes.
- Assessment of current limitations and skills at home and in other settings.
- Screening of the child's willingness to accept liquids and a variety of foods.
- Evaluation of the child's dependence on nutritional supplements to meet dietary needs.
- Evaluation of the child's level of independence and the need for supervision and assistance with feeding and other self-help skills.

Instrumental Evaluation

When additional information is needed to determine the nature of a swallowing disorder, we must conduct an *instrumental evaluation*. Instrumental assessments provide us with specific information about a child's anatomy and physiology that might not otherwise be accessible.

Instrumental examinations might be necessary for infants and toddlers when the pharyngeal and esophageal physiology needs to be delineated objectively to determine safety and efficiency for oral feeding (Arvedson, 2006). Instrumental evaluation also helps us determine if a child's swallow safety can be improved by modifying food textures, liquid consistencies, positioning, or the implementation of treatment strategies.

Criteria for an instrumental examination of a young child's swallowing can include, but are not limited to the following (Arvedson, 2006):

- Wet or gurgly voice quality.
- Need to define oral, pharyngeal, and upper esophageal phases of swallowing.
- Observation of infants demonstrating incoordination of sucking, swallowing, and breathing during oral feedings at breast or bottle.
- Prior aspiration pneumonia or similar pulmonary problems that could be related to aspiration.
- Risk for aspiration based on history and clinical observation.
- Suspicion of a pharyngeal or laryngeal problem based on etiology.

Instrumental methods for evaluation of swallowing include *videofluoroscopic swallow study*, *flexible endoscopic examination of swallowing*, and *ultrasonography*. These evaluations are completed in a medical setting and involve a team that could include a radiologist, radiology technician, and trained SLP. The SLP or radiology technician typically prepares and presents the barium items for the studies; the SLP then works with the radiologist, who records the swallow for visualization and analysis. Our role in the instrumental evaluation of swallowing and feeding disorders is dependent on the training we have had in this specialty area. Based on our knowledge, skills, and experience, we might participate in decisions made by the interprofessional medical team regarding the appropriateness of these procedures, conduct the videofluoroscopic swallow study or flexible endoscopic examination of swallowing, interpret and apply data from the instrumental evaluations to determine the severity and nature of the swallowing disorder and the child's potential for safe oral feeding. We may also formulate feeding and swallowing treatment plans, including recommendations for optimal feeding techniques (ASHA, n.d.). To engage in these responsibilities, we must be familiar with and know how to use information from these diagnostic procedures to yield information about a young child's swallowing function (ASHA, n.d.).

Developing IFSP Outcomes

As we discussed in detail in Chapter 5, once EI eligibility is determined, the IFSP is written with the parents or caregivers. This plan includes desired functional outcomes based on a family's priorities for their child's feeding development. In collaboration with the family, the IFSP team documents specific outcome-related strategies that will be implemented during ongoing treatment. Simione et al. (2020) found that parents who have children with feeding challenges prefer a treatment plan with a holistic approach, incorporating family-centered principles, to improve their child's quality of life. The DEC (2014) Recommended Practices also direct providers to work together with families to produce individualized intervention strategies that can easily be embedded into a family's daily mealtime routines.

According to ASHA (n.d.), the primary goals of feeding and swallowing intervention for young children are as follows:

- Support safe and adequate nutrition and hydration.
- Determine the best practices in feeding methods and techniques to maximize swallowing safety and feeding efficiency.
- Collaborate with the family to incorporate dietary preferences.
- Attain age-appropriate eating skills in the most natural setting and manner possible (i.e., mealtime with the family, eating meals with peers at the child-care center).
- Minimize the risk of pulmonary complications.
- Maximize the quality of life.
- Prevent future issues with positive feeding-related experiences to the extent possible.

Embedding Evidence-Based Approaches in Treatment of Feeding and Swallowing Disorders

As we have discussed throughout this text, the DEC Recommended Practices supports the implementation of interprofessional teams in EI to identify and prioritize the concerns of parents and caregivers from the point of referral and intake, view these concerns through the lens of typical development, support a child's skill development within the context of family relationships and routines in their natural environment, and use a strengths-based approach (DEC, 2014). Each of these recommendations can and should be embedded within our assessment and treatment of feeding and swallowing disorders in EI as well. ASHA (n.d.) confirms that our selection of treatment strategies will depend on the child's age, cognitive, communication, and physical abilities, and specific swallowing and feeding problems, and could involve environmental or indirect treatment approaches to improve the child's safety and efficiency of feeding, but we must do our best to implement and honor the evidence-based approaches we know are most effective with the families we serve.

Serving Families Within the Natural Environment

As EI providers, it is within our scope of practice to provide individualized services within the context of a family's routines and everyday activities; these include feeding activities and mealtime routines (Cohen & Dilfer, 2022). By asking questions, learning about the routines in which families engage, and communicating effectively about their everyday activities, we also learn more about how each family works. Services can then be implemented that include opportunities for families and caregivers to directly participate in intervention (DEC, 2014). Utilizing the evidence-based practices that have been discussed throughout this textbook, including routines-based intervention, the strength-based approach, and practice-based coaching, provides us with the opportunity to connect with families, meet their needs, and build their capacities.

Routines-Based Intervention

Routines-based intervention (RBI), in which professionals and families collaborate to support a child's participation in routines in the home while working toward a family's goals, has also been shown to support improved functioning in feeding routines (Hwang et al., 2013). We can engage in joint problem-solving with family members during mealtimes to increase parents' responsivity to their child. The evidence indicates when parents use responsive strategies at mealtimes, the feeding relationship is strengthened. Additionally, the use of responsive strategies at mealtimes has resulted in reduced parental or caregiver stress, decreased conflict, reduced food fussiness, and increased incorporation of fruits and vegetables in a child's diet (Cormack et al., 2020; Coulthard & Sealy, 2017; DeCosta et al., 2017; Henton, 2018; Nicklaus, 2016). When we schedule our EI sessions during a family's regular meal or snack routine, we offer ideal opportunities to embed learning opportunities for all family members and caregivers. Because we know family members and child-care providers can also have a significant impact on feeding practices, mealtime routines, and child eating outcomes, it is important we consider the timing of our sessions and the location in which we implement our services (Farrow, 2014).

Strengths-Based Approach

We have learned the importance of supporting and incorporating the strengths of both children and families as building blocks to promote the emergence and development of new skills (Campbell et al., 2001; Fenton et al., 2015; Swanson et al., 2011; Trute et al., 2010). The strengths-based approach emphasizes the capacity of families to take ownership of their priorities, needs, and preferences and also to identify, value, and mobilize their strengths, capacities, and resources (McCashen, 2005, 2017). Rather than focusing on their deficits and their child's challenges, the approach guides us to work with families to identify their social, personal, cultural, and structural constraints, it empowers them to focus on what is working, and to take control of their goals (Cohen & Dilfer, 2022; McCashen, 2005). According to Cohen & Dilfer (2022), we help parents reflect and reframe their child's needs; when we do this, they begin to focus more on their child's progress and engage more effectively in intervention with their children (Hewetson & Singh, 2009 as cited in Cohen & Dilfer, 2022).

Practice-Based Coaching Model

We are now clearly aware that practice-based coaching is a strategy we use in EI to support parents and caregivers by encouraging development and reflection of their actions to plan how they might approach situations with their child in which we are not present (Rush & Shelden, 2019). Through observation and reflective questioning, we understand parents' concerns, their unique perspectives, and their observations regarding past and present mealtime experiences (Rush & Shelden, 2005). We can support parents as they learn to recognize their child's strengths and needs and understand why their child might be struggling with feeding and at mealtimes. Through the coaching process, parents and caregivers learn to respond to their children's needs and abilities to make more appropriate, developmentally supportive modifications at mealtimes. As an approach intended to build the capacity of the parents and caregivers, coaching can result in higher levels of competence and has been linked to less frequent conflict and the use of controlling feeding practices during mealtimes (Aviram et al., 2015).

When we provide feedback to the parents and caregivers through practice-based coaching, we help families recognize the child's ability to problem solve and the influence of their own beliefs and behaviors on the child's behaviors when engaged in feeding and mealtimes (Hamby et al., 2019). Practice-based coaching will lead to more long-term success because it empowers parents to recognize and respond to their child's cues, even as they change over time.

Strategies to Address Feeding and Swallowing Disorders in Early Intervention

Difficulties with feeding and swallowing in EI can be the result of multiple causes, concerns, and factors. We also know now that the research supports our use and inclusion of the evidence-based approaches we have been discussing throughout the text when addressing feeding and swallowing issues with infants, toddlers, and their families. In the following sections, we discuss a variety of strategies to directly address the needs of this population of young children. As long as we consistently focus on the family's priorities, strengths, and needs; consider the child from a holistic perspective; embed treatment into the everyday routines and activities in which the child engages; and coach the parents and caregivers to use the knowledge and skills we bring to them beyond our sessions, we can effectively address the unique needs of each child's feeding and swallowing difficulties with the following techniques.

Postural and Positioning Techniques

According to ASHA (n.d.), postural and positioning techniques involve the adaptation of the child's posture or position to establish alignment and stability for safe feeding. These techniques are intended to protect the child's airway and offer safe transit of food and liquid. Although no single posture will result in improvement for all individuals, the purpose of these techniques is to redirect the movement of the bolus in the oral cavity and pharynx and modify the pharyngeal dimensions. They can be used prior to or during the swallow. Several of the most common postures or positions in which we might adjust the child include the following (ASHA, n.d.):

- *Chin-down posture:* We tuck the child's chin down toward their neck to contain and control the bolus prior to initiating the swallow to potentially reduce penetration or aspiration.

- *Chin-up posture:* We tilt the child's chin up to facilitate bolus movement to the pharynx.

- *Head rotation:* We turn the child's head to either the left or the right to direct the bolus toward the stronger side.

- *Head tilt:* We tilt the child's head toward their stronger side to keep the food on the chewing surface.

Diet Modifications

When we consider *diet modifications*, we are talking about altering the viscosity, texture, temperature, portion size, or taste of a food or liquid to facilitate safety and ease of swallowing (ASHA, n.d.). Typical modifications include thickening thin liquids and softening, cutting, chopping, or pureeing solid foods. We can also alter the taste or temperature of a food to provide a child with additional sensory input for swallowing. In collaboration with parents and caregivers, we need to consider and incorporate both child and family preferences when we modify the diet of an infant or toddler. We should also consider the nutritional needs of the child when engaging in this strategy to avoid undernutrition and malnutrition.

Equipment and Utensils

Adaptive equipment and utensils can be used with young children who have feeding issues to foster independence with eating. This can also improve their swallow safety by controlling bolus size or achieving optimal flow rate of liquids. Adaptive equipment includes modified nipples, cut-out cups, weighted forks and spoons, angled forks and spoons, sectioned plates, non-tip bowls, and materials to prevent plates and cups from sliding (ASHA, n.d.). As SLPs, we work with the oral and pharyngeal implications of adaptive equipment, but we frequently need to collaborate with OTs, who work with those variables related to motor control of infants and toddlers to determine which adaptive equipment works best to meet the children's needs.

Oral-Motor and Sensory Stimulation Strategies

Oral-motor therapy involves the stimulation and exercise of the oral musculature related to a deficit. *Sensory stimulation* could target any of the relevant oral structures involved in feeding, including a child's lips, jaw, tongue, soft palate, pharynx, larynx, and respiratory muscles. Oral motor strategies may vary across a spectrum from passive (e.g., tapping, stroking, and vibration) to active (e.g., range-of-motion activities, resistance exercises, or chewing and swallowing exercises). We can use toys, feeding utensils, or our own gloved hand, accompanied by various tastes, temperatures, and textures, to engage in this form of stimulation. These techniques are intended to influence the physiological underpinnings of the infant's or toddler's oropharyngeal mechanism to improve its functions. Some of these interventions might also incorporate sensory stimulation.

Sensory stimulation might be necessary when young children present with reduced responses, overactive responses, or limited opportunities to engage in sensory experiences.

Young children who demonstrate aversive responses to stimulation might need us to implement oral-motor strategies that initially reduce the level of sensory input, with incremental increases as they demonstrate tolerance (ASHA, n.d.).

Pacing

Pacing involves moderating a child's intake by controlling the rate of presentation of food or liquid and the time between their bites or swallows. Pacing with young children could include alternating bites of food with sips of liquid or encouraging them to swallow two to three times per bite or sip. For infants, pacing can be accomplished by limiting the number of consecutive sucks. Strategies that slow the feeding rate allow for more time between swallows to clear the bolus and could support more timely breaths (ASHA, n.d.).

Cue-Based Feeding for Infants

Cue-based feeding is primarily used with infants who are still unable to effectively communicate their needs and wants (Shaker, 2013b). When we implement cue-based feeding, we coach the parents and caregivers to observe and rely on cues from the infant, including lack of active sucking, passivity, pushing the nipple away, or a weak suck. These cues typically indicate when an infant is disengaging from feeding and attempting to communicate the need to stop eating or drinking. They also provide information about the infant's physiological stability, which serves as the foundation from which a child coordinates breathing and swallowing, and they guide the parent or caregiver to intervene and support safe feeding. When we respond to infants' cues, their quality of feeding begins to take priority over the quantity they are ingesting; when this shift happens, infants can set their own pace and are able to enjoy their mealtime experience (Shaker, 2013b).

Based on the recent research presented by Ross and Arvedson (2022), it is important to note that most NICUs are beginning to move away from volume-driven feeding toward cue-based feeding (Ross & Arvedson, 2022; Shaker, 2013a). As SLPs, we play a critical role in the NICU by supporting and educating parents and caregivers to understand and respond accordingly to their infant's communication during feeding. Cue-based feeding is one way in which we can coach families to learn their child's cues and to safely and enjoyably feed them.

Responsive Feeding

Responsive feeding therapy practices are evidence-informed and align well with family-focused EI principles and methods. These practices prioritize a child's autonomy and emphasize and empower the parent or caregiver as the primary mealtime partner facilitating their child's emerging self-regulation, development, and growth (Cormack et al., 2020; Klein, 2012). Like cue-based feeding, responsive feeding focuses on the caregiver–child dynamic. When parents and caregivers serve as responsive feeders, their goal is to understand and read their child's cues for both hunger and satisfaction and acknowledge their communication signals. Responsive feeding emphasizes communication during mealtime, rather than volume, and it can be used with both infants and toddlers (Cormack et al., 2020; Klein, 2012).

Behavioral Feeding Strategies

Once the feeding assessment has been completed, the EI team develops outcomes with the family; this is when we match strategies to specified treatment outcomes. *Behavioral feeding strategies* are based on principles of behavior modification and focus on increasing appropriate actions or behaviors and reducing maladaptive behaviors. When we choose behavioral feeding strategies, we are typically connecting them to outcomes related to increasing a child's oral intake or variety of oral foods, decreasing their behavioral problems at meals, increasing positive parent–child interactions at meals, decreasing parent stress at meals, and advancing a child's developmentally appropriate intake (e.g., moving from purees and smooth foods to chewable solids).

The essential elements of behavior management for feeding with young children are to identify the targeted behavior for change, select techniques to increase or decrease behaviors congruent with feeding goals, and develop a treatment plan that consistently pairs a contingency (positive or negative) with the targeted behavior. Strategies to improve parent or caregiver influence during meals include environmental controls that involve modifications to the schedule of intake and characteristics of meals. Strategies to increase desirable feeding behaviors include the use of both positive and negative reinforcement as well as discrimination training, while those intended to reduce negative feeding behaviors include extinction, satiation, punishment, and desensitization (Linscheid, 2006). When we choose behavioral treatment strategies to address feeding in EI, we typically include a combination of these techniques (Lukens & Silverman, 2014).

Behavioral Strategies to Share With Families. When a family's concerns and priorities are focused on increasing their child's oral intake or variety of oral foods, decreasing their behavioral problems at meals, increasing positive interactions with their child at meals, decreasing their own stress at meals, and advancing their child's developmentally appropriate intake, there are a variety of behavioral techniques we can coach to support these goals.

To begin, it is important to coach the parents and caregivers to set reasonable expectations. Their goal might be to have their child be in the same room as a new food (or any food at all). It might be to simply touch a new or different food or to play with it. Let them know that smelling, or even touching, a new food is a win when we are addressing an extraordinarily choosy infant or toddler. One of the most important pieces of advice we can offer is to let the children touch and play with the food the family wants them to eat. Let them know this process might be messy, but it really does help when we let an infant or toddler explore their food, even before encouraging them to put it anywhere near their mouth. Young children often put everything near or in their mouths to explore; therefore, our hope is that this happens naturally during their play with the textures and colors of food as well. Often, families will avoid messy or dirty activities. Coach them this way: "Make it fun! Play! A big mess is a positive step in the right direction!" If they can embrace messy food play, the infant or toddler should also recognize the opportunity to enjoy this type of exploration. Supporting children when they attempt to touch and smell different foods is a natural developmental stage. Coaching the parents and caregivers to recognize messy play (like painting or play dough) can encourage sensory development and improve their child's willingness and ability to touch new foods.

We also want to coach parents to avoid forcing their child to eat. Children should be offered a variety of choices, but we do not want to demand that they eat anything. If they feel comfortable doing so, encourage them to let the child watch other family members eat, and offer them small bites of what others are eating. We can also instruct the parents to put the bites in front of and within arm's length of the child. If children sweep the food off the tray, encourage the parents to ignore the behavior. If children do not want to be in the highchair, let them play and roam around nearby while others eat. We can coach the parents and caregivers to leave tiny pieces of food around for the infant or toddler to pick up later, when it is not an official "mealtime." The desired outcome is to create a positive experience for the child to engage in eating. Remind family members and caregivers that the goal is to encourage their child to choose and want to eat, rather than attempt to force them to do so. Table 11–4 offers additional behavioral strategies, with a focus on specific food consistencies and scenarios, for us to share with families.

Table 11–4. Behavioral Strategies for Families to Address Feeding Difficulties

---

Liquids
- Play with liquids!
- Blow bubbles in water, milk, or juice with a straw.
- Infants and toddlers often love this and find it entertaining.

Purees
- Pureed foods are a great choice for messy play.
- Consider using a rubber training toothbrush (instead of a spoon) for teething infants to chew on and play while they are presented with the puree. If a young child is already using it as a teether, we can see if they might dip or eat from it (this is handy for infants who are scared of spoons).
- For infants who are particularly sensitive to lumps, use store-bought purees. There is a wide range of available purees that cater to most food sensitivities as well as organic ranges.
- We can also offer purees to older infants or toddlers who refuse mixed textures. Consider offering solid finger foods first, then serve the puree later in the meal so the harder foods can be used as dippers.

Lumpy solids
- Some infants will skip this texture altogether. That is okay!
- It can be useful to create the mixed texture from something solid that might already be in the child's diet (e.g., rice with a mild puree, such as pears or avocado).

- Let them play and mix them together independently.

Eating in other locations
- Some infants and toddlers will actually eat more when they are outside the home, particularly when there are other people to distract them from their discomfort.
- When they can see other people eating naturally (not overacting for the purpose of encouraging the child to eat), some infants and toddlers will be more inclined to do the same.

Administration of oral medication
- Encourage parents and caregivers to avoid administering any oral medications around food or with the same utensils as used for food.
- Try to give medicines in a different room (e.g., bathroom) and by using things other than spoons (e.g., medication syringe).
- Even infants catch on pretty quickly. Trying to hide medicine in food for infants or toddlers with feeding aversions can become a dangerous game. They tend to figure it out and then refuse another food or utensil we have worked hard to maintain or reintroduce.

Tube Feeding

Tube feeding includes alternative avenues of intake such as a nasogastric tube; a transpyloric tube, which is placed in the duodenum or jejunum; a gastrostomy tube, which is placed in the stomach; or a gastrostomy–jejunostomy tube, which is placed in the jejunum. Even when an infant or toddler is fed through an alternate intake, it is still important that we provide feeding-related treatment. These approaches could be considered by the EI team, in close collaboration with the child's medical team, if the child's swallowing safety and efficiency do not reach a level of adequate function or do not adequately support nutrition and hydration. In these cases, the interprofessional team considers the tube-feeding method that most effectively meets the child's needs, and also determines the length during which the child will need tube feeding (ASHA, n.d.).

Treatment Considerations for Infants in the Neonatal Intensive Care Unit

As SLPs in the NICU, we tend to focus our efforts on facilitating infant-led feedings and working with the medical team to minimize the infant's stay in the unit. Recent research presents strong evidence that these two goals are connected: Appropriate support of early feeding skills leads to quality feeding experiences and discharge to home (Ross & Arvedson, 2022). Our role in the NICU is, therefore, integral to successful outcomes for the infants and the families we serve.

When and if we work in the NICU as SLPs, we must remain cognizant of the multidisciplinary nature of this site, the variables that influence at-risk infant feeding, and the process for developing appropriate treatment plans in this setting. In all cases, we must have an accurate understanding of the anatomy and physiology of feeding and swallowing. This understanding gives us the knowledge we need to choose appropriate treatment interventions and support our rationale for their use with the fragile infants we serve in this setting (Ross & Arvedson, 2022).

Developmental Care Standards for Infants in Intensive Care

In 2014 and 2015, an international group of professionals from speech-language pathology, physical therapy, medicine, psychology, and nursing, along with family representatives, worked together to develop an evidence-based framework with guidelines to optimize the NICU environment, including a focus on facilitating feeding. Based on their work, the Developmental Care Standards for Infants in Intensive Care (Browne et al., 2020) were published in 2021. These best practices include the categories of feeding, eating, and nutrition; positioning and touch; skin-to-skin holding; reducing and managing pain and stress; and sleep and arousal. An additional section focuses on implementation of practice and guides hospitals and clinicians to consider the scope of the problem(s) and create processes for change (Browne et al., 2020).

The following guidelines in the Feeding, Eating, and Nutrition section provide us with a roadmap to build the family's capacity and support their competence and confidence in feeding their infant (Browne et al., 2020).

- *Standard 1:* Feeding experiences in the intensive care unit shall be behavior-based and baby-led. Baby-led principles are similar whether applied to enteral, breast, or bottle-feeding experience.

- *Standard 2:* Every mother shall be encouraged and supported to breastfeed or offer human milk to her baby.

- *Standard 3:* Nutrition shall be optimized during the intensive care unit period.

- *Standard 4:* Mothers shall be supported to be the primary feeders of their baby.

- *Standard 5:* Caregiving activities shall consider baby's response to input, especially around face and mouth, and aversive non-critical-care oral experiences shall be minimized.

- *Standard 6:* Professional staff shall consider smell and taste experiences that are biologically expected.

- *Standard 7:* Support of baby's self-regulation shall be encouraged, especially as it relates to sucking for comfort.

- *Standard 8:* Environments shall be supportive of an attuned feeding for both the feeder and the baby.

- *Standard 9:* Feeding management shall focus on establishing safe oral feedings that are comfortable and enjoyable.

- *Standard 10:* Intensive care units shall include interprofessional perspectives to provide best feeding management.

- *Standard 11:* Feeding management shall consider short-term and long-term growth as well as feeding outcomes.

The primary focus of these feeding, eating, and nutrition standards is to bring the parent or primary caregiver to the center of safe, enjoyable feeding experiences with their child (Ross & Arvedson, 2022). We can use these standards and competencies to guide our practice, help our EI team members work toward more developmentally supportive care, and help our colleagues in other disciplines understand the rationale behind our family-centered, strengths-based approach.

The Importance of Communication With the Family

As SLPs, we know it is our responsibility to coach parents and caregivers to recognize and interpret their child's communication signals. When we are working with preterm and medically fragile infants, we must be competent in our knowledge of typical infant behavior and development and be skilled in recognizing and interpreting changes in their behavior. These changes can provide us with cues that signal an infant's well-being or distress during feeding. The behaviors we monitor include changes in the infant's autonomic system (e.g., patterns of respiration, color changes, visceral signs); their movements, postural alignment, muscle tone, and level of motor activity; states of consciousness, clarity of their expression, and transition between states; and ability to attend, orient, and focus on stimuli in their environment (ASHA, n.d.). As SLPs, we are experts in communication and feeding skills. It is important we remember to voice and reinforce our observations and responses to the infant and place the family in the center of the decision-making process. Families are our partners in the NICU and their infants will only be as successful as our communication and collaboration with each other.

Culturally Responsive Practice With Feeding and Swallowing

In Chapter 8, we discussed our responsibility as providers in EI to be cognizant of and provide culturally responsive services. As such, we must honor the diverse experiences and expectations of each family to provide the highest quality of services possible. When addressing the feeding and swallowing needs of the young children we serve, cultural variables also influence our perceptions and behaviors. We know children and families receiving EI supports and services are increasingly diverse, and represent different cultures, ethnicities, traditions, values, and belief systems. Cultural responsiveness is necessary to ensure our success, and the success of the child and family, in every step of the EI process; the assessment and intervention of feeding and swallowing is no exception.

When we assess an infant or toddler with a focus on their feeding and swallowing development and skills, we must be sensitive and responsive to the family's cultural background; religious beliefs; dietary beliefs, practices, and habits; history of disordered eating behaviors; and preferences for medical intervention (ASHA, n.d.). We should encourage them to bring food and drinks that are common to their household and utensils typically used by the child (ASHA, n.d.). We also need to include the family's typical feeding routines, practices, and positioning in our evaluation. Cultural, religious, and individual beliefs about food and eating practices could affect a family member's comfort level or willingness to participate in an assessment and, on occasion, eating habits that appear to be a sign or symptom of a feeding disorder (e.g., avoiding certain foods or refusing to eat in front of others) might actually be related to cultural differences in meal habits or symptoms of an eating disorder (ASHA, n.d.; National Eating Disorders Association, n.d.).

Additionally, families might have strong beliefs about the medicinal value of some foods or liquids. These beliefs and their holistic healing practices might not be consistent with recommendations we have made or that medical professionals have made with regard to their child's health. When these situations arise, it is within our scope of practice and code of ethics to work with the family and determine alternatives that provide their child with the opportunity to engage as safely as possible (ASHA, 2016a, 2016b).

By now, there is no doubt that providing support to families in EI in a manner that is sensitive and responsive to cultural, linguistic, and socioeconomic diversity can build their capacity to help their children; taking an active and responsive role in mealtime routines is one of the ways in which we can empower the families with whom we work (DEC, 2014). As well-trained SLPs, we can use the methods we have learned to consider and respond effectively to the impact of cultural practices, socioeconomic factors, and resources with each child and family we serve (Harris et al., 2018; Hughes et al., 2006; Worobey et al., 2013).

Summary

The information in this chapter provides a foundation on which to build our confidence and competence in providing assessment and treatment in the areas of infant and toddler feeding and swallowing. We were presented with a review of basic definitions and processes, development milestones, characteristics, and causes of feeding and swallowing disorders in infants and toddlers. We reviewed our own roles and responsibilities as SLPs working with young children and families faced with feeding difficulties, dysphagia, or both. We discussed the application of evidence-based approaches that serve as the foundation of EI, as well as specific evaluation and treatment strategies to assess and treat the needs of infants and toddlers with feeding and swallowing difficulties or disorders. The knowledge and skills presented here are not intended to be comprehensive. Research in the areas of feeding and swallowing continues to evolve; we must, therefore, engage in continuous professional development to remain confident and competent in this area of service delivery.

Critical Thinking Questions

1. What is the difference between feeding and swallowing?

2. What is the difference between a feeding disorder and a swallowing disorder? Provide a list of characteristics of a pediatric feeding disorder and a swallowing disorder.

3. What are the possible long-term consequences of feeding and/or swallowing disorders?

4. List the basic development milestones associated with and necessary for safe and engaging feeding and swallowing in infants and toddlers. Do we need to memorize these milestones? Why or why not?

5. What are the differences between a pediatric feeding disorder and an Avoidant/Restrictive Food Intake Disorder? Why is it important we are aware of these differences?

6. What is a tethered oral tissue (TOT)? What is our role in discussing and addressing an infant or toddler who presents with a TOT?

7. What is our scope of practice as SLPs, according to ASHA, related to feeding difficulties and/or dysphagia in EI?

8. As members of an interprofessional team, what are our roles and responsibilities, related to evaluating, assessing, and providing evidence-based intervention in the areas of feeding and swallowing? Why might our roles and responsibilities vary, depending on the composition (membership) of our EI team or the state in which we practice?

9. How can we use family-centered and routines-based behavioral strategies to support and coach parents and caregivers who are concerned about their child's feeding development and skills?

10. Describe at least 10 specific protocols we might utilize to assess feeding and swallowing disorders with the infants and toddlers we serve.

11. What are the primary goals of feeding and swallowing intervention for young children (according to ASHA)?

12. Describe at least 6 specific treatment strategies we might utilize to address specific feeding and swallowing needs of the infants and toddlers we serve.

13. How might we embed the evidence-based, guiding practices of EI into treatment focused on feeding and/or swallowing? How might we implement these practices when providing feeding/swallowing-focused services?

14. What are the Developmental Care Standards for Infants in Intensive Care? When and

why might we need to be familiar with these standards?

References

Adamson, M., & Morawska, A. (2017). Early feeding, child behaviour and parenting as correlates of problem eating. *Journal of Child and Family Studies, 26*, 3167–3178. https://doi.org/10.1007/s10826-017-0800-y

American Psychiatric Association. (2016). *Feeding and eating disorders: DSM-5 selections.* https://www.psychiatry.org/File%20Library/Psychiatrists/Practice/DSM/APA_DSM-5-Eating-Disorders.pdf

American Speech-Language-Hearing Association. (2016a). *Code of ethics.* https://www.asha.org/policy/et2016-00342/

American Speech-Language-Hearing Association. (2016b). *Scope of practice in speech-language pathology.* https://www.asha.org/policy/sp2016-00343/

American Speech-Language and Hearing Association. (n.d.). *Pediatric feeding and swallowing.* https://www.asha.org/practice-portal/clinical-topics/pediatric-feeding-and-swallowing/

Arvedson, J. (2006). Swallowing and feeding in infants and young children. *GI Motility Online.* http://doi:10.1038/gimo17

Arvedson, J. C. (2008). Assessment of pediatric dysphagia and feeding disorders: Clinical and instrumental approaches. *Developmental Disabilities Research Reviews, 14*(2), 118–127. https://doi.org/10.1002/ddrr.17

Arvedson, J. C, Brodsky, L. (2002). *Pediatric swallowing and feeding: Assessment and management* (2 nd ed.). Singular–Thomson Learning.

Arvedson, J. C., Brodsky, L., & Lefton-Greif, M. A. (2020). *Pediatric swallowing and feeding: Assessment and management* (3rd ed.). Plural Publishing.

Atzaba-Poria, N., Meiri, G., Millikovsky, M., Barkai, A., Dunaevsky-Idan, M., & Yerushalmi, B. (2010). Father–child and mother–child interaction in families with a child feeding disorder: The role of paternal involvement. *Infant Mental Health Journal, 31*(6), 682–698. https://doi.org/10.1002/imhj.20278

Aviram, I., Atzaba-Poria, N., Pike, A., Meiri, G., & Yerushalmi, B. (2015). Mealtime dynamics in child feeding disorder: The role of child temperament, parental sense of competence, and paternal involvement. *Journal of Pediatric Psychology, 40*(1), 45–54. https://doi.org/10.1093/jpepsy/jsu095

Beckett, C., Bredenkamp, D., Castle, J., Groothues, C., O'Connor, T. G., Rutter, M., & the English and Romanian Adoptees (ERA) Study Team. (2002). Behavior patterns associated with institutional deprivation: A study of children adopted from Romania. *Journal of Developmental & Behavioral Pediatrics, 23*(5), 297–303.

Benfer, K. A., Weir, K. A., Bell, K. L., Ware, R. S., Davies, P. S. W., & Boyd, R. N. (2014). Oropharyngeal dysphagia in preschool children with cerebral palsy: Oral phase impairments. *Research in Developmental Disabilities, 35*(12), 3469–3481. https://doi.org/10.1016/j.ridd.2014.08.029

Benfer, K. A., Weir, K. A., Bell, K. L., Ware, R. S., Davies, P. S. W., & Boyd, R. N. (2017). Oropharyngeal dysphagia and cerebral palsy. *Pediatrics, 140*(6), e20170731. https://doi.org/10.1542/peds.2017-0731

Black, M. M., & Aboud, F. E. (2011). Responsive feeding is embedded in a theoretical framework of responsive parenting. *The Journal of Nutrition, 141*(3), 490–494. https://doi.org/10.3945/jn.110.129973

Black, M. M., Dubowitz, H., Krishnakumar, A., & Starr, R. H., Jr. (2007). Early intervention and recovery among children with failure to thrive: Follow-up at age 8. *Pediatrics, 120*(1), 59–69. https://doi.org/10.1542/peds.2006-1657

Brackett, K., Arvedson, J. C., & Manno, C. J. (2006). Pediatric feeding and swallowing disorders: General assessment and intervention. *SIG 13 Perspectives on Swallowing and Swallowing Disorders (Dysphagia), 15*(3), 10–15. https://doi.org/10.1044/sasd15.3.10

Browne, J. V., Jaeger, C. B., & Kenner, C., on behalf of the Gravens Consensus Committee on Infant & Family Centered Developmental Care. (2020). Executive summary: Standards, competencies, and recommended best practices for infant- and family-centered developmental care in the intensive care unit. *Journal of Perinatology, 40*(Suppl. 1), 5–10. https://doi:10.1038/s41372-020-0767-1

Calis, E. A. C., Veuglers, R., Sheppard, J. J., Tibboel, D., Evenhuis, H. M., & Penning, C. (2008). Dysphagia in children with severe generalized cerebral palsy and intellectual disability. *Developmental Medicine & Child Neurology, 50*(8), 625–630. https://doi.org/10.1111/j.1469-8749.2008.03047.x

Campbell, P. H., Milbourne, S. A., & Silverman, C. (2001). Strengths-based child portfolios: A professional development activity to alter perspectives of children with special needs. *Topics in Early Childhood Special Education, 21*, 152–161. https://doi.org/10.1177/027112140102100303

Caron, C. J. J. M., Pluijmers, B. I., Joosten, K. F. M., Mathijssen, I. M. J., van der Schroeff, M. P., Dunaway, D. J., . . . Koudstaal, M. J. (2015). Feeding difficulties in craniofacial microsomia: A systematic review. *International Journal of Oral & Maxillofacial Surgery, 44*(6), 732–737. https://doi.org/10.1016/j.ijom.2015.02.014

Carruth, B. R., & Skinner, J. D. (2002). Feeding behaviors and other motor development in healthy children (2–24 months). *Journal of the American College of Nutrition, 21*(2), 88–96. https://doi.org/10.1080/07315724.2002.10719199

Cerniglia, L., Cimino, S., & Ballarotto, G. (2014). Mother–child and father–child interaction with their 24-month-old children during feeding, considering paternal involvement and the child's temperament in a community sample. *Infant Mental Health Journal, 35*(5), 473–481. https://doi.org/10.1002/imhj.21466

Cohen, S. C., & Dilfer, K. (2022). Pediatric feeding disorder in early intervention: Expanding access, improving outcomes, and prioritizing responsive feeding. *Perspectives of the ASHA Special Interest Groups, 7*, 829–840. https://doi.org/10.1044/2022_PERSP-20-00259

Cormack, J., Rowell, K., & Postăvaru, G. I. (2020). Self-determination theory as a theoretical framework for a responsive approach to child feeding. *Journal of Nutrition Education and Behavior, 52*(6), 646–651. https://doi.org/10.1016/j.jneb.2020.02.005

Coulthard, H., & Sealy, A. (2017). Play with your food! Sensory play is associated with tasting of fruits and vegetables in preschool children. *Appetite, 113*, 84–90. https://doi.org/10.1016/j.appet.2017.02.003

Davis-McFarland, E. (2008). Family and cultural issues in a school swallowing and feeding program. *Language, Speech, and Hearing Services in Schools, 39*, 199–213. https://doi.org/10.1044/0161-1461(2008/020)

de Vries, I. A. C., Breugem, C. C., van der Heul, A. M. B., Eijkemans, M. J. C., Kon, M., & Mink van der Molen, A. B. (2014). Prevalence of feeding disorders in children with cleft palate only: A retrospective study. *Clinical Oral Investigations, 18*(5), 1507–1515. https://doi.org/10.1007/s00784-013-1117-x

Division for Early Childhood. (2014). *DEC recommended practices in early intervention/early childhood special education 2014.* http://www.dec-sped.org/recommendedpractices

Dunst, C. J., Bruder, M. B., & Espe-Sherwindt, M. (2014). Family capacity-building in early childhood intervention: Do context and setting matter. *School Community Journal, 24*(1), 37–49.

Farrow, C. (2014). A comparison between the feeding practices of parents and grandparents. *Eating Behaviors, 15*(3), 339–342. https://doi.org/10.1016/j.eatbeh.2014.04.006

Fenton, A., Walsh, K., Wong, S., & Cumming, T. (2015). Using strengths-based approaches in early years practice and research. *International Journal of Early Childhood, 47*(1), 27–52.

Francis, D. O., Krishnaswami, S., & McPheeters, M. (2015). Treatment of ankyloglossia and breastfeeding outcomes: A systematic review. *Pediatrics, 135*(6), e1458–e1466. https://doi.org/10.1542/peds.2015-0658

Franklin, L., & Rodger, S. (2003). Parents' perspectives on feeding medically compromised children: Implications for occupational therapy. *Australian Occupational Therapy Journal, 50*(3), 137–147. https://doi.org/10.1046/j.1440-1630.2003.00375.x

Goday, P. S., Huh, S. Y., Silverman, A., Lukens, C. T., Dodrill, P., Cohen, S. S., . . . Phalen, J. A. (2019). Pediatric feeding disorder: Consensus definition and conceptual framework. *Journal of Pediatric Gastroenterology and Nutrition, 68*(1), 124–129. https://doi.org/10.1097/MPG.0000000000002188

Grantham-McGregor, S. M., & Ani, C. C. (2001). Undernutrition and mental development. *Nestle Nutrition workshop series. Clinical & performance programme, 5*, 1–18. https://doi.org/10.1159/000061844

Greer, A. J., Gulotta, C. S., Masler, E. A., & Laud, R. B. (2008). Caregiver stress and outcomes of children with pediatric feeding disorders treated in an intensive interdisciplinary program. *Journal of Pediatric Psychology, 33*(6), 612–620. https://doi.org/10.1093/jpepsy/jsm116

Gueron-Sela, N., Atzaba-Poria, N., Meiri, G., & Yerushalmi, B. (2011). Maternal worries about child underweight mediate and moderate the relationship between child feeding disorders and mother–child feeding interactions. *Journal of Pediatric Psychology, 36*(7), 827–836. https://doi.org/10.1093/jpepsy/jsr001

Hamby, C. M., Lunkenheimer, E. S., & Fisher, P. A. (2019). The potential of video feedback interventions to improve parent-child interaction skills in parents with intellectual disability. *Children and Youth Services Review, 105,* Article 104395. https://doi.org/10.1016/j.childyouth.2019.104395

Harris, H. A., Jansen, E., Mallan, K. M., Daniels, L., & Thorpe, K. (2018). Concern explaining nonresponsive feeding: A study of mothers' and fathers' response to their child's fussy eating. *Journal of Nutrition Education and Behavior, 50*(8), 757–764. https://doi.org/10.1016/j.jneb.2018.05.021

Henton, P. A. (2018). A call to reexamine quality of life through relationship-based feeding. *American Journal of Occupational Therapy, 72*(3), 7203347010p1–7203347010p7. https://doi.org/ 10.5014/ajot.2018.025650

Hewetson, R., & Singh, S. (2009). The lived experience of mothers of children with chronic feeding and/or swallowing difficulties. *Dysphagia, 24*(3), 322–332. https://doi.org/10.1007/ s00455-009-9210-7

Hughes, S. O., Anderson, C. B., Power, T. G., Micheli, N., Jaramillo, S., & Nicklas, T. A. (2006). Measuring feeding in low-income African-American and Hispanic parents. *Appetite, 46*(2), 215–223. https://doi.org/10.1016/j.appet.2006.01.002

Hurley, K. M., Black, M. M., Papas, M. A., & Caufield, L. E. (2008). Maternal symptoms of stress, depression, and anxiety are related to nonresponsive feeding styles in a statewide sample of WIC participants. *The Journal of Nutrition, 138*(4), 799–805. https://doi.org/10.1093/jn/138.4.799

Hwang, A. W., Chao, M. Y., & Liu, S. W. (2013). A randomized controlled trial of routines-based early intervention for children with or at risk for developmental delay. *Research in Developmental Disabilities, 34*(10), 3112–3123. https://doi.org/10.1016/j.ridd.2013.06.037

Jaffal, H., Isaac, A., Johannsen, W., Campbell, S., & El-Hakim, H. G. (2020). The prevalence of swallowing dysfunction in children with laryngomalacia: A systematic review. *International Journal of Pediatric Otorhinolaryngology, 139,* 110464. https://doi.org/10.1016/j.ijporl.2020.110464

Johnson, D. E., & Dole, K. (1999). International adoptions: Implications for early intervention. *Infants & Young Children, 11*(4), 34–45.

Klein, M. D. (2012, October 26–27). *Tube feeding with love* [Paper presentation]. The Pathways Center at University of Illinois Urbana-Champaign, Glenview, IL.

Klein, M. D. (2019). *Anxious eaters, anxious mealtimes: Practical and compassionate strategies for mealtime peace.* Archway.

Lefton-Greif, M. A. (2008). Pediatric dysphagia. *Physical Medicine and Rehabilitation Clinics of North America, 19*(4), 837–851. https://doi.org/10.1016/j.pmr.2008.05.007

Lefton-Greif, M. A., Carroll, J. L., & Loughlin, G. M. (2006). Long-term follow-up of oropharyngeal dysphagia in children without apparent risk factors. *Pediatric Pulmonology, 41*(11), 1040–1048. https://doi.org/10.1002/ppul.20488

Lefton-Greif, M. A., McGrattan, K. E., Carson, K. A., Pinto, J. M., Wright, J. M., & Martin-Harris, B. (2017). First steps towards development of an instrument for the reproducible quantification of oropharyngeal swallow physiology in bottle-fed children. *Dysphagia, 33*(1), 76–82. https://doi.org/10.1007/s00455-017-9834-y

Linscheid T. R. (2006). Behavioral treatments for pediatric feeding disorders. *Behavior Modification, 30*(1), 6–23. https://doi.org/10.1177/0145445505282165

Logemann, J. A. (1998). *Evaluation and treatment of swallowing disorders.* PRO-ED.

Lucarelli, L., Ammaniti, M., Porreca, A., & Simonelli, A. (2017). Infantile anorexia and co-parenting: A pilot study on mother–father–child triadic interactions during feeding and play. *Frontiers in Psychology, 8,* 376. https://doi.org/10.3389/fpsyg.2017.00376

Lukens, C. T., & Silverman, A. H. (2014). Systematic review of psychological interventions for pediatric feeding problems. *Journal of Pediatric Psychology, 39*(8), 903–917. https://doi.org/10.1093/jpepsy/jsu040

Manikam, R., & Perman, J. A. (2000). Pediatric feeding disorders. *Journal of Clinical Gastroenterology, 30*(1), 34–46. https://doi.org/10.1097/00004836-200001000-00007

Martin, C. I., Dovey, T. M., Coulthard, H., & Southall, A. M. (2013). Maternal stress and problem-solving skills in a sample of children with nonorganic feeding disorders. *Infant Mental Health Journal, 34*(3), 202–210. https://doi.org/10.1002/imhj.21378

McComish, C., Brackett, K., Kelly, M., Hall, C., Wallace, S., & Powell, V. (2016). Interdisciplinary feeding team: A medical, motor, behavioral approach to complex pediatric feeding problems. *MCN: The American Journal of Maternal/Child Nursing, 41*(4), 230–236. https://doi.org/10.1097/NMC.0000000000000252

Merkel-Walsh, R., & Overland, L. (2018). *The functional assessment and remediation of tethered oral tissues.* TalkTools.

Morris, S. E., & Klein, M. D. (2000). *Pre-feeding skills: A comprehensive resource for mealtime development* (2nd ed.). PRO-ED.

National Center for Health Statistics. (2010). *Number of all-listed diagnoses for sick newborn infants by sex and selected diagnostic categories* [Data file]. https://www.cdc.gov/nchs/data/nhds/8newsborns/2010new8_numbersick.pdf

National Eating Disorders Association. (n.d.). *Warning signs and symptoms.* https://www.nationaleatingdisorders.org/warning-signs-and-symptoms

Newman, L. A., Keckley, C., Petersen, M. C., & Hamner, A. (2001). Swallowing function and medical diagnoses in infants suspected of dysphagia. *Pediatrics, 108*(6), e106. https://doi.org/10.1542/peds.108.6.e106

Nicklaus, S. (2016). The role of food experiences during early childhood in food pleasure learning. *Appetite, 104*, 3–9. https://doi.org/10.1016/j.appet.2015.08.022

Owens, R. (2018). *Early language intervention for infants, toddlers, and preschoolers.* Pearson Education.

Pados, B. F., & Hill, R. (2019). Parents' descriptions of feeding their young infants. *Nursing for Women's Health, 23*(5), 404–413. https://doi.org/10.1016/j.nwh.2019.08.001

Reid, J., Kilpatrick, N., & Reilly, S. (2006). A prospective, longitudinal study of feeding skills in a cohort of babies with cleft conditions. *The Cleft Palate–Craniofacial Journal, 43*(6), 702–709. https://doi.org/10.1597/05-172

Robea, M. A., Luca, A. C., & Ciobica, A. (2020). Relationship between vitamin deficiencies and co-occurring symptoms in autism spectrum disorder. *Medicina (Lithuania), 56*(5), 245. https://doi.org/10.3390/medicina56050245

Ross, E., & Arvedson, J. (2022, November/December). From volume-driven to developmentally appropriate feeding in the NICU. *ASHA LeaderLive.*

https://leader.pubs.asha.org/do/10.1044/leader.OTP.27112022.slp-nicu-feeding.28/full/

Rowell, K., & McGlothlin, J. (2015). *Helping your child with extreme picky eating*. New Harbinger.

Rush, D. D., & Shelden, M. L. (2005). Evidence-based definition of coaching practices. *CASEInPoint, 1*(6), 1–6.

Rush, D. D., & Shelden, M. (2019). *The early intervention coaching handbook* (2nd ed.). Brookes.

Seiverling, L., Towle, P., Hendy, H. M., & Pantelides, J. (2018). Prevalence of feeding problems in young children with and without autism spectrum disorder: A chart review study. *Journal of Early Intervention, 40*(4), 335–346. https://doi.org/10.1177/1053815118789396

Shaker, C. S. (2013a). Cue-based feeding in the NICU: Using the infant's communication as a guide. *Neonatal Network, 32*(6), 404–408. https://doi.org/10.1891/0730-0832.32.6.404

Shaker, C. S. (2013b, February 1). Reading the feeding. *The ASHA Leader, 18*(2), 42–47. https://doi.org/10.1044/leader.FTRI.18022013.42

Sharp, W. G., Berry, R. C., McCracken, C., Nuhu, N. N., Marvel, E., Saulnier, C. A., . . . Jaquess, D. L. (2013). Feeding problems and nutrient intake in children with autism disorders: A meta-analysis and comprehensive review of the literature. *Journal of Autism and Developmental Disorders, 43*(9), 2159–2173. https://doi.org/10.1007/s10803-013-1771-5

Simione, M., Dartley, A. N., Cooper-Vince, C., Martin, V., Hartnick, C., Taveras, E. M., & Fiechtner, L. (2020). Family centered outcomes that matter most to parents: A pediatric feeding disorders qualitative study. *Journal of Pediatric Gastroenterology and Nutrition, 71*(2), 270–275. https://doi.org/10.1097/MPG.0000000000002741

Simione, M., Harshman, S., Cooper-Vince, C. E., Daigle, K., Sorbo, J., Kuhlthau, K., & Fiechtner, L. (2023). Examining health conditions, impairments, and quality of life for pediatric feeding disorders. *Dysphagia, 38*(1), 220–226. https://doi.org/10.1007/s00455-022-10455-z

Speyer, R., Cordier, R., Kim, J.-H., Cocks, N., Michou, E., & Wilkes-Gillan, S. (2019). Prevalence of drooling, swallowing, and feeding problems in cerebral palsy across the lifespan: A systematic review and meta-analyses. *Developmental Medicine & Child Neurology, 61*(11), 1249–1258. https://doi.org/10.1111/dmcn.14316

Swanson, J., Raab, M., & Dunst, C. J. (2011). Strengthening family capacity to provide young children everyday natural learning opportunities. *Journal of Early Childhood Research, 9*, 66–80. https://doi.org/10.1177/1476718X10368588

Thomlinson, E. H. (2002). The lived experience of families of children who are failing to thrive. *Journal of Advanced Nursing, 39*(6), 537–545. http://doi.org/10.1046/j.1365-2648. 2002.02322.x

Thompson, K. L., McComish, C., & Thoyre, S. (2023). Dynamic systems theory: A primer for pediatric feeding clinicians. *ASHA Special Interest Groups, 8*(3), 519–532. https://doi.org/10.1044/2023_PERSP-22-00233

Trute, B., Benzies, K. M., Worthington, C., Reddon, J. R., & Moore, M. (2010). Accentuate the positive to mitigate the negative: Mother psychological coping resources and family adjustment in childhood disability. *Journal of Intellectual and Developmental Disability, 35*, 36–43. https://doi.org/10.3109/13668250903496328

Velayutham, P., Irace, A. L., Kawai, K., Dodrill, P., Perez, J., Londahl, M., . . . Rahbar, R. (2018). Silent aspiration: Who is at risk? *The Laryngoscope, 128*(8), 1952–1957. https://doi.org/10.1002/lary.27070

Webb, A. N., Hao, W., & Hong, P. (2013). The effect of tongue-tie division on breastfeeding and speech articulation: A systematic review. *International Journal of Pediatric Otorhinolaryngology, 77*(5), 635–646. https://doi.org/10.1016/j.ijporl.2013.03.008

Wilken, M. (2012). The impact of child tube feeding on maternal emotional state and identity: A qualitative meta-analysis. *Journal of Pediatric Nursing, 27*(3), 248–255. https://doi.org/ 10.1016/j.pedn.2011.01.032

World Health Organization. (2001). *International classification of functioning, disability and health.*

Worobey, J., Borrelli, A., Espinosa, C., & Worobey, H. S. (2013). Feeding practices of mothers from varied income and racial/ethnic groups. *Early Child Development and Care, 183*(11), 1661–1668. https://doi.org/10.1080/03004430.2012.752735

Zimmerman-Pine, P. (2018). *Please release me: The tethered oral tissue (TOT) puzzle* (2nd ed.). MiniBuk.

Chapter 12

Special Populations

Learning Outcomes

When we have completed this chapter, we will be able to:

- List diagnoses and disorders often addressed in EI by the SLP.

- Define and describe characteristics of an infant or toddler at risk for or diagnosed with the following:

  - Autism spectrum disorder.

  - Intellectual disability.

  - Cerebral palsy.

  - Down syndrome.

  - Fragile X syndrome

  - Sensory and perceptual disorders including hard of hearing or deaf, loss of vision, or blindness.

  - Preterm and low birth weight.

  - Child abuse and neglect.

  - Fetal alcohol spectrum disorders.

  - Neonatal abstinence syndrome.

  - Traumatic brain injury.

  - Shaken baby syndrome.

- Describe the developmental expectations and types of echolalia; explain how echolalia can often serve a purpose in both evaluation and treatment processes in EI.

- Present considerations for working as an SLP in the NICU with children born preterm or with low birth weight and their families.

- Discuss implications for assessment and intervention when working with a young child with suspected or diagnosed autism spectrum disorder, intellectual disability, CP, Down syndrome, Fragile X syndrome, sensory and perceptual disorders including hard of hearing or deafness, loss of vision or blindness, preterm and low birth weight, child abuse and neglect, fetal alcohol spectrum disorders, neonatal abstinence syndrome, traumatic brain injury, and shaken baby syndrome.

What Will We Learn and How Can We Apply It?

In EI, each child with whom we work is unique; each family is diverse. Their needs, priorities, and expectations are diverse, and their diagnoses are endless. If we serve in EI long enough, however, there are a variety of disorders we will most likely encounter. In this chapter, we introduce and provide an overview of these conditions to serve as a starting point for our practice.

Because our purpose is to present an introduction and overview of diagnoses and disorders we often face when working with infants and toddlers, this chapter is not intended to be comprehensive. Instead, we focus on autism spectrum disorder (ASD); CP; the most common disorders associated with intellectual disabilities, including Down syndrome and Fragile X; sensory perceptual disorders; and delays and disorders that are a result of substance exposure, preterm and low birth weight, and adverse childhood experiences. Although each of these considerations could potentially fill an entire chapter, we present the information needed to inform our practice, initiate an evaluation or assessment, consider appropriate consultations with or referrals to other providers and professionals, develop intervention plans with families, and explore or acquire additional information as and when needed.

Review of Eligibility for Services

When we consider a young child's eligibility for EI services, we are now aware that we follow Part C of IDEA (2004) requirements. This legislature states that systems must serve any child "under 3 years of age who needs EI services" (IDEA, 2004, §632(5)(A)) because the child "(i) is experiencing developmental delays, as measured by appropriate diagnostic instruments and procedures in one or more of the areas of cognitive development, physical development, communication development, social or emotional development, and adaptive development; or (ii) has a diagnosed physical or mental condition which has a high probability of resulting in developmental delay" (IDEA 2004, §632(5)(A)). Each state also has the option of serving children who do not demonstrate a delay but are considered at risk for developmental challenges secondary to biological or environmental factors (ASHA, 2023b). If a child is not found eligible for Part C services, families can also choose to seek EI services through private, community, or other federal or state-funded early childhood programs.

As we discussed in detail in Chapter 7, our process of determining eligibility is based on whether a child meets the criteria, as just stated, to receive EI services. This process includes the evaluation of the child's skills and needs through the review of information, including medical and developmental reports, assessment reports, observations, and parent report. All areas of a child's development are considered to determine whether they present a delay or differences in development that might make them eligible for Part C services. Determination is based on whether the infant's or toddler's needs are being met within their natural environment, and as needed, the informed clinical opinion of the EI team must be considered (IDEA, 2011).

Although diagnostic categories should not be the primary variable when making decisions in EI, our knowledge of different diagnoses, disorders, and impact of environmental conditions can certainly be useful to us. In addition to determining a child's eligibility for EI, as SLPs, we often play an integral role on the interprofessional team in evaluation and assessment, consultation, and treatment of the young children and families who need our services. As we plan to implement each of these components, we must also have a solid foundation regarding, at the very least, those diagnoses, disorders, and conditions infants and toddlers often face to guide our decisions and effectively support their families.

Autism Spectrum Disorder

According to Autism Navigator (2024), "ASD is a neurodevelopmental disorder defined by persistent deficits in social communication and social interaction, accompanied by restricted, repetitive patterns of behavior, interests, or activities." It is characterized by unique social interactions, diverse ways of learning, intense interests in specific subjects, strong preference for routines, challenges with typical communication, and often different ways of processing sensory information (Centers for Disease Control and Prevention [CDC], n.d.; United Nations General Assembly, n.d.). According to the United Nations General Assembly (n.d.), autism is a lifelong condition that manifests during early childhood, regardless of gender, race or socioeconomic status. This description is consistent with the diagnostic criteria for ASD described in the *Diagnostic and Statistical Manual of Mental Disorders* (5th ed.; *DSM-5*; American Psychiatric Association, 2013). According to the *DSM-5*, individuals who meet the specified criteria are assigned the diagnosis of ASD with one of three severity levels. Each severity level specifies the amount of support needed to function in the general community, given the individual's social communication skills and degree of restricted, repetitive behaviors. Severity can vary by context and might change over time. Severity ratings are intended to be used for descriptive purposes only and are not intended to diagnose or determine eligibility for services (American Psychiatric Association, 2013). It is also important to differentiate between ASD and social communication disorder (Rosin, 2016). As SLPs in EI, we play a significant role in making this differential diagnosis and ensuring young children with ASD and those with social communication disorder have access to services.

The Autism and Developmental Disabilities Monitoring (ADDM) Network is an active surveillance program that provides estimates of the prevalence of ASD among children 8 years old. According to the most recent ADDM findings, 1 in 36 children 8 years old (approximately 4% of boys and 1% of girls) was estimated to have ASD (Maenner et al., 2023). For the first time among 8-year-old children, the prevalence of ASD was lower among White children than among other racial and ethnic groups. Black children with ASD are still more likely than White children with ASD to have a cooccurring intellectual disability. Among the children with ASD with information on cognitive ability, 37.9% were classified as having an intellectual disability. Intellectual disability was present among 50.8% of Black children, 41.5% of non-Hispanic Asian or Pacific Islander children, 37.8% of children who presented with two or more races, 34.9% of Hispanic children, 34.8% of non-Hispanic American Indian or Alaska Native children, and 31.8% of White children with ASD. Children with intellectual disability tend to be diagnosed with ASD earlier (at 43 months of age) than those children without intellectual disability, who were diagnosed, on average, at 53 months of age (Maenner et al., 2023).

For both EI providers and families, ASD can be a puzzling and complex disorder. It can be difficult to diagnose because there are no medical or blood tests for ASD. Instead, the diagnosis of ASD is based on a child's behaviors, as well as delay in, or absence of, typical developmental milestones. The diagnosis often involves a two-stage process. The first stage focuses on screening, which is often conducted by a pediatrician at a well-child visit using validated screening checklists completed by parents or primary caregivers. The American Academy of Pediatrics (2016) recommends developmental and behavioral screening for all children during regular well-child visits at 9 months, 18 months, and 30 months. They further recommend all children are screened specifically for ASD during regular well-child visits at 18 months and 24 months. Should concerns arise during any of these screenings, a second stage of the diagnostic process involves a comprehensive evaluation, typically conducted by an interprofessional team who gathers information from both interview and structured observation.

Implications for Assessment and Intervention

According to ASHA (2023), characteristics of ASD are often evident in very young children. Research focused on children with ASD indicates families and caregivers often report observing symptoms within the first 2 years of their children's lives and express their initial concerns by the time their child reaches 18 months of age (ASHA, 2023a). Parents of children with ASD reported first noticing abnormalities in their children's development, particularly in language development and social relatedness, at around 14 months of age (Chawarska et al., 2007). Although not observed in typically developing infants, infants at risk for and later diagnosed with ASD demonstrated a decline, from previous normative levels, in eye fixation within the first 2 to 6 months of age (Jones & Klin, 2013). By 12 months of age, infants at risk for and later diagnosed with ASD demonstrated atypical eye gaze, passive social smiling, decreased positive affect, and delayed language (Zwaigenbaum et al., 2005). Infants at risk for and later diagnosed with ASD tended to use more distress-based vocalizations (e.g., cries, whines, screams, and squeals) than did children who were typically developing and children who were otherwise developmentally delayed (Plumb & Wetherby, 2013). Children with ASD used fewer joint attention gestures and behaviors as infants and toddlers than typically developing, age-matched peers (Watson et al., 2013; Werner & Dawson, 2005). They also showed subtle differences in sensorimotor and social behavior at 9 to 12 months of age and presented with lower rates of canonical babbling and fewer speech-like vocalizations across the 6- to 24-month age range than did typically developing peers (Baranek, 1999; Patten et al., 2014).

We work with infants and toddlers every day. We are trained to observe their development, behavior, and engagement within and beyond their natural environment, to listen to the concerns of the families, and to use our knowledge and skills to effectively assess and serve these children. As SLPs engaging in EI with families who have concerns about their child, it is within our scope of practice to support the screening and possible diagnosis of young children with ASD as early as possible and to provide the services and supports needed for them to reach their full potential (ASHA, 2023a; Hyman et al., 2020).

Assessment and Diagnosis of ASD

The question of who is responsible for the assessment and diagnosis of ASD is common in our field. Due to the complexity of the disorder, the variety in affected functioning, and the need to differentiate ASD from other disorders or medical conditions, interprofessional collaboration among multiple providers is an integral element of assessment and diagnosis of ASD in young children (Hyman et al., 2020). Ideally, as SLPs, we serve as key members of the EI team in diagnosing ASD. When there is no appropriate team available, and we have been trained in the clinical criteria for ASD and are experienced in diagnosing developmental disorders, as SLPs, we might be qualified to independently make an initial diagnosis of ASD (ASHA, 2023a). It is important, however, to recognize state speech-language pathology licensing boards do not always specify whether diagnosing ASD and other conditions is specifically within our scope of practice. Further, licensing agencies for other health professions, such as a state medical boards, might set rules that prohibit us, as SLPs, from diagnosing ASD independently. Payers such as Medicare, Medicaid, commercial, or private insurers typically require a diagnosis by a physician, psychiatrist, or other medical professional for coverage of services. We are responsible for understanding the requirements in place in our own state, setting, and by payer regarding our options and roles in supporting a young child's diagnosis of ASD.

Regardless of how a diagnosis is determined, it is within our scope of practice and our professional responsibility to ensure that we are aware of the signs of ASD in young children and, when observed, share our concerns and collaborate with the EI team, including the parents and caregivers, to comprehensively assess and accurately diagnosis the infants and toddlers in our care. Table 12–1 provides key characteristics we might observe in a young child for whom a diagnosis of ASD could present.

Table 12–1. Characteristics of Possible Autism Spectrum Disorder in Toddlers

Social Interaction and Communication
- Does not respond when their name is called
- Lack of joint attention and/or attempt to engage in activities with peers or adults
- Limited use of gestures
- Uses people as tools to get their needs met (e.g., puts caregiver's hand on a book to turn the page)
- Difficulty recognizing nonverbal cues (e.g., accurately interpreting facial expressions, body posture, or tone of voice)
- Delayed or complete lack of speech and/or expressive language skills
- Repeats words or phrases verbatim out of context and that do not make sense within a conversation

Patterns of Behavior
- Difficulty with coordination or odd physical patterns that might include odd, stiff, or exaggerated movements of hands, head, or the entire body
- Engages in specific and often rigid routines or rituals (e.g., lining up objects, repeating activities or words)
- Becomes focused on or attached to unusual and/or inanimate objects
- Demonstrates excessive interest in particular objects, actions, or activities that then interfere with social interaction
- Presents unusual sensitivities or sensory interests (e.g., hypersensitive to light, sound, or touch; indifference to pain or temperature)
- Present over- or underreactions to specific sounds, textures, or other sensory input

Note. Adapted from "Autism spectrum disorder," by the American Speech-Language and Hearing Association, 2023 (https://www.asha.org/practice-portal/clinical-topics/autism/communication-about-autism/); "Red Flags of Autism in Toddlers," by Florida State University, 2024 (https://www.readingrockets.org/topics/autism-spectrum-disorder/articles/red-flags-autism-toddlers); "Signs and symptoms of autism spectrum disorder," by the Centers for Disease Control and Prevention, n.d. (https://www.cdc.gov/ncbddd/autism/signs.html).

If we suspect a young child might have ASD, our interprofessional assessment should include the following components (ASHA, 2023a):

- Case history including information related to the child's health, developmental and behavioral history, and current medical status.
- Family history, including siblings with ASD, which includes both medical and mental health.

- Medical evaluations, including a general physical, neurodevelopmental examination, and vision testing.

- Formal and informal assessments conducted by an SLP, including language, speech, motor speech abilities, feeding and swallowing, as needed, and AAC to determine potential benefits for improving functional communication.

- An audiologic assessment conducted by an audiologist.

The comprehensive assessment might also include genetic testing, if there is a family history of intellectual disability or genetic conditions associated with ASD or if the child exhibits physical features that suggest a possible genetic syndrome, and metabolic testing if the child exhibits lethargy, cyclic vomiting, pica, or seizures (ASHA, 2023a).

The outcomes of the assessment could result in any or all of the following actions (ASHA, 2023a):

- A diagnosis of ASD.

- A description of the characteristics and severity of communication-related symptoms.

- Recommendations for intervention, outcomes, and supports and services.

- A referral for an AAC assessment, if this was not completed as part of the comprehensive assessment.

- Referral to other professionals for additional testing to either confirm a diagnosis of ASD or to determine if other disorders or conditions are suspected.

Intervention Strategies for ASD

The goal of treatment for young children with ASD is to facilitate and improve their social communication, language skills, and behaviors to support their ability and capacity to develop relationships, function effectively in social settings, and actively participate in natural, everyday activities and routines with their family and peers. As is the case in any EI situation, we often collaborate with other providers to design and implement effective treatment plans to meet the needs of an infant or toddler with ASD and their family. IFSP outcomes tend to target core challenges of ASD and focus on a child's ability to initiate spontaneous communication in functional activities, engage in reciprocal communication interactions, and generalize skills across activities, environments, and communication partners (ASHA, 2023a).

Family-centered practice, always integral to our services in EI, is often even more important when working with the parents and caregivers of a young child with ASD. We need to create a partnership with each family to ensure they feel empowered and supported. When we consider treatment methods and modalities, we must remember each child, and their family, is unique. Some families might want their child to appear "normal" and will prioritize IFSP outcomes that focus on eye contact, facial expressions, or stim behaviors. Other parents and caregivers might choose to use identity-first language and will want to learn about strategies and programs to support their own improved understanding of their child's individual differences (ASHA, n.d.).

Using the strategies presented in Chapter 9, we should collaborate with parents and caregivers to ensure our supports and services are based on the developmental profile and needs of each child; a broad rather than narrow range of learning opportunities to foster their communication, language, and social engagement; and the family's involvement in intervention through practice-based coaching to maximize their child's language and social engagement (ASHA, 2023a; Paul et al., 2018; Pye et al., 2021).

What About Echolalia?

Echolalia is one of the characteristics we frequently equate with children who have ASD. Researchers have determined up to 85% of individuals with ASD who are verbal exhibit echolalia in some form (Foxx et al., 2004). *Echolalia* is defined as repeating or imitating what another person has said. Children who are echolalic might imitate what they have heard someone say in everyday life, lines they have heard when listening to a book, lyrics to a song, or a script from a television show or movie. Echolalia could also include the exact imitation of a person's inflection, tone of voice, and volume. There are two classifications of echolalia, each with unique characteristics. *Immediate echolalia* involves the repetition of words or phrases that occur immediately or soon after the original words are spoken. An example of immediate echolalia is the child who repeats a question, such as "Do you want a cookie?" rather than responding with a yes or no. *Delayed echolalia* involves the repetition of words or phrases repeated hours, days, weeks, or months after the initial model. An example of delayed echolalia is a child who might sing "The Wheels on the Bus" when someone enters their home. Children with echolalia use what many of us describe as "more advanced language" than they generate independently. For example, a toddler who is exhibiting echolalia might quote long segments from a favorite television show or sing every lyric to a song but seems unable to ask for milk or answer a question in response to their parent or caregiver (Mize, 2008).

Echolalia is considered a normal stage in the development of a young child's expressive language. When children do not move past this stage, however, or will only repeat what others have said and very rarely expresses their own thoughts or sentences, this behavior becomes a concern. This type of echolalia is not part of typical development and could indicate the child is having difficulty learning to use language effectively (ASHA, 2023a).

Between the age of 1 and 2 years, we expect a toddler to echo or imitate us frequently. This phase begins around 18 months of age when a child has mastered the ability to imitate words and is just beginning to imitate phrases. Although they might continue to imitate their parents or caregivers or use echolalia when we ask complex questions, by 2 years of age, children should begin using their own utterances as well to communicate their needs and wants. Echolalia typically peaks at around 30 months of age and declines significantly by the time a toddler turns 3 years old. This decline coincides with the point in time when children become conversational and truly begin to talk on their own, generating original thoughts, asking new questions, and responding to questions appropriately. By 3 years of age, the use of echolalia should be minimal, and children should be creating and initiating their own simple sentences to communicate with those around them (Prizant, 1983; Prizant & Rydell, 1984).

When we work with young children with ASD, however, we might observe that echolalia occurs with greater frequency and lasts for a longer window of time than it does in children with typically developing language (Prizant, 1983; Prizant & Rydell, 1984). At one time, we considered echolalia a behavior that should be eliminated; we now know many children with ASD use echolalia to learn to communicate. For example, a child who wants to go outside might say to their mother, "Let's put your shoes on," as their way of requesting this activity; the child likely heard their mother say this many times, just before they leave the house together. A child could verbalize "Want me to hold you?" while they are crying, or "It's okay Ben," when they are upset; their parents have said this to them many times in this context and the language is meaningful.

Prizant and colleagues (Prizant, 1983; Prizant & Rydell, 1984) reported echolalia as evidence of "gestalt" processing in children with ASD to acquire language. The young children have learned these phrases or sentences as language "chunks," instead of learning language one word at a time. In EI, parents might share that their child "was not talking at all, and then they suddenly started speaking in full sentences." These children did not start talking by using single words and then work their way up; instead, they started talking with phrases or even complete sentences by echoing utterances they heard on television shows, movies, and/or lyrics of songs. Later, they break these sentences down and rearrange the words to create new sentences. Children with ASD often learn language through this method. We should be encouraged, and encourage families, if this is the way their child is naturally developing language. As SLPs, we can help a child who uses echolalia learn to create their own unique utterances as well, either spontaneously or by utilizing the verbal scripts they share with others.

Sometimes echolalia does not serve an identifiable purpose (Mize, 2008). For example, it is difficult to determine an expectation by the child who repeats every line from a book with no apparent reason while in the grocery store. We can coach parents with children who seem to be stuck in a stage of echolalia to look at this as an opportunity to determine what they are having difficulty learning. In this way, echolalia serves an evaluative purpose for us. For example, the child who walks around and aimlessly quotes a movie or book might need help finding an appropriate activity; they might be feeling stressed or anxious and using this routine to calm themselves. A young child who asks their mother "Do you want a cookie?" might need help learning to initiate requests in a more appropriate way. The toddler who repeatedly echoes a question could need support learning the meaning of the words to accurately process the question, or a child might need specific cues or words to learn how to respond appropriately. A child who repeats, "Good job [their own name]" might need a model to learn a declarative phrase, such as "I did it!" The young child who repeats a sibling's words could be attempting to take a turn in the conversation but does not have the words to interject appropriately.

By taking the time to communicate, ask targeted questions, and collaborate with the family to determine if the echolalic utterance serves a purpose, we can discover what the child's intent is, and then find ways to teach the child what to say in this context. By modeling and shaping the utterance into one that is functional for the child, we will be much more responsive and effective than if we are constantly attempting to eliminate the use of their scripts or echolalia (Mize, 2008; Prizant, 1983; Ryan et al., 2022; Sterponi & Shankey, 2014).

Intellectual Disability

Intellectual disability is one of the most common developmental disabilities. It is estimated that 7 to 8 million people in the United States have an intellectual disability; this is equal to 1 in 10 families who are affected (U.S. Department of Education, 2016). Intellectual disability is a term used when an individual presents limits in their ability to learn at an expected level and function in everyday life (IDEA, 2011). Young children with an intellectual disability could have a difficult time communicating their wants and needs. They might learn and develop more slowly than other children of the same age. An infant or toddler with an intellectual disability could take longer to learn to speak, walk, dress, or eat independently; eventually, they could face learning challenges in school.

Diagnostic criteria of an intellectual disability require childhood onset, either prior to birth or any time before a child turns 18 years old (U.S. Department of Education, 2016). It can be caused by injury, disease, or a neurological problem. The etiology of an intellectual disability is often unknown, and the level of impairment varies significantly from one child to the next. Some of the most well-known causes of intellectual disability include the diagnoses we discuss in this chapter (e.g., Down syndrome, fetal alcohol spectrum disorder, Fragile X syndrome, genetic conditions, birth defects, infections), which happen before birth. Others, such as CP, can occur as the infant is being born or soon after their birth. Other causes of intellectual disability may not occur until a child is older and might include traumatic brain injury, stroke, or infections (CDC, 2022b).

Implications for Assessment and Intervention

All young children who are at risk for or who have been identified with intellectual disabilities should have access to high-quality EI services in their natural environments. As always, our services should be based on and build upon the strengths of the child and family, address their needs, be responsive to their priorities, and be delivered through evidence-based practices.

Infants and toddlers with cognitive or intellectual disabilities often present unique developmental differences that require specific supports and services. Determining appropriate programs, how often they will be provided, and which intervention strategies we implement and coach families to embed must be tailored specifically to the needs of each child.

Cerebral Palsy

As we established in Chapters 10 and 11, CP is the most common childhood physical disability (Rosenbaum et al., 2007). Because CP is a diagnosed physical or mental condition with a high probability of resulting in developmental delay, infants and toddlers who have been diagnosed are automatically eligible for EI services (CDC, 2022c). As such, we will most likely connect with and serve children with CP and their families.

What do we need to know about CP to effectively support and serve these families? According to the CDC (2022c), CP is a group of disorders that affect an individual's ability to move and maintain balance and posture. The disability is caused by abnormal brain development or damage to the developing brain that affects a person's ability to control their muscles. The symptoms of CP vary. A child with severe CP might need special equipment to walk or might not be able to walk at all and require lifelong care. Although a child with mild CP might walk awkwardly, they might not need any special assistance over their lifetime. Although CP is permanent and nonprogressive, clinical presentation of symptoms can certainly change over time (Rosenbaum et al., 2007).

All children with CP have difficulties with movement and posture. Many also have related conditions, including intellectual disability; seizures; problems with vision, hearing, or speech; changes in their spine (e.g., scoliosis); or issues with their joints (CDC, 2022c).

Types of Cerebral Palsy

The medical field classifies CP according to the main type of movement involved. Depending on which areas of the brain are affected, spasticity (stiff muscles), dyskinesia (uncontrollable movements), or ataxia (poor balance and coordination) can occur. The four main types of CP are based on these movement issues and include spastic, dyskinetic, ataxic, and mixed CP.

The most common type is spastic CP. Spastic CP affects about 80% of individuals with CP (CDC, 2022c). Children with spastic CP have increased muscle tone; their muscles are stiff and their movements may be awkward. Spastic CP usually is typically described by the parts of the body that are affected (CDC, 2022c).

- *Spastic diplegia/diparesis*: Muscle stiffness is mainly in the legs and the arms are either less affected or not affected at all. Children with spastic diplegia could have difficulty learning to walk or walking with ease because tight hip and leg muscles cause their legs to pull together, turn inward, and cross at the knees (i.e., scissoring).

- *Spastic hemiplegia/hemiparesis:* This type of CP affects only one side of a child's body; the arm is usually more affected than the leg.

- *Spastic quadriplegia/quadriparesis:* This is the most severe form of spastic CP and affects all four limbs, the trunk, and the face. Children with spastic quadriparesis will usually be unable to walk; they tend to have other developmental disabilities (i.e., intellectual disability; seizures; issues with vision, hearing, or speech).

Children with dyskinetic CP have issues controlling the movement of their hands, arms, feet, and legs. They have difficulty sitting and walking. Their movements are uncontrollable and can be slow and writhing or rapid and jerky. The child's face and tongue are sometimes affected, and they could have a difficult time sucking, swallowing, and talking. The muscle tone of a child with dyskinetic CP can frequently change and vary, from too tight to too loose, within even a single day (CDC, 2022c).

Children with ataxic CP have difficulty with balance and coordination. They could be unsteady when they walk and have a hard time with quick movements or movements that require significant muscle control. These children often have trouble controlling their hands or arms when they reach for something. We might also work with children who have symptoms of more than one type of CP. The most common type of mixed CP is spastic-dyskinetic CP (CDC, 2022c).

Causes and Risk Factors

According to the CDC (2022c), CP is caused by abnormal development of the brain or damage to the developing brain that affects a child's muscle control. There are several possible causes of abnormal development or damage. It can happen before birth, during birth, within a month after birth, or during the first years of an infant's life, while the brain is still developing. When CP is related to abnormal development of the brain or damage that occurred before or during birth, it is called *congenital CP*; most cases of CP are congenital (Yang & Wusthoff, 2023). In many cases, the specific cause is unknown. A small percentage of CP cases is caused by abnormal development of the brain or damage that occurs more than 28 days after birth. This is called *acquired CP* and is usually associated with an infection or head injury (Yang & Wusthoff, 2023).

Implications for Assessment and Intervention

The signs of CP vary greatly secondary to the many different types and levels of disability. The main sign that a child might have CP is a delay reaching motor or movement milestones. Because infants and toddlers who present with delays in cognitive development, physical development, communication development, social-emotional development, or adaptive development are eligible for EI services, we might serve children with CP prior to their diagnosis. If we are working with an infant or toddler and observe any of the symptoms presented in Table 12–2, we must discuss our concerns with the EI team, including the parents and caregivers, to determine whether further evaluation or referrals to medical professionals for differential diagnosis are merited.

Table 12–2. Signs and Symptoms of Possible Cerebral Palsy

In infants younger than 6 months of age: • Their head lags when we pick them up while they are lying on their back. • They feel stiff. • They feel floppy. • When held cradled in arms, they seem to overextend their back and neck and constantly act as if they are pushing away from us. • When we pick them up, their legs get stiff, and they cross or scissor them.
In infants older than 6 months of age: • They do not roll over in either direction. • They are unable to bring their hands together. • They have difficulty bringing their hands to their mouth. • They keep one hand fisted while reaching out with the other hand.
In infants older than 10 months of age: • They crawl by pushing off with one hand and leg, dragging the opposite hand and leg. • They scoot around on their buttocks or hop on their knees but do not crawl on all fours.

Note. Adapted from "Cerebral palsy in children," by J. Yang & C. Wusthoff, 2023 (http://www.healthychildren.org/English/health-issues/conditions/developmental-disabilities/pages/Cerebral-Palsy.aspx); "What is CP?" by the Centers for Disease Control and Prevention, 2022f (https://www.cdc.gov/ncbddd/cp/facts.html#:~:text=Cerebral%20palsy%20(CP)%20is%20a, problems%20with%20using%20the%20muscles).

When we provide EI services and supports to young children with CP and their families, it is important to consider the range of disabilities that can affect their motor, cognitive, communication, and feeding development. We need to be aware of the weakness or spasticity with which the children are dealing and must consider their possible inability to control the muscles they need to produce speech and to eat and drink safely and enjoyably. We can address the child's communication needs by focusing on prelinguistic skills (vocalizations), manual sign language, gestures, picture communication boards, and voice output communication devices. If children struggle to produce speech sounds and have difficulty communicating their needs and wants verbally, we might need to consider and discuss AAC options with the family. We can effectively support parents and caregivers by providing them with information and facilitating their children's communication through any possible means and modalities.

Morgan et al. (2021) recently conducted a systematic review of the best available evidence for effective intervention with children from birth to 2 years old who were at high risk of or diagnosed with CP. Their findings indicate, among the best available evidence across the domains of motor function, cognitive skills, communication, eating and drinking, vision, sleep, managing muscle tone, musculoskeletal health, and parental support, building parental and caregiver capacity for attachment with their child is one of the most effective strategies towards best practice regarding CP-specific early interventions (Morgan et al., 2021).

Down Syndrome

Down syndrome is a chromosomal condition associated with intellectual disability, developmental delays, and characteristic facial features. The disorder is caused by the presence of an extra copy of chromosome 21 in the cells of the body. Down syndrome continues to be the most common chromosomal condition diagnosed in the United States. Each year, approximately 6,000 (1 in every 700) newborns in the United States have Down syndrome (Mai et al., 2019).

Types of Down Syndrome

The three types of Down syndrome include trisomy 21, mosaic Down syndrome, and translocation Down syndrome (Shin et al., 2010).

- *Trisomy 21*: About 95% of people with Down syndrome have trisomy 21 (Shin et al., 2010). With this type, each cell in the body has three separate copies of chromosome 21 instead of the typical two copies.

- *Translocation Down syndrome:* This type accounts for approximately 3% of individuals with Down syndrome (Shin et al., 2010). The syndrome occurs when an extra part or an entire extra chromosome 21 is present and is attached to a different chromosome instead of developing as its own chromosome.

- *Mosaic Down syndrome*: This type affects approximately 2% of individuals with Down syndrome (Shin et al., 2010). In children with mosaic Down syndrome, some of their cells have three copies of chromosome 21, whereas other cells have the typical two copies of chromosome 21. Children with mosaic Down syndrome might have the same features as other children with Down syndrome; however, they could have fewer features of the condition, secondary to the presence of some (or many) cells with a typical number of chromosomes.

Causes and Risk Factors

We know Down syndrome is caused by an extra chromosome; we do not know, however, why the chromosomal abnormality occurs or how many different factors play a role. Although women who are 35 years or older when they become pregnant are more likely to have a pregnancy affected by Down syndrome, most babies with Down syndrome are born to mothers younger than 35 years old (Allen et al., 2009; Ghosh et al., 2009; Olsen et al., 1996).

Several procedures are available to screen for and diagnose Down syndrome. Screening tests often include a combination of a blood test, which measures the number of specific substances in the mother's blood, and an ultrasound, which creates a picture of the baby. During an ultrasound, the technician looks for fluid behind the baby's neck as extra fluid in this region could indicate a genetic problem (CDC, 2022c). These screening tests can help determine the baby's risk of Down syndrome. Rarely, screening tests give an abnormal result even when there is nothing wrong. On occasion, the test results are normal and yet they miss an issue that does exist. Diagnostic tests are typically performed after a positive screening test to confirm Down syndrome. These diagnostic tests could include the following and look for changes in chromosomes indicative of Down syndrome (CDC, 2022c).

- Chorionic villus sampling, which examines material from the placenta.

- Amniocentesis, which examines the amniotic fluid (the fluid from the sac surrounding the baby).

- Percutaneous umbilical blood sampling, which examines blood from the umbilical cord.

Despite the different types, all individuals with Down syndrome have an increased risk of certain health problems, including heart defects, respiratory problems, and gastrointestinal issues. Most individuals have mild to moderate intellectual disabilities; many, although not all, individuals with Down syndrome also experience chronic ear infections, hearing loss, eye diseases, and obstructive sleep apnea (CDC, 2022c). Physical symptoms of Down syndrome can include a small head and flattened face, short neck, slanted eyes, low muscle tone, abnormal skin fold at the inside corner of the eye, small stature, and short hands with a single crease in the palm. Many of these physical features become less noticeable as individuals with Down syndrome get older (CDC, 2022c).

Implications for Assessment and Intervention

Although there are common speech and language issues, young children with Down syndrome do not present with a single pattern of communication, speech, and language development. Most children with Down syndrome do, however, face challenges related to their speech and language development. Many children with Down syndrome have more difficulty with expressive language than they do with their comprehension of speech and language; as a result, their receptive language skills are often more advanced than their expressive language skills. Vocabulary acquisition tends to be easier for these children than the acquisition of grammatical structures and sequencing in sentences. Additionally, sequencing sounds and words might be more difficult. Research also indicates children with Down syndrome present with difficulties related to complex organizational processes of executive function, social-cognition, and task motivation (Cebula et al. 2010; Gilmore et al. 2009), which are all characteristics that operate in conjunction with expected delays in expressive language, particularly focused on morphosyntactic weaknesses (Abbeduto et al., 2007; Chapman & Bird, 2012). Our awareness of these challenges supports the competence with which we conduct evaluation and assessment services for these infants and toddlers.

As we have just discovered, in addition to several unique concerns, the speech and language difficulties children with Down syndrome demonstrate are the same as those that challenge other infants and toddlers with developmental delays (Kumin, 1998). Therefore, the knowledge and skills we acquired in Chapters 6 and 9 can also be applied to infants and toddlers with Down syndrome, with a focus on their specific areas of need. We can choose functional outcomes and use treatment strategies that address the strengths of the infant or toddler and focus on their unique developmental patterns.

Although young children with Down syndrome might not say their first words until 2 or 3 years of age, there are multiple cognitive and prelinguistic skills they must acquire before they learn to use words; as SLPs in EI, we can contribute to the development of these skills by addressing them in our sessions and coaching parents and caregivers to embed them in their routines and activities. These include the ability to imitate sounds and gestures, turn-taking skills, visual skills (e.g., looking at the speaker and objects), auditory skills (e.g., listening to music, speech, or speech sounds for increasing periods of time), tactile skills (e.g., learning about touch, exploring objects in the mouth), oral motor skills (e.g., using the tongue, moving the lips), and cognitive skills (e.g., object permanence, cause and effect).

Ultimately, recent research indicates when we focus on language, communication, and feeding within a naturalistic setting, and provide family-centered, coaching-based services, EI results in positive outcomes and effectively supports both children with Down syndrome and their families (Seager et al., 2022). Studies have shown that EI can improve cognitive abilities, speech and language skills, social skills, and self-care skills in children with Down syndrome. Additionally, EI can help children with Down syndrome develop a positive self-image and sense of belonging and can prepare them to lead productive and fulfilling lives. Families who receive EI services report higher levels of satisfaction with their child's development than those who do not receive such services (Seager et al., 2022). Finally, it is important for us to recognize our role in supporting and empowering parents; those who have participated in EI report feeling more confident in their parenting skills and are more prepared to handle the challenges of raising a child with Down syndrome (Seager et al., 2022).

The Importance of Interprofessional Services

Because of the many challenges they face, infants and toddlers with Down syndrome will likely experience delays in multiple areas of development. Each of these potential difficulties can affect a child's communication, language, and feeding development. It is more important than ever that we serve on an interprofessional team in EI and collaborate with our colleagues to most effectively serve these children and their families. Potential EI team members include the family, other health-care providers, social workers, infant mental health specialists, physicians, caregivers, and preschool teachers. In addition to our role, an EI service team often also consists of an OT and PT. PTs offer services to address the physical aspects of the child's development, including gross motor development and mobility. OTs work in the development of occupations such as play, social participation, and activities of daily living. We often collaborate with OTs to facilitate feeding and play development, whereas OTs and PTs often collaborate to encourage the development of motor skills and positioning for play.

In the first months of life, physical development serves as the foundation for all future progress and infants learn through interactions with their environment. To learn, therefore, an infant must have the ability to move freely and purposefully. An infant's ability to explore their surroundings, reach and grasp toys, turn their head while watching a moving object, or roll over and crawl are all dependent on gross and fine motor development. These physical, interactive activities foster an understanding and mastery of the environment and ultimately stimulate cognitive, language, and social development. Physical therapy focuses primarily on the motor development of a young child. During the first 3 to 4 months of life, an infant is expected to gain head control and the ability to pull to sitting positions (with help) with adequate neck support and enough strength in the upper torso to maintain an erect posture. A PT, therefore, could assist a baby with Down syndrome who has low muscle tone to work toward and achieve this milestone. A PT could support an infant or toddler with Down syndrome to physically navigate their environment by helping them learn to crawl, walk, and climb. In the long term, physical therapy can also focus on the prevention of an infant or toddler's use of compensatory movement patterns that children with Down syndrome are prone to developing; these patterns, if not corrected, can lead to orthopedic and functional problems (CDC, 2022b, 2022c).

Occupational therapy is also important to ensure young children with Down syndrome develop and master skills for independence. An OT can support children's development of skills that allow them to open and close objects, pick up and release toys of various sizes and shapes, stack and build, manipulate knobs and buttons, and experiment with crayons. OTs also help children learn to feed and dress themselves; they teach them skills to play and interact socially with other children (CDC, 2022b, 2022c). These skills are all necessary to ensure children with Down syndrome, and all infants and toddlers, are empowered to play, communicate, and engage with others. To effectively support every family within their child's natural environment and to support the child's relationship with their family, teamwork is essential. When we deliver EI supports and services to children with Down syndrome, this is more important than ever.

Fragile X Syndrome

Fragile X syndrome is a genetic disorder caused by changes in a gene called Fragile X Messenger Ribonucleoprotein 1 (FMR1). FMR1 usually makes a protein called FMRP needed for brain development. Individuals who have Fragile X syndrome do not make this protein. The syndrome affects both males and females, although females tend to present milder symptoms than males. A review of research studies estimates that approximately 1 in 4,000 males and 1 in 10,000 females have been diagnosed with Fragile X syndrome (Davidson et al., 2022).

Fragile X is noted as the leading cause of inherited intellectual disabilities. Males with the full mutation demonstrate features of ASD in about 90% of cases; 60% of these individuals meet diagnostic criteria for ASD (Abbeduto et al., 2019). Approximately 17% of females with Fragile X syndrome meet diagnostic criteria for ASD (Abbeduto et al., 2019). Physical symptoms include a long and narrow face, prominent ears and jaw, and microcephaly. Individuals with the syndrome can also present with multiple comorbid medical issues, including strabismus, hearing loss because of recurrent ear infections, obesity, joint hypermobility, and seizures. In addition to physical conditions and comorbid medical issues, children with Fragile X syndrome tend to display a wide range of psychological and behavioral symptoms, including attention deficits, hyperactivity, aggressiveness, and anxiety and tend to have delays in all areas of their development, both early on and throughout life (Abbeduto et al., 2019; Hagerman & Hagerman, 2002). Table 12–3 provides a full range of common symptoms of Fragile X syndrome.

Table 12–3. Common Symptoms of Fragile X Syndrome

Physical features
• Flat feet
• High-arched palate
• Long, narrow face
• Large forehead
• Large jaw
• Large ears and crossed/lazy eyes
• Low muscle tone
• Soft skin
• Flexible or double-jointed fingers
Behavior
• Attention-deficit/hyperactivity disorder (ADHD)
• Flapping or biting hands
• Poor eye contact
• Sensitivity to crowds, touch, sounds, foods, and textures
• Social anxiety or shyness
Intelligence and cognitive development
• Delayed early developmental milestones
• Delayed development of nonverbal communication (e.g., using gestures, body language, facial expressions)
• Difficulty learning new skills
• Language processing
Mental health issues
• Anxiety
• Depression
• Obsessive-compulsive behaviors
Other health conditions
• Aggressiveness or irritability
• Obesity
• Seizures
• Self-injury behaviors
• Sleep difficulties

Note. Adapted from "Epidemiology of Fragile X syndrome: a systematic review and meta-analysis," by J. Hunter et al., 2014; *Fragile X syndrome: Diagnosis, treatment, and research,* by R. J. Hagerman & P. J. Hagerman, 2002.

Implications for Assessment and Intervention

Young children with Fragile X syndrome are often referred to EI for delays in communication and language development. As SLPs, we are often the first providers to see them. We will likely work with an infant or toddler who has not yet been diagnosed with the syndrome. It is important that we are aware of the signs and symptoms presented earlier and work with our EI team if we suspect a child has Fragile X. The only way to diagnose the syndrome is with a special blood test called the FMR1 DNA Test for Fragile X. The American Academy of Pediatrics recommends that children diagnosed with general developmental delays, intellectual disability, or ASD receive a genetic test for Fragile X syndrome (Hersh & Saul, 2011).

Although there is no cure for Fragile X syndrome, the symptoms can be treated medically and, as EI providers, we can address a child's developmental delays and support and empower the family. Roberts et al. (2008) suggested several useful language intervention strategies to address the needs of young children with Fragile X syndrome, including responsive treatment techniques and milieu teaching. Recall from our introduction to these strategies in Chapter 9 that responsive strategies involve us modeling a target communication behavior without an expectation of a child's response (ASHA, 2008). In milieu teaching, we simply combine these strategies within natural, play-based, or routines-based activities. These techniques include self-talk, parallel talk, modeling, serve-and-return, and expansion or recasting of the child's verbalizations. Linguistic mapping is also a powerful strategy because it offers the family easily accessible opportunities to respond to their child's interests. They consistently expose their child to vocabulary to communicate something in which they have already shown an interest. We coach them to watch for their child's communication acts and to respond with language that will eventually empower them. When parents or caregivers embrace and embed this form of responsive modeling in their everyday activities and routines, they demonstrate how much they value their role as their child's first and most important teacher. When we coach parents and caregivers to engage in these responsive strategies with their child with Fragile X syndrome, we teach them to understand their child's intentional communicative behaviors and attend to their child's focus. It is also important that we ensure intervention is applicable to real-life activities. As is the case with all infants and toddlers in EI, when our time with the family and the strategies we share with them are relevant to their child, they are more likely to embed and generalize this information outside of and between our sessions with them.

Sensory and Perceptual Disorders

When we consider how infants interact with their environment, most of their engagement with parents, caregivers, and their environment is connected to the sensory and perceptual stimuli to which they respond. Early bonding with a parent or caregiver is related to an infant's ability to make eye contact and sustain gaze with their parents, respond to their voices by gurgling and cooing, and receive comfort through the sight, sound, and touch of others. Infants often attempt to move because they see or hear something that intrigues them. They learn that people and objects exist in the world primarily because they become aware of them in their environment. Early infant development is typically linked to their vision and hearing abilities. When these senses do not develop as expected, their development is affected.

Under IDEA Part C (2004), infants and toddlers who are deaf, blind, or have hearing or vision loss are considered at risk for experiencing serious developmental delays without EI services; these children are at particular risk for developing delayed communication, speech, and language skills. In some states, children with these diagnoses automatically qualify for EI services; this is not, however, always the case.

Hard of Hearing or Deaf

Hard of hearing refers to any degree of hearing loss, mild to severe, and can occur when there is a problem with the inner, middle, and/or outer ears, or the nerves needed for hearing. According to the CDC (2022a), more than 6,000 infants were identified as deaf or hard of hearing in 2020 alone. Approximately 1.9% of children have difficulty hearing, and permanent hearing loss is diagnosed in more than 1 out of every 1,000 children screened for hearing loss, regardless of whether they have symptoms (Shah, 2022).

There are many causes of hearing loss, including those that are congenital, or present at birth, and those that can be acquired after birth. *Congenital hearing loss* means hearing loss that is present at birth. Causes of hearing loss in newborns include infections (e.g., rubella or herpes simplex virus), premature birth, low birth weight, birth injuries, maternal drug and alcohol use while pregnant, jaundice and Rh factor problems, maternal diabetes, maternal high blood pressure while pregnant (preeclampsia), anoxia, or genetics (CDC, 2022a; Shah, 2022). *Acquired hearing loss* appears at any time after birth and can be the result of a disease, a condition, or an injury. Conditions that can cause acquired hearing loss in young children include ear infections, ototoxic drugs, meningitis, measles, encephalitis, chicken pox, influenza, mumps, head injury, or noise exposure (CDC, 2022a; Shah, 2022).

The four types of hearing loss are *conductive hearing loss*, which is caused by something that stops sounds from getting through the outer or middle ear; *sensorineural hearing loss*, which occurs when there is a problem in the way the inner ear or hearing nerve works; *mixed hearing loss*, which includes both a conductive and a sensorineural hearing loss; and *auditory neuropathy spectrum disorder*, which occurs when sound enters the ear normally, but because of damage to the inner ear or the hearing nerve, it is not organized in a way that the brain can understand (CDC, 2022a; Shah, 2022).

The degree of hearing loss an individual experiences can range from mild, where a child might hear some speech sounds but struggle to hear all sounds, to profound, in which a child will not hear any speech or sounds. Finally, a child with hearing loss can be described via several points of comparison (CDC, 2022a):

- *Unilateral or bilateral:* Hearing loss is in one ear or both ears.

- *Prelingual or postlingual:* Hearing loss happened before or after a person learned to talk.

- *Symmetrical or asymmetrical*: Hearing loss is the same in both ears or is different in each ear.

- *Progressive or sudden:* Hearing loss worsens over time or happens quickly.

- *Fluctuating or stable*: Hearing loss gets either better or worse over time or stays the same over time.

- *Congenital or acquired/delayed onset*: Hearing loss is present at birth or appears sometime later in life.

Screening and Diagnosis

Most states now require that newborns undergo routine screening tests to detect hearing loss. Newborns are usually screened in two stages. First, newborns are tested for echoes produced by healthy ears in response to soft clicks made by a handheld device (i.e., evoked otoacoustic emissions testing). If the results of this test raise questions about the infant's hearing, a second test is administered to measure electrical signals from the brain in response to sounds (i.e., auditory brainstem response test [ABR]). The ABR is painless and typically conducted while the infant is asleep. If the results of the ABR are abnormal, the test is repeated in 1 month. If hearing loss is still detected, the infant might be fitted with hearing aids and referred for EI services (National Institute on Deafness and Other Communication Disorders [NIDCD], 2021; Shah, 2022).

Cochlear Implants

A cochlear implant is a small, complex electronic device that issues a sense of sound to a person who is profoundly deaf or severely hearing impaired. The implant consists of an external portion that sits behind the ear and an internal portion surgically placed under the skin. A cochlear implant is different from a hearing aid. Hearing aids amplify sounds so they can be detected by damaged ears, whereas cochlear implants bypass the damaged portions of the ear to directly stimulate the auditory nerve. Signals generated by the implant are sent through the auditory nerve to the brain, which then recognizes the signals as sound. It is important for us to recognize hearing through a cochlear implant is different from normal hearing and infants, and toddlers need time to learn or relearn how to hear (NIDCD, 2021).

The U.S. Food and Drug Administration (FDA) first approved cochlear implants in the mid-1980s to treat hearing loss in adults. Since 2000, cochlear implants have been FDA-approved for use in eligible children as early as 12 months of age. Cochlear Americas Corporation recently received approval to lower the age of cochlear implantation to 9 months for children with bilateral, profound sensorineural hearing loss (The Hearing Journal, 2020). Children and adults who are deaf or severely hard-of-hearing can be fitted for cochlear implants. As of December 2019, approximately 736,900 registered devices have been implanted worldwide. In the United States, roughly 118,100 devices have been implanted in adults and 65,000 in children (NIDCD, 2021).

Young children who are deaf or severely hard-of-hearing and use a cochlear implant while they are young are exposed to sounds to develop speech and language skills during a critical window of time. According to Leigh and colleagues (2016), when children receive a cochlear implant followed by intensive therapy before they are 18 months old, they are better able to hear, comprehend sound and music, and speak than peers who receive implants when they are older. Additionally, eligible children who receive a cochlear implant before 18 months of age develop language skills at a rate comparable to children with normal hearing and are more likely to succeed in mainstream classrooms (Leigh et al., 2016).

Implications for Assessment and Intervention

Through the implementation of early hearing detection and intervention programs in the United States, there is an unprecedented demand for SLP services with infants and toddlers with hearing loss. There is no doubt SLPs contribute valuable knowledge and skills on EI teams when serving infants and toddlers with hearing loss and their families. Many of us, however, have limited experience working with these young children. According to Robbins (2009), there are several clinical needs about which we need to be knowledgeable to implement supportive services for infants and toddlers with hearing loss and their families.

We need to help families manage their infant's hearing aids or cochlear implants. Aids or implants are the means by which the young child's developing brain accesses sound. If parents or caregivers have included auditory and spoken language development among their IFSP outcomes for their child, one of our goals is to support the family in ensuring their child uses an appropriate hearing device all the time. Although an audiologist will fit the devices and monitor the hearing loss, we play a crucial role in providing ongoing support to parents related to issues such as inserting the devices, working quickly toward full-time use, and responding if or when the infant or toddler pulls out the devices (Robbins, 2009).

We must also be able and willing to discuss communication options with the family and encourage parents and caregivers to see communication along a continuum. As do all parents, those of infants with hearing loss balance the demands of everyday family life with the extraordinary demands of supporting their child's communication development at home. Parents and caregivers of these young children also have the additional and stressful task of making decisions about communication methodology, including American Sign Language, manually coded English signs, auditory-oral approaches, or some combination of these. We find parents and caregivers have often made an initial decision about methodology when the first IFSP is developed. They need our reassurance that if their child's needs change over time, their initial decision is not a lifelong commitment to one approach over another. Communication methodologies fall along a continuum; what might have been appropriate in the early months of EI could require alteration as the child develops and grows. This issue is of particular importance for families of infants with profound hearing loss who have chosen cochlear implants for their children but are waiting for surgery. Most babies awaiting implant surgery wear traditional hearing aids. In these cases, some families struggle with whether to use sign language as a temporary communication method prior to the surgery. They often rely on us for advice and information. It is important that we continue to explore current literature on this topic to ensure we are able to offer these families evidence-based information (Robbins, 2009).

Considering the Family

When a family finds out their newborn or infant is deaf or hard of hearing, they are launched onto a journey during which multiple decisions need to be made. They are wrapping their heads around their child's hearing loss and are faced with information and conversation about hearing aids, cochlear implants, spoken language, sign language, and total communication. As EI providers, we know every family is dealing with many different emotions and concerns when we meet them; we must do our best to keep this in mind, particularly with families who are confronted with a diagnosis of hearing loss, as we begin to share information with them. The evidence-based approaches that serve as the foundation of EI are also effective when we engage with families of children who are deaf or have hearing loss. Our primary goal is to foster families' abilities to embed an abundance of age-appropriate communication and language opportunities, joint engagement routines, and regular conversational turns throughout natural, daily interactions. Access to communication and language by their child is often a priority for these families (DesJardin et al., 2014; Quittner et al., 2013). Therefore, we can coach parents and caregivers to promote the development of their infant or toddler by providing an engaging social-emotional environment, creating and maximizing natural language, and developing learning opportunities within everyday routines and activities. Ensuring that families understand their efforts to stimulate their child's language development and provide access to language early in their development is a critical step in addressing the child's need and opportunity to benefit from social, cognitive, and linguistic outcomes (Joint Committee on Infant Hearing, 2019).

Parent choice is crucial as it relates to communication options and choices. How parents communicate with their child is a personal and individual choice. Within these choices, we work with families who choose to speak, then add sign later; who choose to sign without speech; who speak and never use sign; and who choose, as medically appropriate, to pursue cochlear implants. Each time a new decision or choice is made regarding their communication with their infant or toddler, the needs of the child and family change, too. Our ability to remain flexible as the parents attempt to chart their course through what is, for them, uncharted territory, allows us to support them throughout their process while respecting the decisions they are making.

Loss of Vision or Blind

Nearly 3% of children younger than 18 years are blind or visually impaired (CDC, 2022c). Loss of vision can range from no vision (i.e., blindness) or very low vision to an inability to see particular colors. It can happen at any age. Although most vision conditions in children stay the same throughout life, some could result in vision problems for only a short time. Other conditions get worse over time, resulting in poorer vision or blindness as children get older. Low vision is when a child is unable to see all the things they should be able to see for their age. A child might have low to no vision, blurred vision, or loss of peripheral vision; they might have color blindness and may not be able to see some colors. A child is considered legally blind when they are unable to see at 6 meters what a child with typical vision can see at 60 meters or their field of vision is less than 20 degrees in diameter, in comparison to an individual with typical vision who sees 180 degrees in diameter (American Academy of Pediatrics, 2016).

Infants can be born with impaired vision, or the loss of vision can also happen later due to disease, injury, or a medical condition. The most common causes of vision loss include the following (American Academy of Pediatrics, 2016):

- Neurological conditions that affect the parts of the brain that control sight (e.g., cortical vision loss).
- Genetic conditions (e.g., albinism, retinitis pigmentosa).
- Prematurity or prenatal conditions.
- Conditions like pediatric glaucoma, cataracts, and cancers (e.g., retinoblastoma).
- Infections with viruses during pregnancy (e.g., rubella, cytomegalovirus, sexually transmitted infection, toxoplasmosis).
- Structural problems with the eyes that limit vision (e.g., microphthalmia or anophthalmia).
- Damage or injury to the eye, to the pathways connecting the eye to the brain, or to the visual center of the brain.

Early Signs and Symptoms

Most infants begin to focus on faces and objects by 4 to 5 weeks of age. By about 8 to 12 weeks, most infants will smile at and track familiar faces and objects. An infant who does not demonstrate these milestones could have a loss of vision. If we observe any of the following signs or symptoms related to a child's vision, we should communicate our concerns with the parents or caregivers (American Academy of Pediatrics, 2016).

- Their eyes move quickly from side to side (nystagmus), jerk, or wander randomly.
- Their eyes do not follow familiar faces or objects.
- They do not seem to make eye contact with parents or caregivers.
- Their eyes do not react to a bright light being turned on in the room.
- Their pupils seem white or cloudy rather than black.
- Their eyes turn in toward their nose or drift out toward the side of their face; this movement might happen consistently or on occasion.

Implications for Assessment and Intervention

When working with a young child who cannot see, we must consider the important role their hands play in relation to their language development (Miles, 2003). The hands of children who are visually impaired or blind are often extremely expressive, and tend to take the place of their smile, eye gaze, and facial expressions. Young children who are blind often move excitedly in response to pleasure and interest, even before they find themselves able to explore or intentionally reach out. Fraiberg (1977) discovered that parents and caregivers who were coached to notice the hands of their blind children reported stronger relationships with their infants. Teaching parents to recognize and accurately interpret their children's use of their hands as smiles and signs of interest helped them maintain positive turn-taking interactions and reinforced the early bonding necessary for healthy development (Fraiberg, 1977). With this information in mind, we need to remind families that pointing and gesturing will not have the same meaning for their child as they do for a child who can see. Mutual touch should replace pointing, as it represents the development and establishment of joint attention between an adult and child who is visually impaired or blind (Miles, 2003).

Researchers have determined several additional consistent characteristics across infants and toddlers who are blind or visually impaired, specific to their communication and language development, about which we should be aware when assessing current levels of functioning and developing IFSP outcomes. Although there is evidence that most children overcome this delay, these children tend to have a slight delay in the acquisition of their first meaningful words (Bigelow, 2005; Brambring, 2007). Toddlers who are blind or have a loss in vision could also be delayed in their use of single words and two-word combinations (McConachie, 1990; McConachie & Moore, 1994). Additional research indicates these children demonstrate longer periods of echolalia, a period of incorrect use of pronouns, differences in the use of spatial prepositions, and the extensive use of questions (Anderson et al., 1984; Brambring, 2006; Urwin, 1984). Each of these skills is acquired by young children as they explore their environments and learn to connect words with concepts.

It is important to remember that vision loss and blindness will affect how a child learns (Ferrell, 1997). As we assess the communication and language development of infants and toddlers who have loss of vision or are blind, the following three factors must be considered.

- The child will have reduced opportunities to engage in incidental learning through observation and imitation (Raver & Childress, 2015).

- The child will have to use other sensory information to understand the world around them; this means they will learn concepts by examining and exploring items piece by piece rather than holistically (Ferrell, 2000).

- The child will face additional challenges when faced with experiences and concepts traditionally visual and abstract in nature (e.g., colors, images in a book or on a computer screen, birds or airplanes or butterflies flying overhead).

We should also be mindful of these factors as we work with families, choose strategies to implement in our sessions, and coach them to address their children's unique needs. Using a strengths-based assessment and intervention approach, in which we collect information about the things each child likes to do, activities in which they participate, and skills they have acquired, addresses these considerations and effectively serves as our foundation for engaging the visually impaired or blind child in everyday learning activities that focus on their strengths, supporting their participation in activities, and interacting with the child in a way that builds on their strengths to promote new learning (Early Childhood Technical Assistance Center, 2020). To use the strengths-based approach with children who experience loss of vision or blindness, we need to embed authentic and functional strategies that must include both family-centered and routines-based evaluation and assessment instruments.

Additional suggestions for engaging children who are blind or have a loss of vision and coaching their parents and caregivers include the following (Miles, 2003; Raver & Childress, 2015):

- Consistently connect objects, people, and actions in the child's environment with verbal labels.

- Create consistent routines and maintain daily schedules to impart predictability.

- Encourage and support the child's movement and exploration within and beyond their immediate reach.

- Engage in self-talk and parallel talk; talk about imminent and upcoming activities to prepare the child for the transition.

- Foster the child's independence and teach new skills related to eating, drinking, and everyday activities.

- Provide a variety of experiences and encourage the child to explore with their hands.

- Offer toys and materials with a variety of textures, weights, and temperatures.

- Reduce auditory distractions.

Use of Hand-Under-Hand Prompting With Children Who Have Sensory and Perceptual Disorders

We were introduced to hand-under-hand prompting in Chapter 9. This strategy involves physical prompting during which an adult guides a child's hands from beneath; it is less intrusive than manipulating the child's hands. Hand-under-hand prompting is particularly beneficial for young children who are tactilely defensive, have sensory processing disorders, or are deaf and blind (National Center on Deaf-Blindness, 2021).

When we use the hand-under-hand technique, our hands perform the activity while the child's hands rest on top of ours; the infant or toddler can feel what our hands are doing by guiding them in this noninvasive way. When we use hand-under-hand prompting, the child is not forced to comply but can move their hands at will. If the activity is new to the child and they are at all hesitant to engage, they might feel more secure touching our hands rather than the unknown object or activity. Additionally, this strategy gives children the opportunity to focus their energy on feeling the movements of our hands, rather than on an object or action, because their palms are on our hands. With hand-under-hand prompting, it is common for young children to feel more comfortable and in control; they can move their hands freely with this placement. We need to connect our hand-under-hand prompting with a verbal description of the activity or task in which we are engaging with the child (Miles, 2003; National Center on Deaf-Blindness, 2021).

Preterm and Low Birth Weight

Preterm birth, classified as birth before 37 weeks gestational age, accounts for nearly 1 in 10 live births in the United States annually (Osterman et al., 2022). The rate of preterm births in 2020 was 10.09%; the rate of infants born with low birth weight in the same year was 8.24% (Osterman et al., 2022).

Significant medical conditions, including CP, sensory impairments, and other disabilities can be the result of preterm birth or low birth weight. Infants who are born extremely premature and the smallest infants born with low birth weight have the poorest outcomes, particularly if they have severe respiratory distress or major brain bleeds during the neonatal period (Ambalavanan et al., 2012). All children born preterm or low birth weight are at increased risk for adverse neurodevelopmental outcomes including language, cognitive and executive function, social-emotional, and motor delays. There is a plethora of research supporting the relationship between preterm and low-birth-weight infants and long-term difficulties with language acquisition (Barre et al., 2011). In addition to the development of vocabulary, these children often demonstrate persistent difficulties with language processing, grammatical issues, and phonological working memory challenges (Ramon-Casas et al., 2013; Sansavini et al., 2007). They also present delays in social engagement, particularly in their awareness and development of joint attention, as early as 6 to 9 months of age (De Schuymer et al., 2011). Social-emotional development is also affected in children who were born preterm or low birth weight. Research indicates these toddlers often present difficulties and delays with compliance, attention, imitation, and play skills (Boyd et al., 2013; Spittle et al., 2009).

Preterm and low birth weight as conditions for EI eligibility vary significantly from state to state. In some states, these conditions are considered for automatic eligibility; in others, these infants are considered at risk and EI services are delayed until the infant or toddler demonstrates observable developmental delays or disabilities. Based on these discrepancies and the concern that timely services are not being provided to children born low birth weight or preterm and their families, the DEC (2018) endorsed the development of national guidelines for the identification and eligibility for Part C services of children born low birth weight and preterm in the United States. The following are the core principles of this endorsement and the DEC recommendations (DEC, 2018).

- Children born with low birth weight and preterm are at high risk for neurodevelopmental concerns including language, cognitive and executive function, social-emotional, and motor delays.

- There are marked inconsistencies in terms of practices and policies regarding services for children born low birth weight and preterm that vary widely from state to state, leading to complications in identification and referral of these children.

- Practitioners would benefit from increasing knowledge and skills to support their work with infants, toddlers, and young children who were born low birth weight or preterm and their families.

- There is consistent evidence dating back to the 1980s indicating EI can improve outcomes for children born low birth weight and preterm, as evidenced on increased performance on follow-up tests of cognitive and verbal skills at 8 and 18 years of age.

- Family involvement and low-risk environments were important contributors to positive outcomes starting in the NICU.

- Low birth weight of less than or equal to 1,500 grams (3.3 pounds) and less than 37 weeks gestational age should be considered a diagnosed physical or mental condition for an infant to be determined eligible to receive EI services.

Assessment and Intervention in the NICU

Children born preterm or low birth weight typically spend their first days or weeks of life in the NICU. Their stay could extend anywhere from 2 days to multiple months, depending on their medical status. During this time, families benefit tremendously from the expertise of the medical staff as well as EI providers. As SLPs in the NICU, we often address an infant's feeding and swallowing difficulties. The first thing we typically do with a newborn in this environment is to conduct an assessment. We might conduct an Apgar test in order to determine a point of comparison of the infant's muscle tone, reflex, irritability, and other developmental factors. We visually assess the physical development of the infant and can conduct a series of neurological tests to evaluate brain development. We often use ultrasound, videofluoroscopy, endoscopic examination, and auscultation to determine the physiology of the infant's mouth and throat structures. Once we have diagnosed any feeding issues, we typically collaborate with the rest of the care team to develop a treatment plan. This plan might include goals for the infant to improve food intake, shorten the length of feeding sessions, or increase comfort, as assessed by various visual or behavioral signals offered during feedings. It is also imperative that we assess the infant's ability to coordinate the suck–swallow–breathe reflex, as a failure to engage these motor skills in the correct sequence can lead to aspiration and further breathing complications or pneumonia (García-Tormos et al., 2013).

Although feeding is the most immediate goal for neonates in the NICU, we also keep long-term developmental goals in mind. Infants' care in the NICU can affect the long-term development of their ability to communicate. As SLPs, we can implement multiple intervention approaches, including those that address the infant's vestibular, auditory, visual, and tactile systems. Areas of intervention that could affect an infant's communication include activities to promote prolonged periods of sleep, adaptation of the environment, and postural changes (Rossetti, 2001). Physical and environmental adaptations include positioning or swaddling (e.g., snugly wrapping the infant in a blanket to restrict limb movement) to support their motor system, and controlling external stimuli, such as lighting and noise (Arvedson et al., 2010). Studies have revealed that even mundane aspects of infant care in the NICU, including how the infants are positioned in their isolettes and the amount of noise in the room, can affect their muscle development and ability to perceive and develop communication, language, and speech sounds (Blackburn, 1998; Nair et al., 2003; Rossetti, 2001). As SLPs, we now recommend low-noise environments in the NICU and the use of physical supports, such as swaddling and the establishment of skin-to-skin contact between infants and their parents, to help reduce the potential impacts on their development (Blackburn, 1998; Nair et al., 2003; Rossetti, 2001). Finally, we have an important role to play in the infant's long-term development by sharing our knowledge with parents and caregivers. Although our immediate interaction revolves around the most effective ways to feed their infant at home, we also discuss their transition to EI in their own natural environments, what the supports and services might involve, and how they will continue to be involved in their child's growth, development, and ability to learn.

Adverse Childhood Experiences

We know prolonged periods of excessive, toxic stress in early childhood can seriously affect the developing brain and contribute to lifelong problems with learning, behavior, and both physical and mental health. *Adverse childhood experiences* (ACEs) are defined as stressful experiences occurring during childhood that directly affect a child or the family environment in which they live. These experiences include physical, sexual, or emotional abuse; neglect; or household adversity as a result of domestic violence, imprisonment, substance abuse, parental mental health problems or family breakdown, child neglect, parental bereavement, and children living in care (Allen & Donkin, 2015; Bellis et al., 2015).

Many children who receive EI services are in situations that hinder their development. As SLPs in EI, we inevitably work with infants and toddlers who have faced or are living with ACEs. It is important for us to be familiar with how these situations can affect early development, learning, and parent–child interactions. Decades of research indicates our early investment in the lives of vulnerable infants and toddlers results in considerable returns for the children, their families, and society. High-quality EI programs contribute significantly to improved outcomes in terms of school success, productivity in the workplace, responsible citizenship, and successful parenting of the next generation.

Child Abuse and Neglect

EI is an essential part of protecting vulnerable children and minimizing the impact of any abuse or trauma they suffer in life. Acting before harm has been done is much easier and often less damaging than working to resolve problems after they have happened. It is useful to understand what is involved in the process and why our role with these infants and toddlers is so important.

There are different forms of child maltreatment. These often coexist, and overlap is considerable. The four main types are physical abuse, sexual abuse, emotional abuse, and neglect.

Physical abuse of children involves a parent or caregiver inflicting physical harm or engaging in actions that create a high risk of harm. Specific forms include shaking, dropping, striking, biting, and burning (e.g., by scalding or touching with cigarettes). Infants and toddlers are the most vulnerable population because their developmental stages (e.g., colic, inconsistent sleep patterns, temper tantrums, toilet training) can be frustrating for parents and caregivers.

Abuse is the most common cause of serious head injury in infants; abdominal injury is also common in toddlers (Pekarsky, 2022). Children in these age groups are at an increased risk of brain and spine injuries because of the relative size of their head to their body and their weaker neck muscles. It is important for us to remember that children could be neglected or abused by parents and other caregivers or relatives, people living in the child's home, or people who are granted child-care responsibilities (Pekarsky, 2022).

Neglect is the failure to provide for or meet a child's basic physical, emotional, educational, and medical needs. Neglect tends to occur without intent to harm. According to Pekarsky (2022), there are several different types of neglect:

- Physical neglect: Failure to provide adequate food, clothing, shelter, supervision, and protection from potential harm.

- Emotional neglect: Failure to provide affection, love, or other kinds of emotional support.

- Educational neglect: Failure to enroll a child in school, ensure attendance at school, or provide home schooling.

- Medical neglect: Failure to ensure a child receives appropriate care or needed treatment for injuries or physical or mental disorders.

Incidence of Child Abuse and Neglect

In 2020, 3.9 million reports of possible child abuse were made to Child Protective Services in the United States, involving 7.1 million children. Of these reports, 2.1 million were investigated in detail and approximately 618,000 abused or neglected children were identified; 76.1% were neglected (including medical neglect), 16.5% were physically abused, 9.4% were sexually abused, and 0.2% were sex trafficked. Many of the children were victims of multiple types of abuse. Also reported in 2020, about 1,750 children in the United States died of neglect or abuse; half were under 1 year of age (USDHHS, 2020). Infants and young children are at an increased risk of abuse, and girls are slightly more likely to be maltreated than boys (USDHHS, 2020).

Risk Factors for Child Abuse and Neglect

As EI providers, our awareness of the signs that child neglect or abuse is happening is an incredibly important part of safeguarding practices. We have an even bigger impact, however, when we know the warning signs and common factors that could lead to a young child being harmed and knowing how to act early to prevent it from happening.

Neglect and abuse are often the result of a complex combination of individual, family, and social factors. Being a single parent, financial stress or food insecurity, substance use disorders, mental health issues, or any combination of these factors increase the likelihood of a parent or caregiver to neglect or abuse their child. Neglect has been identified 12 times more frequently among children who are living in poverty than children who are living above the poverty line (Pekarsky, 2022). Adults who were physically or sexually abused as children are more likely to abuse their own children. First-time parents, adolescent parents, and parents who have several children under the age of 5 are also at increased risk of abusing their children. Occasionally, strong emotional bonds do not develop between parents and their children. This lack of bonding occurs more commonly with premature infants, sick infants who are separated from their parents early in their infancy, and biologically unrelated children (e.g., stepchildren); the lack of these emotional bonds also increases the risk of abuse (Pekarsky, 2022).

Implications for Intervention

Decades of research indicates our early investment in the lives of these vulnerable infants and toddlers results in considerable returns for the children, their families, and society. Our work in EI contributes significantly toward improved outcomes for both children and families in terms of school success, productivity in the workplace, responsible citizenship, and successful parenting of the next generation. Therefore, when engaging in assessment, eligibility determination, and treatment with these young children at risk and their families, we need to consider the following factors.

- High rates of maltreated infants, toddlers, and young children present with significant physical, cognitive, social-emotional, relational, and psychological problems (Barth et al., 2007; U.S. Department of Health and Human Services [DHHS], 2005; Wiggins et al., 2007).

- Data from a nationally representative sample of infants and toddlers who have experienced abuse or neglect suggest approximately 30% of maltreated infants and toddlers demonstrate a delay using narrow Part C eligibility criteria; approximately 47% demonstrate a delay using moderate Part C eligibility criteria (Rosenberg & Robinson, 2005).

- Young children in foster care have higher rates of chronic health conditions and special needs than national estimates for children living at home (American Academy of Pediatrics, 2000; DHHS, 2003, 2005, 2007).

- Seventy-eight percent of children between the ages of 13 and 24 months who had been in foster care for 1 year were at medium or high risk for developmental delay or neurological impairment (DHHS, 2003).

- The COVID-19 pandemic and resulting restrictive measures were associated with increased risk factors for vulnerable children and families, including lack of access to vital services (Wilke et al., 2020).

- Programs that emphasize both high-quality services for children and direct support for their parents can have positive impacts for both young children and their families experiencing significant adversity (Center on the Developing Child at Harvard University, 2007).

- Parents of children in the child welfare system are more likely to participate in EI services if they understand that Part C is a voluntary program separate from Child Protective Services (Dicker & Gordon, 2006).

- Providing us, as EI providers, with special strategies, training, and professional support to engage, retain, and successfully serve child welfare families in Part C services can greatly increase the likelihood of effective service provision, including improved child outcomes (Barth et al., 2007).

- To best serve vulnerable young children, EI providers and Child Protective Services should have a clear understanding of each other's roles, work collaboratively, and coordinate their services. Effective intervention requires interagency collaboration among all relevant agencies (Barth et al., 2007; Child Welfare Information Gateway, 2007; Dicker & Gordon, 2006; DHHS, 2003; Zero to Three, 2005).

We might find ourselves in a situation in which we suspect neglect or abuse is happening to an infant or toddler. As mandated reporters, we are required by law in every state to report incidents of suspected abuse or neglect. Our reports are made to Child Protective Services or another appropriate child protection agency. In most situations, we can choose to tell the parents or caregivers that we are required to make a report and that they will be contacted, interviewed, and likely visited at their home if the report is accepted. In some cases, informing a parent or caregiver before police or other agency assistance is available might create greater risk of injury to the child, ourselves, or both. Under those circumstances, we might choose to delay informing the parent or caregiver. Once our report is made, representatives of child protective agencies and/or social workers conduct an evaluation of the events, and the child's circumstances. They help the physician or other professionals determine the likelihood of subsequent harm and identify the best immediate options for the infant or toddler (Pekarsky, 2022).

Substance Exposure

Prenatal exposure to substances, including alcohol and narcotics, can have significant effects on infant and toddler development. As EI providers, we engage with young children, parents, and caregivers who are affected by prenatal substance exposure through our family-centered approach. By doing so, we can effectively assess the needs of each family member and serve them through coordinated, collaborative teamwork. Families receive support in their parenting roles, and services reflect the needs of parents and caregivers following the birth of their infant, and throughout their child's early development. Infants and toddlers receive our services to prevent and address developmental challenges and trauma they might experience. To support these families and children, we need a strong foundation of knowledge in this area to apply to our practices.

Fetal Alcohol Spectrum Disorder

Fetal alcohol spectrum disorders (FASD) is an umbrella term describing the range of effects that can occur in an individual whose mother consumed alcohol during pregnancy. FASD occurs in approximately 10 per 1,000 live births or about 40,000 babies per year. Fetal alcohol syndrome (FAS), the most recognized condition in the spectrum, is estimated to occur in 0.5 to 2 per 1,000 live births (CDC, 2022e).

FAS consists of a pattern of neurologic, behavioral, and cognitive deficits that can interfere with growth, learning, and socialization. According to the CDC (2022e), FAS involves four major components:

- A characteristic pattern of facial abnormalities (small eye openings, indistinct or flat philtrum, thin upper lip).
- Growth deficiencies, such as low birth weight.
- Brain damage, such as small skull at birth, structural defects, and neurologic signs, including impaired fine motor skills, poor eye–hand coordination, and tremors.
- Maternal alcohol use during pregnancy.

Behavioral or cognitive problems could include intellectual disability; learning disabilities; attention deficits; hyperactivity; poor impulse control; and social, language, and memory deficits (CDC, 2022e).

Fetal alcohol effects (FAEs) is a term that applies to children with prenatal alcohol exposure who do not have all the symptoms of FAS. Many have growth deficiencies, behavior problems, cognitive deficits, and other symptoms. However, they do not have the facial features associated with FAS. Although the term FAE is still used, the Institute of Medicine has coined more specific terms. These include *alcohol-related neurodevelopmental disorder* (ARND) and *alcohol-related birth defects* (ARBD; CDC, 2022e).

ARND refers to various neurologic abnormalities, such as problems with communication skills, memory, learning ability, visual and spatial skills, intelligence, and motor skills. Children with ARND have central nervous system deficits but not all the physical features of FAS. Their problems could include sleep disturbances, attention deficits, poor visual focus, increased activity, delayed speech, and learning disabilities (CDC, 2022e).

ARBD describes defects in the skeletal and major organ systems. Virtually every defect has been described in some patients with FAS, including abnormalities of the heart, eyes, ears, kidneys, and skeleton, such as holes in the heart, underdeveloped kidneys, and fused bones (CDC, 2022e).

Implications for Assessment and Intervention

It is extremely difficult to diagnose FASD. A team of professionals is needed, including a physician, psychologist, PT or OT, and SLP. Diagnostic tests include physical exams, intelligence tests, as well as occupational and physical therapy, psychological, speech and language, and neurologic evaluations. Diagnosis is easier if the birth mother confirms alcohol use during pregnancy. However, FASD can be diagnosed without confirming maternal alcohol use, if all the symptoms are present (CDC, 2022e).

The effects of FASD can include physical, mental, behavioral, and learning disabilities with possible lifelong implications. Flak et al. (2014) conducted a meta-analysis of more than 1,500 studies examining the association between mild, moderate, and binge prenatal alcohol exposure and the development of the child. Findings include the following:

- Based on eight studies that included more than 10,000 children 6 months to 14 years old, any binge drinking during pregnancy was associated with a child having problems with cognition.

- Based on three high-quality studies of approximately 11,900 children between the ages of 9 months and 5 years, moderate drinking during pregnancy was associated with a child having behavior problems.

- Findings support previous findings suggesting harmful effects of binge drinking during pregnancy on child cognition.

- Drinking alcohol during pregnancy at low levels (less than daily drinking) might increase the chance of child behavior problems.

The results of this analysis highlight the need for EI to reduce the impact of FASD and to support the development of infants and toddlers who have been exposed to alcohol prior to birth.

Neonatal Abstinence Syndrome

Neonatal abstinence syndrome (NAS) refers to a group of problems that occur in a newborn because of sudden discontinuation of addictive opioids to which the newborn was exposed prenatally (Patrick et al., 2020). Almost all drugs pass through the placenta and into the fetus when the mother is pregnant and can cause the fetus to become dependent. At birth, the infant continues to be dependent on the drug; because the drug is no longer available, the newborn's central nervous system becomes overstimulated and results in symptoms of withdrawal.

Clinical symptoms of NAS typically begin within the first few days after birth (Patrick et al., 2020). Infants suffering from withdrawal tend to be extremely irritable and often have a difficult time being comforted. Swaddling or wrapping the baby in a blanket could help comfort the newborn. These infants might also need extra calories because of their increased activity. Intravenous fluids are sometimes needed if the infant becomes dehydrated or experiences severe vomiting or diarrhea.

Nonpharmacological care is typically the first level of therapy for infants with NAS at most hospitals. These care strategies include rooming in with the parents, breastfeeding, tight swaddling, and maintaining a low-stimulation environment. These strategies promote infant behavioral regulation, appropriate sleep and wake periods, adequate nutrition and growth, and maintenance of an intact maternal–infant dyad (Mangat et al., 2019). Some babies need medications to treat severe withdrawal symptoms, such as seizures, and to help relieve the discomfort and difficulties associated with withdrawal. The treatment drug is usually in the same family of drugs as the substances from which the baby is withdrawing. Once the signs of withdrawal are controlled, the dosage is gradually decreased to help wean the baby off the drug (Mangat et al., 2019).

Implications for Assessment and Intervention

The number of infants with NAS increased by 300 percent between 2009 and 2013, with an incidence of 6 cases per 1,000 births (CDC, 2022e). With the rise in infants experiencing NAS, it is important that as EI providers, we are aware of signs, symptoms, and intervention strategies that can be shared with families to support the healthy development of their children.

Although research regarding NAS symptoms and detection is well-established, and pharmacological interventions mitigate those symptoms and wean the infant from opioid dependence, we still do not know which drug combinations and maternal health and demographic characteristics predict which infants will get NAS. We also do not know what the best feeding intervention strategies or newborn hearing protocols are for these infants (Proctor-Williams, 2018). Regardless of the dearth of available evidence-based practices, as SLPs, we often work with infants with NAS to assess their difficulties with feeding, and to support the parents.

Once symptoms of NAS are resolved, the infant technically no longer has NAS (CDC, 2022e). We know, however, that young children within utero opioid exposure and NAS are more likely to have cognitive, speech and language, and motor deficits. They tend to have higher rates of behavior problems and impaired executive function. As they get older, they demonstrate poor and deteriorating school performance (Benninger et al., 2020; Conradt et al., 2019; Fill et al., 2018; Hunt et al., 2008; Kim et al., 2021; Larson et al., 2019; Lee et al., 2020; Miller et al., 2020; Monnelly et al., 2019; Nygaard et al., 2016; Oei et al., 2017; Yeoh et al., 2019). It is in the best interests of the child, therefore, to consider their risk for developmental delays and future cognitive, communication, and language disorders. We must use our clinical judgment to determine eligibility for EI supports and services for these families.

Traumatic Brain Injury

According to the CDC (2016), children 4 years old and younger have the highest rates of any age group of emergency department visits secondary to traumatic brain injury (TBI). It is, therefore, important for us, as EI providers, to be aware of the risk factors, signs, and symptoms of TBI in very young children.

The cognitive impairments of young children might not be immediately obvious after the injury but could become apparent as the infant or toddler gets older and faces increased cognitive and social expectations for new learning and more complex, socially appropriate behavior. We can help parents and caregivers understand that TBI in young children is not a one-time event. The delayed effects of TBI can create lifetime challenges related to everyday living and learning for children, their families, schools, and communities. Some children could endure lifelong physical challenges. The greatest challenges many children with brain injury face, however, are changes in their abilities to think, learn, and develop socially appropriate behaviors. Young children who are diagnosed with TBI are often referred for EI services to monitor their development and maximize their long-term cognitive and communication outcomes (Brain Injury Association of America, 2023).

Despite the limited evidence regarding assessment, symptom monitoring, and treatment outcomes for infants and toddlers who have experienced TBI, as SLPs, we are trained to assess and provide intervention to these children. Because their cognitive and communication skills are still developing, symptoms and deficits are difficult to evaluate, especially in preverbal children.

Although there are some TBI assessment scales with sections for young children that consider consciousness, cognitive, communication, and behavioral patterns, most standardized tests for children with TBI are not appropriate for infants and toddlers because of their norms or task demands (Dacy, 2023). Therefore, observation and interviews with family members and caregivers are integral to determining changes in a child's baseline function, identifying subtle deficits, and documenting differences from expected developmental norms.

We cannot predict or make any promises to families regarding the long-term impact of a TBI on their infants or toddlers; we can, however, support the children and their families by keeping a close eye on and tracking any changes in their cognitive, communication, or language skills, hearing acuity, and behavior. Outcomes, intervention strategies, and accommodations will most likely change frequently over time with the child's development and cognitive, communication, social, and preacademic needs. As SLPs, we can ensure recommendations continue to represent the child's needs at individual points in the child's TBI recovery and through their transition to Part B services.

Shaken Baby Syndrome

Shaken baby syndrome is a serious brain injury resulting from the forceful shaking of an infant or toddler. It is also called abusive head trauma, shaken impact syndrome, inflicted head injury, or whiplash shaken infant syndrome (Mayo Clinic, 2023). Shaken baby syndrome destroys a child's brain cells, prevents the brain from getting enough oxygen, and can cause permanent brain damage or death. According to the Mayo Clinic (2023), shaken baby syndrome symptoms and signs include:

- Extreme fussiness or irritability.
- Difficulty staying awake.
- Breathing problems.
- Poor eating.
- Vomiting.
- Pale or bluish skin.
- Seizures.

- Paralysis.
- Coma.

Shaken baby syndrome is difficult to diagnose. A child who has been forcefully shaken needs to be examined by multiple medical specialists and an expert in child abuse. A physician will examine the child and ask questions about the child's medical history. Various medical and instrumental tests might be needed to detect their injuries. In the first year of life, the incidence of abusive head trauma is estimated to be approximately 35 cases per 100,000 infants. The morbidity and mortality from abusive head trauma are significant. Approximately 65% have significant neurological disabilities, and between 5% and 35% of infants die of injuries sustained. Most survivors have both cognitive and neurologic impairment (Joyce et al., 2022; Mayo Clinic, 2023).

Although victims occasionally present with bruising or other injuries on the face, we might not see signs of physical injury to the child's outer body. Injuries that might not be immediately seen include bleeding in the brain and eyes, spinal cord damage, and fractures of the ribs, skull, legs, and other bones (Mayo Clinic, 2023). Many children with shaken baby syndrome show signs and symptoms of prior child abuse. In mild cases of shaken baby syndrome, a child could appear normal after being shaken; regardless, over time, they can develop health or behavioral problems. Even brief shaking of an infant can cause irreversible brain damage. Many children affected by shaken baby syndrome do not survive their injuries. Infants and toddlers who do survive sometimes require medical care for life-altering conditions such as blindness, developmental delays, learning difficulties or behavior issues, intellectual disability, seizure disorders, or CP (Mayo Clinic, 2023).

Implications for Assessment and Intervention

When we work with an infant or toddler who has been diagnosed with shaken baby syndrome, the entire EI team must be committed to working together to provide cohesive, comprehensive services. It is likely children with this condition will require special services for the duration of their lives. We need to rely on our colleagues to ensure we are effectively supporting the parents and caregivers as they navigate this difficult journey with their child.

Summary

We reviewed multiple diagnoses, disorders, and conditions we will face when working with and supporting young children and their families in EI. As stated initially, the information in this chapter is not intended to be comprehensive. Instead, we focused on key considerations regarding ASD; CP; the most common disorders associated with intellectual disabilities, including Down syndrome and Fragile X; sensory perceptual disorders; and delays and disorders that are a result of substance exposure, preterm and low birth weight, and ACEs. We learned what we need to take an initial step forward, inform our services to ensure they are based on evidence and best practices, and recognize when additional information and data are needed. We have covered a great deal of material in this chapter and throughout the textbook, and yet our work is only beginning.

Critical Thinking Questions

1. Define and describe the basic characteristics of an infant or toddler at risk for, or diagnosed with, the following:
    - Autism spectrum disorder.
    - Intellectual disability.
    - Cerebral palsy.
    - Down syndrome.
    - Fragile X syndrome.
    - Sensory and perceptual disorders including hard of hearing or deaf, loss of vision or blindness.
    - Preterm and low birth weight.
    - Child abuse and neglect.
    - Fetal alcohol spectrum disorders.
    - Neonatal abstinence syndrome.
    - Traumatic brain injury.
    - Shaken baby syndrome.
2. Name and describe the 2 types of echolalia. How are they different? What are developmental expectations related to echolalia? How might a young child use their echolalia to communicate with intent? Does their echolalia ever provide us with assessment or intervention information?
3. What variables do we need to consider when working in the neonatal intensive care unit with children born preterm or low birthweight and their families?
4. Present and discuss the implications for assessment and intervention when working with an infant or toddler at risk for, or diagnosed with, the following:
    - Autism spectrum disorder.
    - Intellectual disability.
    - Cerebral palsy.
    - Down syndrome.
    - Fragile X syndrome.
    - Sensory and perceptual disorders including hard of hearing or deaf, loss of vision or blindness.
    - Preterm and low birth weight.
    - Child abuse and neglect.
    - Fetal alcohol spectrum disorders.
    - Neonatal abstinence syndrome.
    - Traumatic brain injury.
    - Shaken baby syndrome.
5. Name at least 3 additional diagnoses, disorders, and/or conditions we may face when working with and supporting young children and their families in EI. Why are these not presented and discussed in this chapter?

References

Abbeduto, L., Thurman, A. J., McDuffie, A., Klusek, J., Feigles, R. T., Brown, W. T., ... Roberts, J. E. (2019). ASD comorbidity in Fragile X syndrome: Symptom profile and predictors of symptom severity in adolescent and young adult males. *Journal of Autism and Developmental Disorders, 49*, 960–977. https://doi.org/10.1007/s10803-018-3796-2

Abbeduto, L., Warren, S. F., & Conners, F. A. (2007). Language development in Down syndrome: From the prelinguistic period to the acquisition of literacy. *Mental Retardation and Developmental Disabilities Research Reviews, 13*, 247–261.

Allen, M., & Donkin, A. (2015). *The impact of adverse experiences in the home on the health of children and young people, and inequalities in prevalence and effects.* UCL Institute of Health Equity.

Allen, E. G., Freeman, S. B., Druschel, C., et al. Maternal age and risk for trisomy 21 assessed by the origin of chromosome nondisjunction: a report from the Atlanta and National Down Syndrome Projects. *Human Genetics, 125*(1), 41-52.

Ambalavanan, N., Carlo, W. A., Tyson, J. E., Langer, J. C., Walsh, M. C., Parikh, N. A., …Subcommittees of the Eunice Kennedy Shriver National Institute of Child Health and Human Development Neonatal Research Network. (2012). Outcome trajectories in extremely preterm infants. *Pediatrics, 130*(1), e115–e125. https://doi.org/10.1542/peds.2011-3693

American Academy of Pediatrics. (2000). Health care of young children in foster care. *Pediatrics, 109*, 536–539.

American Academy of Pediatrics. (2016). *The AAP Parenting Website.* https://www.healthychildren.org/English/Pages/default.aspx

American Psychiatric Association. (2013). *Diagnostic and statistical manual of mental disorders* (5th ed.).

American Speech-Language-Hearing Association. (2008). *Core knowledge and skills in early intervention speech-language pathology practice.* https://doi.org/10.1044/policy.KS2008-00292

American Speech-Language and Hearing Association. (2023a). *Autism spectrum disorder.* https://www.asha.org/practice-portal/clinical-topics/autism/#collapse_2

American Speech-Language-Hearing Association. (2023b). *Early intervention* [Practice portal]. https://www.asha.org/practice-portal/professional-issues/early-intervention/

American Speech-Language and Hearing Association. (n.d.). *Communication about autism: Considerations for ASHA members.* https://www.asha.org/practice-portal/clinical-topics/autism/communication-about-autism/

Anderson, E. S., Dunlea, A., & Kekelis, L. S. (1984). Blind children's language: Resolving some differences. *Journal of Child Language, 11*, 645–664.

Arvedson, J., Clark, H., Frymark, T., Lazarus, C., & Schooling, T. (2010). Evidence-based systematic review: Effects of oral motor interventions on feeding and swallowing in preterm infants. *American Journal of Speech-Language Pathology, 19*, 321–340.

Autism Navigator. (2024). *What is Autism?* https://autismnavigator.com/what-is-autism/

Baranek, G. T. (1999). Autism during infancy: A retrospective video analysis of sensory-motor and social behaviors at 9–12 months of age. *Journal of Autism and Developmental Disorders, 29*(3), 213–224.

Barre, N., Morgan, A., Doyle, L. W., & Anderson, P. J. (2011). Language abilities in children who were very preterm and/or very low birth weight: A meta-analysis. *The Journal of Pediatrics, 158*(5), 766-774.

Barth, R. P., Scarborough, A., Lloyd, E. C., Losby, J., Casanueva, C., & Mann, T. (2007). *Developmental status and early intervention service needs of maltreated children.* http://aspe.hhs.gov/hsp/08/devneeds/index.htm

Bellis, M. A., Ashton, K., Hughes, K., Ford, K. J., Bishop, J., & Paranjothy, S. (2016). *Adverse childhood experiences and their impact on health-harming behaviours in the Welsh adult population.* Public Health Wales NHS Trust.

Benninger, K. L., Borghese, T., Kovalcik, J. B., Moore-Clingenpeel, M., Isler, C., Bonachea, E. M., ... Maitre, N. L. (2020). Prenatal exposures are associated with worse neurodevelopmental outcomes in infants with neonatal opioid withdrawal syndrome. *Frontiers in Pediatrics, 8*, 462. https://doi.org/10.3389/fped.2020.00462

Bigelow, A. E. (2005). Blindness and psychological development of young children. In B. Hopkins (Ed.), *Cambridge encyclopedia of child development* (pp.409-413). Cambridge University Press.

Blackburn, S. (1998). Environmental impact of the NICU on developmental outcomes. *Journal of Pediatric Nursing, 13*(5), 279–289.

Boyd, L. A. C., Msall, M. E., O'Shea, T. M., Allred, E. N., Hounshell, G., & Leviton, A. (2013). Social-emotional delays in 2 years of extremely low gestational age survivors: Correlates of impaired orientation/engagement and emotional regulation. *Early Human Development, 89*, 925–930. https://doi.10.1016/j.earlhumdev.2013.09.019

Brain Injury Association of America. (2023). *Children: What to expect.* https://www.biausa.org/brain-injury/about-brain-injury/children-what-to-expect

Brambring, M. (2006). *Early intervention with infants and preschoolers who are blind. Bielefeld Observation Scales* (BOSBLIND) (J. Harrow, Trans.). Edition Bentheim.

Brambring, M. (2007). Divergent development of verbal skills in children who are blind or sighted. *Journal of Blindness & Visual Impairment, 101*(12), 749–762.

Cebula, K. R., Moore, D. G., & Wishart, J. G. (2010). Social cognition in children with Down's syndrome: Challenges to research and theory building. *Journal of Intellectual Developmental Disability, 54,* 113–134.

Center on the Developing Child at Harvard University. (2007). *A science-based framework for early childhood policy: Using evidence to improve outcomes in learning, behavior, and health for vulnerable children.* http://www.developingchild.net/pubs/persp/pdf/Policy_Framework.pdf

Centers for Disease Control and Prevention. (2022a). *Annual data: Early hearing detection and intervention (EHDI) program.* https://www.cdc.gov/ncbddd/hearingloss/ehdi-data.html

Centers for Disease Control and Prevention. (2022b). *Facts about Down syndrome.* https://www.cdc.gov/ncbddd/birthdefects/downsyndrome.html#ref

Centers for Disease Control and Prevention. (2022c). *Facts about intellectual disability.* https://www.cdc.gov/ncbddd/developmentaldisabilities/facts-about-intellectual-disability.html

Centers for Disease Control and Prevention. (2022e). *Fetal alcohol spectrum disorders (FASDs).* https://www.cdc.gov/ncbddd/fasd/index.html

Centers for Disease Control and Prevention. (2022f). *What is CP?* https://www.cdc.gov/ncbddd/cp/facts.html#:~:text=Cerebral%20palsy%20(CP)%20is%20a,problems%20with%20using%20the%20muscles

Centers for Disease Control and Prevention. (n.d.). *Signs and symptoms of autism spectrum disorder.* https://www.cdc.gov/ncbddd/autism/signs.html

Chapman, R. S., & Bird, E. K.-R. (2012). Language development in childhood, adolescence, and young adulthood in persons with Down syndrome. In J. A. Burack, R. M. Hodapp, G. Iarocci, & E. Zigler (Eds.), *The Oxford handbook of intellectual disability and development* (pp. 167–183). Oxford University Press.

Chawarska, K., Paul, R., Klin, A., Hannigen, S., Dichtel, L. E., & Volkmar, F. (2007). Parental recognition of developmental problems in toddlers with autism spectrum disorders. *Journal of Autism and Developmental Disorders, 37*(1), 62–72. https://doi.org/10.1007/s10803-006-0330-8

Child Welfare Information Gateway. (2007). *Addressing the needs of young children in child welfare: Part C—Early intervention services.* http://www.childwelfare.gov/pubs/partc/index.cfm

Conradt, E., Flannery, T., Aschner, J. L., Annett, R. D., Croen, L. A., Duarte, C. S.,… Lester, B. M. (2019). Prenatal opioid exposure: Neurodevelopmental consequences and future research priorities. *Pediatrics, 144*(3), e20190128. https://doi.org/10.1542/peds.2019-0128

Davidson, M., Sebastian, S. A., Benitez, Y., Desai, S., Quinonez, J., Ruxmohan, S., ... & Cueva, W. (2022). Behavioral problems in Fragile X syndrome: A review of clinical management. *Cureus, 14*(2), e21840. https://doi:10.7759/cureus.21840

De Schuymer, L., De Groote, I., Beyers, W., Striano, T., & Roeyers, H. (2011). Preverbal skills as mediators for language outcome in preterm and full term children. *Early Human Development, 87*(4), 265–272. https://doi.org/10.1016/j.earlhumdev.2011.01.029

DesJardin, J. L., Doll, E. R., Stika, C. J., Eisenberg, L. S., Johnson, K. J., Ganguly, D. H., Colson, B. G., & Henning, S. C. (2014). Parental support for language development during joint book reading for young children with hearing loss. *Communication Disorders Quarterly, 35*(3), 167–181. https://doi.org/10.1177/1525740113518062

Dicker, S., & Gordon, E. (2006). Critical connections for children who are abused and neglected: Harnessing the new federal referral provisions for early intervention. *Infants & Young Children, 19*(3), 170–178.

Division for Early Childhood. (2018). *New position statement: DEC position statement on low birth weight, prematurity & early intervention.* https://www.decdocs.org/position-statement-low-birth-weight

Early Childhood Technical Assistance Center. (2020). *Identifying child strengths.* https://ectacenter.org/~pdfs/decrp/PG_Asm_IdentifyingChildStrengths_prac_print_2017.pdf

Ferrell, K. A. (1997). What is it that is different about a child with blindness or visual impairment? In P. Crane, D. Cuthbertson, K. A. Ferrell, & H. Scherb (Eds.), *Equals in partnership: Basic rights for families of children with blindness or visual impairment* (pp. v–vii). Hilton/Perkins Programs of Perkins School for the Blind and the National Association for Parents of the Visually Impaired.

Ferrell, K. A. (2000). Growth and development of young children. In M. C. Holbrook & A. J. Koenig (Eds.), *Foundations of education: Vol. 1. History and theory of teaching children and youths with visual impairments* (2nd ed., pp. 111–134). AFB Press.

Fill, M.-M. A., Miller, A. M., Wilkinson, R. H., Warren, M. D., Dunn, J. R., Schaffner, W., & Jones, T. F. (2018). Educational disabilities among children born with neonatal abstinence syndrome. *Pediatrics, 142*(3), e20180562. https://doi.org/10.1542/peds.2018-0562

Flak, A. L., Su, S., Bertrand, J., Denny, C. H., Kesmodel, U. S., & Cogswell, M. E. (2014). The association of mild, moderate, and binge prenatal alcohol exposure and child neuropsychological outcomes: A meta-analysis. *Alcoholism, Clinical and Experimental Research, 38*(1), 214–226. https://doi.org/10.1111/acer.12214

Florida State University. (2024). *Red flags of autism in toddlers.* Reading Rockets. https://www.readingrockets.org/topics/autism-spectrum-disorder/articles/red-flags-autism-toddlers

Fraiberg, S. (1977). *Insights from the blind: Comparative studies of blind and sighted infants.* Basic Books.

Foxx, R. M., Schreck, K. A., Garito, J., Smith, A., & Weisenberger, S. (2004). Replacing the echolalia of children with autism with functional use of verbal labeling. *Journal of Developmental and Physical Disabilities, 16*(4), 307–320.

García-Tormos, L. I., García-Fragoso, L., & García-García, I. E. (2013). El rol del patologo del habla: Lenguaje dentro de la Unidad de Cuidado Intensivo Neonatal [Role of the speech pathologist: Language in the neonatal intensive care unit]. *Boletin de la Asociacion Medica de Puerto Rico, 105*(4), 56–59.

Ghosh, S., Feingold, E., Dey, S. K. (2009). Etiology of Down syndrome: Evidence for consistent association among altered meiotic recombination, nondisjunction, and maternal age across populations. *American Journal of Medical Genetics Annals, 149A*(7), 1415-20.

Gilmore, L., Cuskelly, M., Jobling, A., & Hayes, A. (2009). Maternal support for autonomy: Relationships with persistence for children with Down syndrome and typically developing children. *Research in Developmental Disabilities, 30,* 1023–1033.

Hagerman, R. J., & Hagerman, P. J. (2002). *Fragile X syndrome: Diagnosis, treatment, and research.* Johns Hopkins University Press.

The Hearing Journal. (2020, May). *FDA lowers cochlear implantation age to 9 months.* https://journals.lww.com/thehearingjournal/blog/breakingnews/pages/post.aspx?PostID=381#:~:text=Cochlear%20Americas%20has%20received%20approval,bilateral%2C%20profound%20sensorineural%20hearing%20loss

Hersh, J. H., & Saul, R.A. (2011). Committee on Genetics: Health supervision for children with Fragile X syndrome. *Pediatrics, 127*(5), 994–1006. https://doi.org/10.1542/peds.2010-3500

Hunt, R. W., Tzioumi, D., Collins, E., & Jeffery, H. E. (2008). Adverse neurodevelopmental outcome of infants exposed to opiate in utero. *Early Human Development, 84*(1), 29–35. https://doi.org/10.1016/j.earlhumdev.2007.01.013

Hunter, J., Rivero-Arias, O., A., Kim, E., Fotheringham, I., & Leal, J. (2014). Epidemiology of Fragile X syndrome: A systematic review and meta-analysis. *American Journal of Medical Genetics Part A, 164A*(7), 1648–1658. https://doi.org/10.1002/ajmg.a.36511

Hyman, S. L., Levey, S., & Myers, S. M. (2020). Identification, evaluation, and management of children with autism spectrum disorder. *Pediatrics, 145*(1), e20193447.

Individuals With Disabilities Education Improvement Act of 2004, Pub. L. No. 108-446, § 632, 118 Stat. 2744 (2004). http://idea.ed.gov/

Individuals With Disabilities Education Improvement Act. (2011). Part C Final Regulations. 34 C.F.R. §§ 303 (2011). https://www.gpo.gov/fdsys/pkg/FR-2011-09-28/pdf/2011-22783.pdf

Joint Committee on Infant Hearing. (2019). Year 2019 position statement: Principles and guidelines for early hearing detection and intervention programs. *The Journal of Early Hearing Detection and Intervention, 4*(2), 1–44.

Jones, W., & Klin, A. (2013). Attention to eyes is present but in decline in 2–6-month-old infants later diagnosed with autism. *Nature, 504*(7480), 427–431. https://doi.org/10.1038/nature12715

Joyce, T., Gossman, W., & Huecker, M. (2022). *Pediatric abusive head trauma.* StatPearls. https://www.ncbi.nlm.nih.gov/books/NBK499836/

Kim, H. M., Bone, R. M., McNeill, B., Lee, S. J., Gillon, G., & Woodward, L. J. (2021). Preschool language development of children born to women with an opioid use disorder. *Children, 8*(4), 268. https://doi.org/10.3390/children8040268

Kumin, L. (1998). *Comprehensive speech and language treatment for infants, toddlers, and children with Down syndrome.* www.ds-health.com/speech.htm

Larson, J. J., Graham, D. L., Singer, L. T., Beckwith, A. M., Terplan, M., Davis, J. M., … Bada, H. S. (2019). Cognitive and behavioral impact on children exposed to opioids during pregnancy. *Pediatrics, 144*(2), e20190514. https://doi.org/10.1542/peds.2019-0514

Lee, S. J., Bora, S., Austin, N. C., Westerman, A., & Henderson, J. M. T. (2020). Neurodevelopmental outcomes of children born to opioid-dependent mothers: A systematic review and meta-analysis. *Academic Pediatrics, 20*(3), 308–318. https://doi.org/10.1016/j.acap.2019.11.005

Leigh, J. R., Dettman, S. J., & Dowell, R. C. (2016). Evidence-based guidelines for recommending cochlear implantation for young children: Audiological criteria and optimizing age at implantation. *International Journal of Audiology, 55*(Suppl. 2), S9–S18. https://doi.org/10.3109/14992027.2016.1157268

Maenner, M. J., Warren, Z., Williams, A. R., Amoakohene, E., Bakian, A. V., Bilder, D. A., …Shaw, K. A. (2023). Prevalence and characteristics of autism spectrum disorder among children aged 8 years—Autism and Developmental Disabilities Monitoring Network, 11 sites, United States, 2020. *Morbidity and Mortality Weekly Report, 72*(SS-2), 1–14. http://dx.doi.org/10.15585/mmwr.ss7202a1

Mai, C. T., Isenburg, J. L., Canfield, M. A., Meyer, R. E., Correa, A., Alverson, C. J., … Kirby, R. S. (2019). National population-based estimates for major birth defects,

2010–2014. *Birth Defects Research, 111*(18), 1420–1435.

Mangat, A. K., Schmolzer, G. M., & Kraft, W. K. (2019). Pharmacological and non-pharmacological treatments for the neonatal abstinence syndrome (NAS). *Seminars in Fetal & Neonatal Medicine, 24*(2), 133–141. https://doi.org/10.1016/j.siny.2019.01.009

Mayo Clinic. (2023). *Shaken baby syndrome.* https://www.mayoclinic.org/diseases-conditions/shaken-baby-syndrome/symptoms-causes/syc-20366619

McConachie, H. R. (1990). Early language development and severe visual impairment. *Child: Care, Health, and Development, 16,* 55–61.

McConachie, H. R., & Moore, V. (1994). Early expressive language of severely visually impaired children. *Developmental Medicine and Child Neurology, 36,* 230–240.

Miles, B. (2003). *Talking the language of the hands to the hands.* The National Information Clearinghouse on Children Who Are Deaf-Blind.

Miller, J. S., Anderson, J. G., Erwin, P. C., Davis, S. K., & Lindley, L. C. (2020). The effects of neonatal abstinence syndrome on language delay from birth to 10 years. *Journal of Pediatric Nursing, 51,* 67–74. https://doi.org/10.1016/j.pedn.2019.12.011

Mize, L. (2008). *Echolalia…What it is and what it means.* Teach Me to Talk. https://teachmetotalk.com/2008/06/01/echolaliawhat-it-is-and-what-it-means/

Monnelly, V. J., Hamilton, R., Chappell, F. M., Mactier, H., & Boardman, J. P. (2019). Childhood neurodevelopment after prescription of maintenance methadone for opioid dependency in pregnancy: A systematic review and meta-analysis. *Developmental Medicine and Child Neurology, 61*(7), 750–760. https://doi.org/10.1111/dmcn.14117

Morgan, C., Fetters, L., Adde, L., Badawi, N., Bancale, A., Boyd, R. N., … Novak, I. (2021). Early intervention for children aged 0 to 2 years with or at high risk of cerebral palsy: International clinical practice guideline based on systematic reviews. *JAMA Pediatrics, 175*(8), 846–858. https://doi.org/10.1001/jamapediatrics.2021.0878

Nair, C., Gupta, G., & Jatana, S. (2003). NICU environment: Can we be ignorant? *Medical Journal Armed Forces India, 12,* 22–38.

National Center on Deaf-Blindness. (2021). *Hand-under-hand technique: NCDB practice guide.* https://www.nationaldb.org/media/doc/HandUnderHandTechnique_a.pdf

National Institute on Deafness and Other Communication Disorders. (2021). *Cochlear implants.* https://www.nidcd.nih.gov/health/cochlear-implants

Nygaard, E., Slinning, K., Moe, V., & Walhovd, K. B. (2016). Behavior and attention problems in eight-year-old children with prenatal opiate and poly-substance exposure: A longitudinal study. *PLoS ONE, 11*(6), e0158054. https://doi.org/10.1371/journal.pone.0158054

Oei, J. L., Melhuish, E., Uebel, H., Azzam, N., Breen, C., Burns, L., … Wright, I. M. (2017). Neonatal abstinence syndrome and high school performance. *Pediatrics, 139*(2), e20162651. https://doi.org/10.1542/peds.2016-2651

Olsen, C. L., Cross, P.K., Gensburg, L.J., & Hughes, J.P. (1996). The effects of prenatal diagnosis, population ageing, and changing fertility rates on the live birth prevalence of Down syndrome in New York State, 1983-1992. *Prenatal Diagnosis, 16*(11), 991-1002.

Osterman, M., Hamilton, B., Martin, J., Driscoll, A., & Valenzuela, C. (2022). *Births: Final data for 2020 National Vital Statistics Report*. National Center for Health Statistics. https://www.cdc.gov/nchs/data/nvsr/nvsr70/nvsr70-17.pdf

Patrick, S. W., Barfield, W. D., & Poindexter, B. B. (2020). Committee on fetus and newborn, committee on substance use and prevention: Neonatal opioid withdrawal syndrome. *Pediatrics, 146*(5), e2020029074. https://doi.org/10.1542/peds.2020-029074

Patten, E., Belardi, K., Baranek, G. T., Watson, L. R., Labban, J. D., & Oller, D. K. (2014). Vocal patterns in infants with autism spectrum disorder: Canonical babbling status and vocalization frequency. *Journal of Autism and Developmental Disorders, 44*(10), 2413–2428.

Paul, R., Norbury, C., & Gosse, C. (2018). *Language disorders from infancy through adolescence* (5th ed.). Elsevier.

Pekarsky, A. (2022). *Overview of child neglect and abuse*. https://www.merckmanuals.com/professional/pediatrics/child-maltreatment/overview-of-child-maltreatment

Plumb, A. M., & Wetherby, A. M. (2013). Vocalization development in toddlers with autism spectrum disorder. *Journal of Speech, Language, and Hearing Research, 56*(2), 721–734. https://doi.org/10.1044/1092-4388(2012/11-0104)

Prizant, B. M. (1983). Language acquisition and communicative behavior in autism: Toward an understanding of the "whole" of it. *Journal of Speech and Hearing Disorders, 48*(3), 296–307.

Prizant, B. M., & Rydell, P. J. (1984). Analysis of functions of delayed echolalia in autistic children. *Journal of Speech and Hearing Research, 27*(2), 183–192.

Proctor-Williams, K. (2018, November). The opioid crisis on our caseloads. *The ASHA Leader*. https://doi.org/10.1044/leader.FTR1.23112018.42

Pye, K., Jackson, H., Iacono, T., & Shiell, A. (2021). Early intervention for young children with autism spectrum disorder: Protocol for a scoping review of economic evaluations. *Systematic Reviews, 10*(1), 295. https://doi.org/10.1186/s13643-021-01847-7

Quittner, A. L., Cruz, I., Barker, D. H., Tobey, E., Eisenberg, L. S., & Niparko, J. K. (2013). Effects of maternal sensitivity and cognitive and linguistic stimulation on cochlear implant users' language development over four years. *Journal of Pediatrics, 162*(2), 343–348. https://doi.org/10.1016/j.jpeds.2012.08.003

Ramon-Casas, M., Bosch, L., Iriondo, M., & Krauel, X. (2013). Word recognition and phonological representation in very low birth weight preterms. *Early Human Development, 89*(1), 55–63. https://doi.org/10.1016/j.earlhumdev.2012.07.019

Raver, S. A., & Childress, D. C. (2015). *Family-centered EI: Supporting infants and toddlers in natural environments.* Brookes.

Robbins, A. M. (2009, March). The SLP and early intervention with infants and toddlers with hearing loss. *The ASHA Leader.* https://doi.org/10.1044/leader.FTR3.14042009.16

Roberts, J. E., Chapman, R. S., & Warren, S. F. (2008). *Speech and language development and intervention in Down syndrome and Fragile X syndrome.* Brookes.

Rosenbaum, P., Paneth, N., Leviton, A., Goldstein, M., Bax, M., Damiano, D., … Jacobsson, B. (2007). A report: The definition and classification of cerebral palsy April 2006. *Developmental Medicine & Child Neurology, 49*(Suppl. 109), 8–14. https://doi.org/10.1111/j.1469-8749.2007.tb12610.x

Rosenberg, S., & Robinson, C. (2005). *Implementing Part C provisions under CAPTA and IDEA.* http://www.nectac.org/~ppts/meetings/nationalIDec05/rosenbergSteven054Jan4-handout.ppt

Rosin, S. (2016). *Autism spectrum disorder or social communication disorder?* [Video]. American Speech-Language Hearing Association. https://www.youtube.com/watch?v=OYfX9O1w4Wo&t=4s

Rossetti, L. M. (2001). *Communication intervention: Birth to three.* Delmar Cengage Learning.

Ryan, S., Roberts, J., & Beamish, W. (2022). Echolalia in autism: A scoping review. *International Journal of Disability, Development and Education.* https://doi.10.1080/1034912X.2022.2154324

Sansavini, A., Guarini, A., Alessandroni, R., Faldella, G., Giovanelli, G., & Salvioli, G. (2007). Are early grammatical and phonological working memory abilities affected by preterm birth? *Journal of Communication Disorders, 40*(3), 239–256. https://doi.org/10.1016/j.jcomdis.2006.06.009

Seager, E., Sampson, S., Sin, J., Pagnamenta, E., & Stojanovik, V. (2022) A systematic review of speech, language, and communication interventions for children with

Down syndrome from 0 to 6 years. *International Journal of Language & Communication Disorders, 57*, 441–463. https://doi.org/10.1111/1460-6984.12699

Shah, U. (2022). Hearing impairment in children. *Merck Manual.* https://www.merckmanuals.com/en-ca/home/children-s-health-issues/ear-nose-and-throat-disorders-in-children/hearing-impairment-in-children

Shin, M., Siffel, C., & Correa, A. (2010). Survival of children with mosaic Down syndrome. *Journal of Medical Genetics, 152A*, 800–801.

Spittle, A. J., Treyvaud, K., Doyle, L. W., Roberts, G., Lee, K. J., Inder, T. E., ... Anderson, P. J. (2009). Early emergence of behavior and social-emotional problems in very preterm infants. *Journal of the American Academy of Child and Adolescent Psychiatry, 48*(9), 909–918. https://doi.org/10.1097/CHI.0b013e3181af8235

Sterponi, L., & Shankey, J. (2014). Rethinking echolalia: Repetition as interactional resource in the communication of a child with autism. *Journal of Child Language, 41*(2), 275–304. https://doi:10.1017/S0305000912000682

United Nations General Assembly. (n.d.) *World Autism Awareness Day.* https://www.un.org/en/observances/autism-day/background

U.S. Department of Education. (2016, October). 38*th annual report to Congress on the implementation of the Individuals with Disabilities Education Act, 2016.* Author. https://www2.ed.gov/about/reports/annual/osep/2016/parts-b-c/38th-arc-for-idea.pdf

U.S. Department of Health and Human Services, Administration for Children, Youth and Families. (2003). *National survey of child and adolescent well-being: One year in foster care report.* http://www.acf.hhs.gov/programs/opre/abuse_neglect/nscaw/reports/nscaw_oyfc/oyfc_title.html

U.S. Department of Health & Human Services, Administration for Children and Families, Administration on Children, Youth and Families, Children's Bureau. (2022). *Child maltreatment 2020.* Available from https://www.acf.hhs.gov/cb/dataresearch/child-maltreatment

U.S. Department of Health and Human Services, Administration for Children, Youth and Families. (2005). *National survey of child and adolescent well-being: CPS sample component Wave 1 data analysis report, April 2005.* http://www.acf.hhs.gov/programs/opre/abuse_neglect/nscaw/reports/cps_sample/cps_title.html

U.S. Department of Health and Human Services, Administration for Children, Youth and Families. (2007). *National survey of child and adolescent well-being: Special health care needs among children in child welfare* (Research Brief No. 7). http://www.acf.hhs.gov/programs/opre/abuse_neglect/nscaw/reports/special_health/special_health.html#foot1

Urwin, C. (1984). Communication in infancy and the emergence of language in blind children. In R. Schiefelbusch & J. Picklar (Eds.), *The acquisition of communication competence* (pp. 479–524). University Park Press.

Watson, L. R., Crais, E. R., Baranek, G. T., Dykstra, J. R., Wilson, K. P., Hammer, C. S., & Woods, J. (2013). Communicative gesture use in infants with and without autism: A retrospective home video study. *American Journal of Speech-Language Pathology, 22*(1), 25–39. https://doi.org/10.1044/1058-0360(2012/11-0145)

Werner, E., & Dawson, G. (2005). Validation of the phenomenon of autistic regression using home videotapes. *Archives of General Psychiatry, 62*(8), 889–895. https://doi.org/10.1001/archpsyc.62.8.889

Wiggins, C., Fenichel, E., & Mann, T. (2007). *Literature review: Developmental problems of maltreated children and early intervention options for maltreated children.* http://aspe.hhs.gov/hsp/07/ChildrenCPS/litrev/report.pdf

Wilke, N. G., Howard, A. H., & Pop, D. (2020). Data-informed recommendations for services providers working with vulnerable children and families during the COVID-19 pandemic. *Child Abuse & Neglect, 110*(Pt. 2), 104642. https://doi.org/10.1016/j.chiabu.2020.104642

Yang, J., & Wusthoff, C. (2023). *Cerebral palsy in children.* http://www.healthychildren.org/English/health-issues/conditions/developmental-disabilities/pages/Cerebral-Palsy.aspx

Yeoh, S. L., Eastwood, J., Wright, I. M., Morton, R., Melhuish, E., Ward, M., & Oei, J. L. (2019). Cognitive and motor outcomes of children with prenatal opioid exposure: A systematic review and meta-analysis. *JAMA Network Open, 2*(7), e197025. https://doi.org/10.1001/jamanetworkopen.2019.7025

Zero to Three. (2005). *Restructuring the federal child welfare system: Assuring the safety, permanence and well-being of infants and toddlers in the child welfare system.* http://www.zerotothree.org/site/DocServer/Jan_07_Child_Welfare_Fact_Sheet.pdf?docID=2622

Zwaigenbaum, L., Bryson, S., Rogers, T., Roberts, W., Brian, J., & Szatmari, P. (2005). Behavioral manifestations of autism in the first year of life. *International Journal of Developmental Neuroscience, 23*(2–3), 143–152. https://doi.org/10.1016/j.ijdevneu.2004.05.001

Appendix A

Screening Measures That Include Speech, Language, and Communication

Name	Age Range; Screening Areas	Administration Notes	Language	Publisher
Ages & Stages Questionnaire Third Edition (2009)	0;1–5;6 years Communication, gross motor, fine motor, problem solving, and social-emotional	Parent/caregiver completes in 10–15 minutes. Provider scores in 2–3 minutes.	English, Arabic, Chinese, French, Spanish, Vietnamese	Brookes
Ages & Stages Questionaire SE-2 (2015)	0;1–6;0 years Social-emotional development including self-regulation, compliance, social communication, adaptive functioning, autonomy, affect, and interaction with people	Parent/caregiver completes the questionnaires in 10–15 minutes. Professionals scores it in 1–3 minutes.	English, Arabic, French, Spanish	Brookes
Brigance Early Childhood Screens III (2013)	Core screens for birth–0;11 years; 1;0–1;11 years; Birth–2;11 years Self-help and social-emotional screen for 2;0–2;11 years Physical development, language	Provider completes in 10–15 minutes. Parent/caregiver report form is available. Parent/caregiver report can be used for all sections for birth–2;11 screens.	English, Spanish	Hawker Brownlow

	development, adaptive behavior and self-help, and social-emotional skills Academic skills/cognitive development starting at age 2;0			
The Capute Scales Clinical Linguistic & Auditory Milestone Scale (CLAMS) (2005)	0;1–3;0 years Expressive and receptive language development	Parent/caregiver completes questionnaire and clinical observation. Birth through 18 months based on parent report. At older ages, it is a combination of parent report and clinical observation. The questionnaire is 100 items across ages.	English	Brookes
Communication and Symbolic Behavior Scales Developmental Profile (CSBS DP) (2001)	0;6–2;0 years functional level communication 0;6–6;0 years chronological age if developmental delays are present Measures seven language	Parent/caregiver completes the checklist. Provider scores the checklist. Follow-up questionnaire and behavior sample available for	English	Brookes

	predictors: emotion and eye gaze, communication, gestures, sounds, words, understanding, and object use	use, if indicated. 5–10 min for the Infant-Toddler Checklist (24 multiple-choice questions). It takes 15–25 min for the Caregiver Questionnaire (four pages, parent completes this form for more detail if checklist suggests concern). Norm-referenced		
MacArthur-Bates Communicative Development Inventory (2018)	0;8–2;6 years Short form extension for English-learning children up to 3;1 years Language and communication skills Words and Gestures form for 8–18 months Words and Sentences form for 16–30	Completed by parent/caregiver or as a structured provider interview. Completed in 20–40 min and provider scores in 10–15 min. Percentiles and classifications are provided.	English and Spanish forms; also numerous adaptations for different languages are listed.	Brookes

	months Forms may be used with children outside those age ranges if they have developmental delays Asks about children's developing abilities in early language including vocabulary comprehension, production, gestures, and grammar			
Modified Checklist for Autism in Toddlers Revised with Follow-Up (MCHAT-R/F) (2009)	1;4–2;6 years Screens for autism spectrum disorder or developmental delay	Approximately 20 questions completed by parent/caregiver. No specific qualifications required to score results.	Approximately 70 translations available	
Parents' Evaluation of Developmental Status (PEDS) (2012) Parents' Evaluation of Developmental Status: Developmental	Birth–7;11 years PEDS identifies parental concerns with learning, intellectual, language, mental health, autism spectrum, and motor disorders PEDS:DM provides information	PEDS is 10 items completed by the parent/caregiver or using interview. PEDS: DM is 6–8 items. Recommended to use tools together. Completed in 5–	PEDS available in more than 50 languages PEDS DM available in 12 languages	PEDS-TEST

Milestones (PEDS: DM)	about parent report about key developmental milestones predictive of delays in fine motor, gross motor, expressive language, receptive language, self-help, social-emotional, academic/pre academic A cognitive score also is derived from information collected	15 minutes. Provider scores the predictive/non predictive concerns. <u>Additional information</u> on sensitivity, specificity, and cost.		
Parents' Evaluation of Developmental Status: Developmental Milestones-Assessment Level (PEDS: DM-AL)	Birth–7;11 years Fine motor, gross motor, expressive language, receptive language, self-help, social-emotional, and academic/pre academic A cognitive score also is derived from information collected; see validation for use with groups with more elevated risk for	Options for parent-completed questionnaire, interview, or direct interaction with child. Administration takes about 30–45 min depending on approach. PEDS:DM-AL provides cutoffs for concerns, age equivalents, and percent delay. It can be used for screening and/or	English	PEDSTEST

		developmental delays and has additional items	progress monitoring.		

Appendix B

Authentic and Functional Evaluation and Assessment Instruments in Early Intervention

Ages and Stages Questionnaires: Social-Emotional Second Edition (ASQ-SE-2) (2015)	
Publisher	Brookes
Age range	1–72 months: 9 questionnaires and scoring sheets at 2, 6, 12, 18, 24, 30, 36, 48, and 60 months of age
Purpose	The ASQ-SE-2 is modeled after the ASQ-3 and is tailored to identify and exclusively screen social and emotional behaviors. The ASQ-SE-2 is an easy-to-use tool with all the advantages of ASQ-3. It is cost- effective, parent-completed, photocopiable, and culturally sensitive. With questionnaire results, professionals can quickly recognize young children at risk for social or emotional difficulties, identify behaviors of concern to caregivers, and identify any need for further assessment.
Areas included	Self-regulation, compliance, social-communication, adaptive functioning, autonomy, affect, and interaction with people
Time to administer	A questionnaire takes 10–15 minutes to complete
Scored	1–3 minutes
Type of scores	Total scores in the developmental areas are reported in relation to established cutoff scores that indicate if further assessment or monitoring is required in the specific developmental areas
Age norms	Developed to compliment the ASQ by specifically addressing the social and emotion behavior of children from ages 3–66 months
Age ranges given for Items	Uses cutoff scores
Standardized tasks	Items were written based on setting and time; developmental, health, and family/cultural variables
Based on	Yes

observations in natural settings	
Based on information from parents or Providers	Completed by parent either during an interview or independently; requires a sixth-grade reading level
Other languages	Spanish
Who administers	Parents complete via interview with an early intervention or early childhood professional

The Assessment, Evaluation, and Programming System for Infants and Children (AEPS) 2nd Edition (2002)

Publisher	Brookes
Age range	Birth–3 years; 3 to 6 age range also available
Purpose	- Criterion-referenced to: - Identify children's strengths across developmental areas - Identify functional goals and objectives for IFSPs - Assist in planning and guiding intervention - Monitor children's progress
Areas included	- Fine motor - Gross motor - Adaptive - Cognitive - Social-communication - Social
Time to administer	30–120 minutes
Scored	Area raw scores summarize results from 0, 1, 2 scoring of items and can be converted to percentage scores in each domain per test period.
Type of scores	Developmental levels are estimates of performance.
Age norms	No, but cutoff scores are provided to corroborate eligibility decisions
Age ranges given for items	No, not useful for creating age equivalencies
Standardized tasks	Not a standardized tool
Based on observations in natural settings	Yes

Based on information from parents or providers	Yes
Other languages	Spanish, French, and Korean
Who administers	Early intervention service providers, teachers, specialists, parents, and caregivers

Battelle Developmental Inventory (BDI-2) 2nd edition (2007) (Normative Update 2016)

Publisher	Riverside
Age range	Birth–7 years
Purpose	Norm-referenced • Helps identify relative strengths and opportunities for learning of typically developing children • Assess and identify children with a disability or developmental delay • Plan and provide instruction and intervention by using the behavioral milestone in an item as the targeted objective; scoring criteria can be used to measure attainment • Evaluate the effects of various intervention strategies and educational programs on groups of children
Areas included	Adaptive, personal-social, communication, motor and cognitive
Time to administer	Complete BDI-2: 1–2 hours
Scored	Can be hand scored or scored with the optional software
Type of scores	Total BDI-2 DQ Score-Per author the most reliable score, domain DQ scores, scaled scores, percentile ranks, and age equivalents
Age norms	Caution is suggested in using age-equivalent scores; these should always be interpreted in conjunction with percentile rank or standard score information.
Age ranges given for items	No, single age score given in year and months
Standardized tasks	Structured procedures usually require using specific instruction text. There is some flexibility in the wording: However, the changes should not alter the intent of the item content. BDI-2 provides a variety of accommodations to allow a child with special needs to be able to respond to the item.
Based on observations	No. Includes Test Session Behavioral Observations, which is documentation of any unusual responses or behavior/s by the

in natural settings	child during testing that could affect interpretation of results.
Based on information from parents or providers	The parent, teacher, and caregiver interview is used, especially for many items in the earliest age ranges. Limited information is requested.
Other languages	Spanish
Who administers	Early childhood, kindergarten and primary teachers, special educators, early intervention providers, and related service providers. Educational aides with considerable experience with the children being assessed may use the BDI-2 or parts of it if they have received comprehensive training. General qualifications include an understanding of testing in general and the BDI-2 specifically, and knowledge of development, and experience working with young children.

Brigance Inventory of Early Development III (IED III) (2013)

Publisher	Curriculum Associates
Age range	Criterion referenced: Birth–7 years
Purpose	Norm-referenced and criterion-referenced versions To identify educational strengths and needs and current levels of development, monitor progress, and support IFSP development
Areas included	Physical development (preambulatory, gross motor, and fine motor), language development (receptive language and expressive language), literacy, mathematics and science, daily living, social and emotional development
Time to administer	30–60 minutes
Scored	Generates criterion-referenced data related to curricular objectives or, if using the standardized approach option, provides standardized scores for norm-referenced assessments, including raw scores, age equivalents, percentiles, quotients, age level of instructional range, and total adaptive behavior scores
Type of scores	Raw score, age equivalents, percentiles, and quotients (using standardized administration)
Age norms	Yes, when using the standardized approach option
Age ranges given for items	Yes, for both criterion-referenced and standardized approaches
Standardized tasks	Yes, the directions for administration and for scoring have been field-tested and are explicitly stated so that the test can

	be administered in exactly the same way by different examiners.
Based on observations in natural settings	Yes, some assessments can be administered by observing the child in a natural setting. Specific assessment methods are indicated on the first page of each assessment.
Based on information from parents or providers	Yes, some assessments can be administered by interviewing the parent/caregiver or someone who knows the child well. For these assessments, prescribed directions, specific questions, and exact wording are included.
Other languages	No
Who administers	Designed to be administered by a variety of early intervention providers

The Carolina Curriculum for Infants and Toddlers with Special Need (CCITSN) 3rd edition (2004)

Publisher	Brookes
Age range	CCITSN (3rd edition): Birth–26 months CCPSN (2nd edition): 24–60 months
Purpose	Criterion-referenced; to link assessment to intervention through hierarchies of developmental tasks that are relevant to typical routines for young children and pertinent to long-term adaptation. Considered an "authentic" tool.
Areas included	Personal/social adaptation, cognition, communication, fine motor, gross motor
Time to administer	Manual indicates 60–90 minutes for experienced assessor
Scored	+ = skill mastered +/– = inconsistent or emerging skill – = unable to do skill
Type of scores	Developmental levels are estimates of performance.
Age norms	Scored by looking at pattern of where "plus" scores cluster = Developmental age
Age ranges given for items	3-month increments up to 24 months; 6-month increments from 24–36 months
Standardized tasks	Not a standardized tool; age levels are estimates based on information from other standardized instruments and developmental literature
Based on observations in natural settings	Yes

Based on information from parents or providers	Yes
Other languages	CCITSN has been translated into Portuguese, Russian, Korean, Chinese, Spanish, and Italian.
Who administers	Designed to be administered by a variety of early intervention providers

Developmental Assessment for Young Children-2nd edition (DAYC-2) (2013)

Publisher	PRO-ED
Age range	Birth–5 years;11 months
Purpose	Norm-referenced—To identify developmental delays in children who can benefit from early intervention: Built to measure the 5 areas of assessment mandated by IDEA: Cognition, communication, social-emotional development, physical development, and adaptive behavior
Areas included	Cognition, communication, social-emotional development, adaptive behavior, physical development
Time to administer	Each subtest: 10–20 minutes; total: 50–100 minutes
Scored	Yes. Provides standard scores, percentile ranks, age equivalents, and if all subtests are completed, a general developmental quotient
Type of scores	Norm-referenced instrument, standard scores, percentile ranks, age equivalents, general development quotient
Age norms	Yes
Age ranges given for items	Yes
Standardized tasks	Yes
Based on observations in natural settings	Yes; may use observation in natural environment, but primarily relies on direct assessment and interview
Based on information from parents or providers	Yes; interview is part of the assessment process
Other languages	None

Who administers	Examiners with formal training in assessment and child development

The Early Learning Accomplishment Profile (E-LAP) 3rd Edition (2002)

Publisher	Kaplan Early Learning Company and Chapel Hill Training-Outreach Project
Age range	Birth–3 years
Purpose	The purpose of this criterion-referenced assessment is to assist teachers, clinicians, and parents in assessing individual skill development in six domains of development. The results of the Early LAP can be used to generate a complete picture of a child's developmental progress in the six domains so that individualized, developmentally appropriate activities can be planned and implemented. This assessment can be used with any infant and toddler, including children with disabilities.
Areas included	Gross motor, fine motor, social emotional, cognition, language, self-help
Time to administer	45–90 minutes to administer, updates may be on an ongoing basis
Scored	Yes. Scores represent approximations of developmental ages for use in planning developmentally appropriate instruction. These are not age equivalents because the instrument is not norm-referenced.
Type of scores	Approximation of developmental levels
Age norms	No. Normative developmental ages assigned to items vary among reputable research-based sources. The ELAP data reflect documented norms in research, but the manual suggests it is essential that the developmental ages be viewed as approximate in nature.
Age ranges given for items	Yes. Age ranges provided for items are approximations of developmental ages and not age equivalents.
Standardized tasks	Assessment guidelines do provide information about specific materials, procedures, and criteria to use for scoring each item during administration or appropriate observation of the child's skills.
Based on observations in natural settings	Yes. Depending on the components being evaluated, information from natural observation may be used.
Based on information from parents or providers	Yes. Information from parents may be used.

Other languages	Spanish
Who administers	Teachers, clinicians, or professionals familiar with child development in conjunction with observational information from others
Hawaii Early Learning Profile (HELP) (2004)	
Publisher	Vort Corporation
Age range	Birth–3 years
Purpose	Comprehensive, ongoing, family-centered, curriculum-based assessment process for infants and toddlers and their families to identify needs, tracking growth and development and determining "next steps" (targeting outcomes)
Areas included	Regulatory/sensory organization, cognition, language, gross motor, fine motor, social and self-help skills
Time to administer	On-going observations; summaries to be provided periodically; initial assessment 45–90 minutes
Scored	Yes; obtains approximate developmental levels; does not yield a single age level or score; not norm referenced or standardized. The HELP Strands can provide approximate or estimated developmental levels within and between areas of development.
Type of scores	Approximate age ranges
Age norms	No
Age ranges given for items	Yes
Standardized tasks	No
Based on observations in natural settings	Yes. Observation in multiple sessions is preferred.
Based on information from parents or providers	Yes. Parent report and/or parent facilitation in eliciting targeted skills is encouraged.
Other languages	Spanish
Who administers	One or more childhood specialists (e.g., speech-language pathologist, teacher, nurse, occupational therapist, physical therapist)
Michigan Developmental Programming for Infants and Young Children Early Intervention Developmental Profile (EIDP) (1981)	
Publisher	University of Michigan's Institute for the Study of Mental

	Retardation and Related Disabilities; University of Michigan Press
Age range	Birth–3 years
Purpose	The purpose of this criterion-referenced assessment is to assist teachers, clinicians, and parents in assessing individual skill development in six domains of development.
Areas included	Addresses six areas of development: perceptual/fine motor, cognition, language, social/emotional, self-care, and gross motor
Time to administer	30–90 minutes
Scored	Yes. Scores represent approximations of developmental ages for use in planning developmentally appropriate instruction. These are not age equivalents because the instrument is not norm-referenced. The tool recommends establishing a *basal level* and a *ceiling level* for each scale. The basal and ceiling levels define a range of items on which the child's performance is inconsistent; this range provides a focus for programming efforts. This also provides a zone of proximal developmental level. Not all items are arranged in true order; some items occur concurrently. It requires one to use their training guidance, experience, and informed opinion in determining a present level of development.
Type of scores	Does not provide a developmental age; scores are grouped in 3- or 4-month age ranges. The score sheet is designed to permit small increments in a child's skills to be frequently noted and a child's development to be graphically displayed.
Age norms	No. Normative developmental ages assigned to items vary among reputable research-based sources. The EIPD data reflect documented norms in research, but the manual suggests it is essential that the developmental ages be viewed as approximate in nature.
Age ranges given for items	Yes. Age ranges provided for items are approximations of developmental ages and not age equivalents.
Standardized tasks	Assessment guidelines do provide information about specific materials, procedures, and criteria to use for scoring each item during administration or appropriate observation of the child's skills.
Based on observations in natural settings	Yes. Depending on the components being evaluated, information from natural observation may be used.

Based on information from parents or providers	Yes. Information from parents may be used for most items.
Other languages	Not available
Who administers	Designed to be administered by a multidisciplinary team that includes a psychologist or special educator and early intervention service providers
Receptive-Expressive Emergent Language Test – 3rd Edition (REEL-3) (2003)	
Publisher	PRO-ED
Age range	Birth–3 years
Purpose	The REEL-3 is designed to help clinicians identify infants and toddlers who: 1. Have language impairments 2. Have other disabilities that affect language development
Areas included	Two core subtests: Receptive Language and Expressive Language; optional Vocabulary Inventory form (Forms A and B)
Time to administer	20–30 minutes; no time limits given
Scored	Scores derived from normative data
Type of scores	Raw score, subtest ability score (receptive and expressive) and composite ability score (total language), percentile ranks, age equivalents
Age norms	Age equivalents derived from raw scores
Age ranges given for items	N/A
Standardized tasks	N/A
Based on observations in natural settings	Guidelines given for home/natural environment observation are available in the examiner's manual.
Based on information from parents or providers	The examiner asks a series of questions that require a simple *yes* or *no* response by the caregiver.
Other languages	No
Who administers	Educators, psychologists, speech-language pathologists
Rossetti Infant-Toddler Language Scale (2006)	

Publisher	Linguisystems
Age range	Birth–3 years
Purpose	The Rossetti Infant-Toddler Language Scale is designed to provide the clinician with a comprehensive, easy-to-administer, and relevant tool to assess the pre-verbal and verbal aspects of communication and interaction in the young child. The results reflect the child's mastery of skills in each of the areas assessed at 3-month intervals.
Areas included	Criterion-referenced instrument: Interaction-attachment, pragmatics, gesture, play, language comprehension, and language expression
Time to administer	Time will vary; estimated 10–30 minutes
Scored	• Test items are considered "passed" if the behavior in question is noted through observation or through direct elicitation. When a behavior is not observed or elicited during the assessment, the caregiver is asked about the behavior. Observation, elicitation, and reporting carry equal weight when scoring. • A child must demonstrate all behaviors for a particular developmental area within an age range before a developmental age level can be considered mastered rather than emerging. • Scoring guidelines, suggested questions for caregivers, and testing tips are given for each test item.
Type of scores	The child's performance is compared to known developmental parameters as opposed to a group of typically developing children. Observe (O): Behavior directly observed, child performs spontaneously; Elicit (E): Performed behavior when cued; Report (R): parents confirm that behavior is usually performed by child.
Age norms	Norms were based on a sample of 357 children ages 4–36 months. Each age had 60 children (20 children from each of 3 states). The sample was divided by gender and type of community; attempts were also made to include varying ethnic backgrounds and socioeconomic statuses. Nonverbal children were excluded. 80% of children passed the test at each level. Validity was not reported. Reliability = .88–.99
Age ranges given for items	Yes; results reflect the child's mastery of skills in each of the areas assessed at 3-month intervals.
Standardized tasks	No, criterion-referenced test

Based on observations in natural settings	Yes
Based on information from parents or providers	Yes, but also can be elicited during assessment
Other languages	Spanish
Who administers	The Rossetti Infant-Toddler Language Scale is designed for use by any member of the early intervention assessment team or early childhood intervention team regardless of primary academic discipline. It can be administered by a single administrator or as part of a multi- or transdisciplinary team assessment. The examiner(s) should have a thorough knowledge of child development and communication skills.

Transdisciplinary Play-Based Assessment and Intervention 2 (TPBA/I2) (2008)	
Publisher	Brookes
Age range	Birth–6 years
Purpose	Criterion-referenced: To determine eligibility, write IFSP/IEP outcomes/goals, monitor progress, plan for intervention/instruction, and identify family concerns, priorities, and resources
Areas included	Sensorimotor development (includes daily life and self-care), emotional and social development, communication development (includes American Sign Language), cognitive development
Time to administer	60–90 minutes; requires additional planning time
Scored	Yes
Type of scores	Age scores
Age norms	The child is compared with normal development, accepted by the different professional bodies (physical, occupational, and speech language therapy) as what constitutes typical development within age ranges.
Age ranges given for items	Age tables available for skills in all areas of development
Standardized tasks	Administration is not standardized and no specific tasks are required.
Based on observations	Yes; can be administered in the home or in any play area. Complete administration includes observation of play with a

in natural settings	professional facilitator, peer, and family member(s).
Based on information from parents or providers	Parent input is obtained through questionnaires prior to assessment as well as during administration.
Other languages	Forms/questionnaires available in Spanish. Play-based assessment can be conducted in any language. Contains suggestions for working with interpreters.
Who administers	Team of early intervention professionals (special educators, occupational therapist, physical therapist, speech-language pathologist, psychologist) in conjunction with parents/caregivers; minimum of two disciplines must be represented

Appendix C

Case Studies in Early Intervention

Case Study 1

Tucker: Prenatal with spina bifida

Key Ideas

- Diagnosed condition
- Eligibility
- Family stress
- Marital stress
- Mental health
- Prenatal diagnosis
- Referral sources
- Spina bifida

The Story

Valerie and Malcolm have been married for 3 years and are expecting their first child. During their 16-week obstetric appointment, which included a routine ultrasound, they learned their child would be born with myelomeningocele, a form of spina bifida, in which a portion of the spinal column forms improperly. At their 20-week prenatal visit, they found out that the infant would be a boy. They named him Tucker.

Some spina bifida repairs can occur in utero, but Tucker's condition was not conducive for prenatal surgery. His parents have spent many months learning about spina bifida and preparing for the surgery he will have immediately after his birth. Valerie and Malcolm's obstetrician and Tucker's future pediatrician also shared information about Part C EI services. They learned that a diagnosis of spina bifida qualifies Tucker for services due to a physical condition that has a high probability of resulting in developmental delay.

Although Malcolm and Valerie are trying to learn as much as they can about EI before Tucker's arrival, it is sometimes overwhelming trying to understand everything they can about this program. There are many new terms, uncertainties about what help they might receive, the costs associated, and most important, questions about Tucker's prognosis. Although they feel there is still much to learn and understand, what is even more stressful is trying to answer questions and concerns from extended family members and friends. The emotions of excitement and anticipation to meet their new baby, mixed with anxiety and often sleepless nights, has led to some marital tension. Valerie frequently worries that the amount of stress she is under is bad for Tucker's development.

Case Study 2

Ellie: 3-month-old with cleft lip and palate

Key Ideas

- Cleft palate and lip
- Extended family support
- Family-identified IFSP outcomes
- Financial stressors
- Interim IFSP
- NICU
- Prematurity
- Transition from NICU to EI

The Story

Carl Parker owns his own plumbing business and his wife, Joanne, is the office manager for the company. They have 18 employees and the business is thriving.

The Parkers have two daughters, 4-year-old Cassie and 3-month-old Ellie. Joanne's pregnancy was uncomplicated, but Ellie was born at 28 weeks gestation. She weighed 3.4 pounds and has a cleft palate and cleft lip. Due to significant feeding difficulties, Ellie spent the first 2 months of life in the NICU, where she had a nasogastric (NG) feeding tube placed.

While Ellie was in the NICU, Joanne took time away from work and spent days at a time with Ellie, coming home late in the evenings to sleep. Carl's mother came to live with the family and provided care for Cassie. Carl visited Ellie every weekend, which provided some respite for Joanne. It was a stressful time trying to be good parents and meet the needs of both of their daughters, while also worrying about financial implications from Joanne's absence at work and the extensive medical care for Ellie.

As it came closer to the time of discharge from the NICU, staff shared information about local EI services. Even with the feeding tube, Ellie struggled to gain weight and received a diagnosis of failure to thrive (FTT). Due to the feeding difficulties, diagnosis of FTT, and the urgent need for ongoing support for the Parkers, the service coordinator wrote an interim IFSP. Services, which included visits by the EI SLP, who specialized in feeding, and a nurse, began the day after Ellie came home.

Currently, Carl's mother continues to live with the family, helping with Cassie, cooking meals, and doing light housework. Mrs. Parker has indicated she does not feel she can help with NG feedings and appears to be uncomfortable holding Ellie. Ellie is scheduled for surgery in 2 months to repair the cleft palate and cleft lip. The Parkers have learned that Ellie will probably be hospitalized for 1 to 2 days but recovery could take several weeks. Although Carl and Joanne appreciate Mrs. Parker's help and recognize she will be a much-needed support after Ellie's surgery, they long for a time when the family of four can establish their own routines and everyday life. They also hope that following her surgery, Ellie will be a more successful eater and the NG tube can be removed.

Case Study 3

Faisel: 5-month-old with cytomegalovirus

Key Ideas

- Cytomegalovirus
- Hearing loss
- Microcephaly
- Nutritionist
- Nurse
- Seizures
- Low birth weight

The Story

The CDC reports that cytomegalovirus (CMV) is a common virus that 50% of the adult population has had without any complications. Infants born with congenital CMV usually also have no complications (CDC, 2020). Twenty percent of infants infected with this virus, however, have lifelong medical concerns. The CDC (2020) further noted that "CMV is the most common infectious cause of birth defects in the United States."

Nasir and his wife, Maryam, have a 5-month-old son, Faisel, who was born with congenital CMV. He has microcephaly and continues to struggle with weight gain. He currently is in the 25th percentile for weight and height. Faisel has seizures and takes medication; however, the family does not feel his seizure disorder is under control. Although some infants with congenital CMV can have vision loss, Faisel's vision appears within normal limits, and he visually tracks toys when Nasir and Maryam slowly move them from side to side. He passed his newborn hearing test, as well as a follow-up hearing test at 3 months; regardless, Maryam and Nasir are worried that he does not startle at loud noises and is not turning his head to sounds in his environment. They have also learned that children with congenital CMV can develop hearing loss, so this is an ongoing concern for them.

Due to his difficulty gaining weight and his seizure disorder, Faisel is seen by an EI registered nurse every 2 weeks. He is also followed closely by a developmental pediatrician and a nutritionist.

Nasir and Maryam are uncertain about Faisel's future but their biggest priorities are to get his seizures under control, increase his caloric intake so he gains weight, and closely monitor him for possible hearing loss. They have indicated that if Faisel begins to demonstrate signs of hearing loss, they would be very interested in bringing an SLP into their EI team. For now, however, they want to focus on more of his health concerns.

Case Study 4

Caleb: 9-month-old with Down syndrome

Key Ideas

- American Sign Language
- Developmental and speech services as joint sessions
- Down syndrome
- Family passion
- Family chooses to wait for services
- Referral to EI at birth
- Sibling as model
- Stable middle-class family

The Story

Caleb is a 9-month-old who was born with Down syndrome. He lives with his parents, Kelly and Drew Miller, and his 5-year-old brother, Connor. Kelly and Drew are both musicians. Kelly teaches private piano and violin lessons and Drew is a music professor at the local college. Connor is demonstrating strong musical talents and he already plays multiple songs on the piano.

Caleb was referred to EI at birth. The intake coordinator contacted the Millers and explained that Caleb automatically qualified for EI services due to his diagnosis. Kelly and Drew opted to wait a few months to start services, deciding they just wanted to enjoy Caleb for a little while before starting what they envisioned as a lifetime of supports and services. Following Caleb's 6-month check-up, the Millers decided they were ready to start EI services, so Kelly contacted the intake coordinator who had called a few months earlier.

Caleb began services when he was 7 months old. He currently receives both special instruction and speech-language therapy once per month. Occasionally the special instructor and SLP provide joint sessions. Kelly and Drew take turns participating in services so they both feel fully involved in Caleb's EI. The special instructor and SLP also actively include Connor in all sessions; he is a natural play partner and language role model for Caleb.

Kelly and Drew were interested in learning American Sign Language (ASL) as a bridge to support Caleb's language development. The Millers were provided many ASL resources including online courses, a local community course, and books about "baby signs." The SLP and special instructor both know multiple signs and use them throughout sessions.

The Millers are also very interested in giving Caleb every opportunity to join in their family's passion for music. During EI sessions, Kelly and Drew share many of Caleb's musical toys and all of the signs they use specifically around musical instruments. They are also using signs to communicate about other everyday activities, including eat, drink, milk, sleep, and play. Connor has learned many signs quickly and with ease; he is frequently observed using those signs when he plays with Caleb.

Case Study 5

Aqueelah: 12-month-old with meningitis-induced hearing loss

Key Ideas

- Child-care challenges
- Cochlear implant
- Conflict with medical team
- Frequency of services
- Meningitis-induced hearing loss
- Rural community
- Practice-based coaching

The Story

At birth, Aqueelah passed the newborn hearing screening. When she was 9 months old, she developed meningitis and sustained bilateral hearing loss following the infection. She is currently 12 months old and lives with her mother, Jalisa, and Jalisa's boyfriend, Tyrone. Jalisa works as a full-time dental assistant and Tyrone cares for Aqueelah while Jalisa is at work. Tyrone would really like to return to his job as a marketer, but the couple has had difficulty finding a child-care setting in their rural community that will enroll Aqueelah because of her deafness.

Aqueelah was referred by her pediatrician to the local EI program shortly after her hospitalization with meningitis. At the time of referral, Dr. Walters indicated that Aqueelah should receive speech-language therapy three times a week. During Aqueelah's IFSP meeting, the EI team shared information about coaching and how they work closely with caregivers to build their confidence and competence to support their child's development. This was all new information for Jalisa and Tyrone; however, they really liked the idea that they would be such integral parts of Aqueelah's services. They also discussed their questions regarding whether Aqueelah might be a candidate for a cochlear implant.

Aqueelah currently receives EI services from an SLP twice a month for an hour each session, as well as service coordination once per month. Jalisa and Tyrone are learning many signs as they continue to explore the possibilities of a cochlear implant. Their current long-term IFSP goal is that Aqueelah will be able to sign or verbalize two- to three-word short sentences (e.g., "want juice," "need snack," "pick me up," "want doggie," "go on swing") to express her wants and needs. The service coordinator is assisting the family in locating options for Aqueelah to have opportunities to interact with other children (e.g., library story time, YMCA, swim class) while they continue to investigate child-care options.

Case Study 6

Audelee: 19-month-old with expressive language disorder and social-emotional concerns

Key Ideas

- Adoption
- Emotional trauma
- Expressive language limited
- Same-sex marriage
- Professional parents
- Receptive language good
- Referral and assessment
- Service coordination
- Social-emotional screening
- Work from home

The Story

Carol, a software designer, and Lindsey, an engineer, have been married for 5 years. They both telecommute from their apartment in a large urban area. They had been discussing having a child of their own, but Carol's sister and brother-in-law were killed in a car accident a few months ago and they are now raising their niece, Audelee, who is 19 months old. Audelee was in the car during the accident; she sustained only minor cuts and bruises. Lindsey and Carol are in the process of finalizing all legal adoption proceedings.

Before her parents' death, Audelee was a bubbly child who was babbling and beginning to say a few single words, including "Mama," "Dada," and "ba" for her bottle. In the 4 months since the accident, Audelee seems to have withdrawn and often appears depressed or disengaged. Carol and Lindsey rarely hear any sounds. Audelee points to things she wants and seems to understand much of what is said to her.

At Audelee's recent 18-month checkup, Lindsey shared their concerns with the pediatrician. They completed a social-emotional screening and talked about language development. The doctor suggested referrals to the local EI program and a developmental pediatric clinic might be important next steps.

Carol and Lindsey were quickly referred to EI, and the intake coordinator made the initial visit. Together, they all agreed to move forward with an assessment to determine if Audelee is eligible for EI services. The intake coordinator will also be the family's service coordinator. There was a long waiting list at the pediatric clinic, so Audelee's appointment is scheduled in 6 weeks. The service coordinator offered to go with Carol and Lindsey to that appointment if they thought the additional support would be helpful.

Case Study 7

Kiana: 23-month-old with shaken baby syndrome

Key Ideas

- Custody/guardianship
- Front loading services
- Global developmental delays
- Grandparent raising child
- IFSP review
- Limited resources
- Shaken baby syndrome
- Volatile/abusive relationships

The Story

Marge is a 59-year-old divorced woman who lives in a small, subsidized apartment in an urban neighborhood. She is retired from a local grocery store where she was a cashier for more than 30 years. Marge has a 28-year-old daughter, June, who has a long history of trouble with the law and involvement in abusive relationships. Marge and June's relationship is significantly strained and they rarely see each other.

June gave birth to a little girl, Kiana, who is now 23 months old. One night when Kiana was 4 months old, June's boyfriend became frustrated with Kiana's incessant crying and shook her vigorously to make her stop. Kiana stopped breathing, but paramedics were able to revive her. Kiana was diagnosed with shaken baby syndrome and spent 6 months in the NICU. June did not visit Kiana while she was hospitalized but Marge took the bus and visited her granddaughter daily. Marge attended meetings with Kiana's medical team and tried to learn all she could about Kiana's development, care, and medical needs. When it was time for Kiana's discharge, Child Protective Services granted guardianship to Marge.

Kiana has global developmental delays as a result of the sustained brain injury. She has limited vision and sees mostly shapes and shadows. She commando crawls or scoots to move around the room. Kiana is a happy, social child. She loves when Marge sings silly songs, dances with her, or reads her short books. Kiana makes babbling sounds and says, "Ma" as Marge's grandmother name.

Kiana has been in EI since she was discharged from the hospital. She currently receives special instructions weekly and OT once a month. At Kiana's recent 6-month IFSP review, Marge shared she thinks Kiana is becoming frustrated because she cannot convey her wants and needs. The team brainstormed strategies to support Kiana's language development. They discussed potential IFSP outcomes and decided they would like to explore possible AAC strategies. They also decided to add speech and language services weekly for 3 months to determine the best AAC option and to support Marge's ability to communicate with Kiana. The team agreed that after 3 months, if all goes smoothly, they will decrease speech and language services to once per month.

Case Study 8

Sally: 24-month-old with limited language and velopharyngeal insufficiency

Key Ideas

- Limited language
- Microtia
- Much older siblings
- No diagnosis
- Referral to ENT
- Submucosal cleft palate
- Velopharyngeal incompetence

The Story

Two-year-old Sally lives with her mother Catherine, father Jack, 15-year old brother Sam, and 17-year old sister Julia. Sally was born with microtia. Her mother made a parent referral to the local EI system when Sally was 21 months old as she was concerned about Sally's limited speech sounds and words. Although Sally's siblings are much older, Catherine clearly remembered their language development, and she was worried Sally was showing signs of a language delay.

During Sally's initial assessment, a developmental educator/special instructor and a nurse comprised the multidisciplinary assessment team. They found Sally eligible for EI services and made a recommendation to have an SLP assess Sally's communication and language skills. During the focused speech-language evaluation, Catherine shared that she and her husband had very different perspectives about Sally's development. Jack felt Sally was the baby of the family and reported Sam and Julia did a lot of "talking for her." Catherine had more concerns that Sally's language was significantly delayed and required a more careful look. She reported that Sally only makes "m" and "n" sounds and the only two-word approximations Catherine had heard were "more" and "no." Catherine shared that neither she nor Jack had concerns about the microtia and "simply delighted in this little one just as she was!"

Following the speech evaluation, the IFSP team, including Catherine, reconvened to discuss next steps. Because Sally has a pediatrician, but has never been seen by an ENT, the IFSP addendum included the recommendation for an ENT consultation and speech-language services once per week for an hour.

While they waited for the ENT appointment, the SLP provided services weekly. As Catherine and the SLP worked together, they discovered some unusual characteristics about Sally, including the fact that her nose was always runny even when she did not appear to have a cold. During one session, the SLP attempted to have Sally blow bubbles and she was unable to blow out through her mouth. On another occasion while the SLP was present, Catherine gave Sally a blue lollipop. The SLP observed that, as Sally was licking the lollipop, blue-hued saliva was running out of Sally's nose.

Sally's development perplexed the SLP; although many of the characteristics they observed were similar to childhood apraxia, Sally was too young for that diagnosis. The runny nose, inability to blow, and only "m" and "n" sounds made it difficult to determine how to proceed with therapy. Prior to Sally's ENT appointment and with Catherine's written permission, the SLP contacted the physician to share her observations and concerns.

Following the ENT appointment, Catherine reported the doctor wanted to do more extensive testing with Sally. Once these appointments were completed, Sally was diagnosed with a submucosal cleft palate and velopharyngeal insufficiency.

Case Study 9

Dustin: 26-month-old with possible autism spectrum disorder and mental health concerns

Key Ideas

- Autism spectrum disorder
- Faith/religion
- Grandparents raising child
- May not have any interest in EI services
- Medicaid
- Mental health
- Poverty
- Transitional homelessness

The Story

Stella and Billy Carter have two children, Tiffany, 18 years old, and Bud, 15 years old. Dustin, who is 26 months old, is Tiffany's child. Stella and Billy have legal custody of Dustin, as Tiffany has ongoing mental health challenges, and she disappears for long periods of time.

Dustin's pediatrician referred him to the local EI system with concerns about possible ASD characteristics. At first, Billy and Stella were concerned he might be deaf or hard of hearing because he was not responding to voices. A hearing test, however, indicated that Dustin's hearing is within normal limits. Stella and Billy both find it difficult to engage with Dustin in play or to communicate with him. He does not physically express affection to anyone and turns away from hugs or kisses. He seldom smiles at people. He likes to sit in the window facing the sunshine and may smile to himself and hum and rock. If his routine is changed, he quickly becomes agitated. One of Dustin's favorite activities is to sit on the landing of the front steps of his home, push his wrestling figurines over the edge, and watch them bump down the steps. He then methodically scooches down the steps, retrieves the figures, lines them up on the landing, and starts over again. He will engage in this activity for hours.

Dustin's language appears to be delayed. He does say some words, often in imitation of a catchy word someone says or a phrase he hears on TV. He does not use those words to communicate; instead, he will point and grunt, or scream, if he wants something.

The Carters have had a long struggle with poverty. They lost their house to a fire a year ago. Thankfully, everyone escaped unharmed, but the belongings they had been able to scrape together were all destroyed. They are currently living with relatives who were already crowded into a two-bedroom house. Given the crowded conditions, it is impossible for anyone to get a decent night's sleep, an adequate meal, or any semblance of privacy. Because there is no working plumbing in the house, proper hygiene is out of the question. Billy is an unskilled laborer, seasonally employed in landscaping, and Stella currently works on the custodial crew in an area hotel. Bud, or other relatives, watch Dustin if Billy and Stella are both working the same hours. The ups and downs of the economy and the unpredictability of their beat-up car have meant that they are both periodically unemployed. The Carters have Medicaid for Dustin, but they have no health or dental insurance for themselves.

The Carters are on the list for a Habitat for Humanity house, and Billy has already contributed his "sweat equity" on other houses in the community. Although Stella believes her faith is being "sorely tested," she does take refuge in her church and attends every Wednesday evening and on Sundays. Both Stella and Billy believe "what goes around comes around" and try to help others who are in need. Stella is fiercely protective of Dustin and very open to accepting him as he is, with all of what she calls "his little ways."

Case Study 10

Javier: 30-month-old with Spanish as native language and expressive language delay

Key Ideas

- Community support
- Expressive language delay
- Frustration/behavior issues
- Intake visit
- Late referral to EI
- Nonnative English speaking
- Parent not physically present frequently
- Undocumented and concern for government involvement
- Possible referral to Part B and transition

The Story

Jorge and Renata are the parents of three children ranging in age from 10 years to 30 months. They moved from Guatemala to the United States about 9 months ago. Spanish is the family's native language although Jorge and the two older children, who are both school-aged, speak English very well. Renata understands some English but is hesitant to try to use any English in conversations.

Jorge is a migrant worker with a work visa; he works on farms in various parts of the state depending on crop season. He is frequently away from home for several months at a time, coming home as often as his job permits. Renata is very busy with three children, especially being the sole caregiver and managing all home responsibilities. She feels fortunate that the family lives in a mobile home park with other migrant worker families as they all share resources, childcare, emotional support, and friendship. Renata is undocumented, and she has concerns about accessing any type of community services. They use a local health clinic for medical care for the children.

Javier (Javi) is 30 months old. Renata and Jorge have both noticed his language development seems much slower than that of his older siblings. One of their neighbors shared information about local Part C services, as her son currently receives EI services. The nurse at the health clinic also mentioned possibly referring Javi to EI services.

Renata was reluctant to contact the EI program, but Javi is becoming more and more frustrated when his family does not understand what he wants or needs. He frequently throws things and falls to the floor crying and kicking. Renata decided to call EI and the intake coordinator will be making an initial visit early next week.

Reference

Centers for Disease Control and Prevention. (2020). *About cytomegalovirus*. https://www.cdc.gov/cmv/overview.html

Appendix D

Case Studies in Early Intervention: Discussion Questions

When considering each case study, the student or service provider will be able to:

1. Describe the evaluation process used to determine eligibility for early intervention services.

2. List the criteria that will be considered to determine whether or not the child is eligible for early intervention supports and services.

3. Based on the information presented in this case, would the child be eligible for early intervention services in our state? On what basis would we make that determination?

4. Describe the importance of the family as the focal point of intervention.

5. Present any considerations we must address to provide culturally and linguistically responsive services for the child and their family.

6. Describe early intervention services that will best support the child and their family.

7. Describe the characteristics of the child's presenting diagnosis.

8. Describe the components of providing services to the child and their family in their natural environment.

9. Consider treatment strategies that may be incorporated into the early intervention services to meet the unique needs of the child and their family.

10. Given the description of the child, who are the service providers (i.e. disciplines) we would want to serve on the family's early intervention team? Why would we choose these providers?

11. What are some questions we might ask that are appropriate in this case in order to obtain more information about the child and the family?

12. Develop a comprehensive care plan that addresses the needs of the child and their family. Include in the plan the services that can be utilized to help meet these needs, who should be assigned responsibility for them, and a timeline for plan implementation.

13. Present two or three possible IFSP outcomes that might be appropriate for the child and their family. Be sure to consider the child's current abilities and development, as well as their family's concerns, needs, and priorities.

14. What services, if any, do we believe would benefit the child and their family? How and why?

15. What other recommendations or referrals should we consider for the child and their family?

Appendix E

Glossary

Acquired hearing loss: Loss of hearing that appears or develops at any time after birth and can be the result of a disease, a condition, or an injury.

Adaptive development: The development of behaviors and self-help skills that assist children in coping with the natural and social demands of their environment, including sleeping, feeding, mobility, toileting, dressing, and higher-level social interactions.

Adaptive equipment and utensils: Any equipment and utensils that improve swallow safety and foster independence when eating; may include modified nipples, cut-out cups, weighted forks and spoons, angled forks and spoons, sectioned plates, non-tip bowls, and materials to prevent plates and cups from sliding.

Adult-based learning: A focus on adult learning principles that provide caregivers with strategies to effectively engage with their children.

Adverse childhood experiences (ACEs): Potentially traumatic events or experiences that occur during childhood (0-17 years).

Alcohol-related neurodevelopmental disorder (ARND): Neurodevelopmental impairment that includes a range of neurologic abnormalities (e.g., problems with cognitive skills, communication skills, memory, learning ability, visual and spatial skills, motor skills) that are the result of prenatal alcohol exposure.

Alcohol-related birth defects: Description of abnormalities in the skeletal and major organ systems cause by prenatal alcohol exposure.

Articulation: How individuals produce speech sounds using the mouth, lips, and tongue.

Articulation disorder: Inability to correctly produce speech sounds (phonemes) due to imprecise placement, timing, pressure, speed, or flow of movement of the oral mechanism.

Assessment: The combination of formal and informal procedures used to identify a child's strengths and needs, the family's priorities, resources, and concerns, and determine services to meet their needs.

Assessment for eligibility: Process in early intervention that is offered/implemented if eligibility for services cannot be determined based on the intake process; involves a thorough review of the child's records, administration of a developmental screening tool, and family interview.

Assessment for service planning: Process in early intervention in which a family-directed assessment of their resources, priorities and concerns is conducted once a child is found eligible for supports and services.

Attachment: The emotional relationship that develops between an infant and the parent or primary caregiver during their first year of life.

Atypical development: Abnormal or questionable sensorimotor responses or an identified affective disorder, that might include abnormal muscle tone, limitations in joint range of motion, abnormal reflex or postural reactions, poor quality of movement patterns or quality of skill performance, and oral-motor skills dysfunction, including feeding difficulties.

Auditory neuropathy spectrum disorder (ANSD): Hearing problem in which the ear detects sound normally, but because of damage to the inner ear or the hearing nerve, it is not organized in a way that the brain can understand it.

Augmentative and alternative communication (AAC): An area of practice that supplements or compensates for impairments in speech-language production, comprehension, or both; AAC can include manual signs, gestures, finger spelling, tangible objects, line drawings, speech-generating devices, and picture communication boards.

Authentic assessment: The systematic recording of developmental observations over time about the naturally occurring behaviors and functional competencies of young children in daily routines by parents or caregivers.

Autism spectrum disorder (ASD): A neurodevelopmental disorder defined by persistent deficits in social communication and social interaction, accompanied by restricted, repetitive patterns of behavior, interests, or activities.

Avoidant/Restrictive food intake disorder (ARFID): An eating or feeding disturbance manifested by persistent failure to meet appropriate nutritional or energy needs associated with one (or more) of the following: Significant weight loss; significant nutritional deficiency; dependence on enteral feeding or oral nutritional supplements; or marked interference with psychosocial functioning.

Behavioral feeding strategies: Strategies based on principles of behavior modification and focus on increasing appropriate actions or behaviors and reducing maladaptive behaviors.

Caregiver practice: Step in practice-based coaching in which the parent or caregiver takes the lead in their interaction with the child, while the service providers observes and supports the interaction, as needed.

Cerebral palsy (CP): Condition marked by impaired muscle coordination and/or other disabilities, typically caused by abnormal brain development or damage to the developing brain.

Childhood apraxia of speech (CAS): A neurological pediatric speech sound disorder in which the precision and consistency of movements underlying speech are impaired in the absence of neuromuscular deficits.

Chin-down posture: Strategy in which the child's chin is tilted down toward their neck to contain and control the bolus prior to initiating the swallow to potentially reduce penetration or aspiration.

Chin-up posture: Strategy in which the child's chin is tilted up to facilitate bolus movement to the pharynx.

Classification: The ability to group, sort, categorize, and connect objects and people according to their attributes.

Cognitive development: The acquisition of knowledge, thoughts, problem solving skills, all of which support children to think about and understand their environment.

Communication: The active process of exchanging information and ideas, including both nonverbal and verbal behavior.

Communication temptations: Strategy in which the service provider structures or manipulates the environment in such a way that the child has to use some form of communication to obtain a desired item or outcome.

Conductive hearing loss: Loss of hearing caused by something that stops sounds from getting through the outer or middle ear.

Congenital hearing loss: Loss of hearing that is present at birth.

Council for Clinical Certification in Audiology and Speech-Language Pathology: The semiautonomous credentialing body of ASHA that defines standards for clinical certification in speech-language pathology and audiology, determines the application of these standards in granting certification to individuals, has final authority to withdraw certification in cases where certification has been granted on the basis of inaccurate information, and administers the certification maintenance program.

Criterion-referenced tests: Standardized assessment tests that measure an individual's performance against a set of predetermined criteria or performance standards.

Cue-based feeding: The process of coaching parents and/or caregivers to observe and rely on cues from the infant (e.g., lack of active sucking, passivity, pushing the nipple away, weak suck) that may indicate when they are disengaging from feeding and attempting to communicate the need to stop eating or drinking.

Cultural responsivity: The ability to interact effectively with all people, regardless of their culture, and to recognize how their cultural dimensions could affect a family's approach to services for their child.

Daily routines: Naturally occurring activities in which a child and their family engages in, on a daily basis.

Delayed echolalia: The repetition of words or phrases echoed after the fact, even hours, days, weeks, or months later.

Demonstration with narration: Intervention strategy in which the service provider demonstrate a strategy with the child while the parent or caregiver observes; during and after the demonstration, the provider narrates their actions with the purpose of modeling how the parent/caregiver may use the strategy.

Developmental delay: When a child does not meet expected developmental milestones in comparison to peers.

Diet modification: The alteration of the viscosity, texture, temperature, portion size, or taste of a food or liquid to facilitate safety and ease of swallowing.

Direct teaching: Intervention strategy in which the family is provided with information about a specific strategy, routine, or developmental milestone; the intention of sharing information is to add to the parents' or caregivers' knowledge and ability to support their child in new ways.

Down syndrome: A congenital condition arising from a defect involving chromosome 21, and characterized by a distinctive pattern of physical characteristics and often associated with intellectual disability and developmental delays.

Duration: Projection of how long an early intervention service will be needed (i.e. includes start and end dates of services).

Dynamic assessment: Evaluation method used to identify a child's skills and their learning potential; may include stimulability testing for a particular behavior, by evaluating independent presentation of the behavior or skill, using cues or models to facilitate the child's use of the behavior/skill, followed by re-evaluation of the behavior/skill.

Early intervention: Evidence-based, specialized supports and services designed to meet the needs of families with infants and toddlers from birth to 36 months of age who have or could be at risk for developmental delays or disabilities.

Echolalia: Repetition or imitation of what another person has said.

Education for All Handicapped Children Act: Federal legislation enacted in 1975 that mandated a free appropriate public education (FAPE) for all children with disabilities from 5 to 21 years of age.

Eligibility determination: The process of establishing whether a child meets the system's eligibility criteria to receive early intervention services.

Emotional development: The development of a young child's feelings about themselves, the people in their lives, and the environment in which they live and play.

Esophageal phase: An involuntary swallowing phase during which the bolus is carried to the stomach through the process of esophageal peristalsis.

Established risk: A condition or situation that has a high probability of resulting in developmental delay if early intervention services are not provided.

Evaluation: The procedures used by qualified personnel to determine a child's initial and continuing eligibility, consistent with each state's definition of infants and toddlers with disabilities.

Executive functioning: Set of mental skills through which children regulate their behavior, attention, persistence, problem-solving, memory, organization, and planning skills.

Expectant delay: An intervention strategy in which the environment is arranged in a way in which the child will require assistance through some form of communication.

Expressive language: The ability to express wants and needs through verbal or nonverbal communication.

Extensions: An intervention strategy in which the adult acknowledges and responds to what the child has said, and adds additional information (e.g., morphological markers, clauses, phrases) to support both language and communication intent.

Family: Group of individuals who have the most influence on a child's growth and development.

Family-centered services: An approach to working with families across service systems to build their capacity to care for, and optimize their child's development; based upon the belief that the best way to meet a person's needs is within their families and that the most effective way to ensure safety, permanency, and well-being is to provide services that engage, involve, strengthen, and support families.

Feeding: The process involving any aspect of eating or drinking, including the gathering and preparing of food and liquid for intake, sucking and/or chewing, and swallowing.

Feeding disorder: Condition related to a range of eating activities, including the avoidance of eating or limitations regarding what or how much an individual will eat; may or may not include difficulty with swallowing.

Fetal alcohol effects (FAEs): A term that applies children with prenatal alcohol exposure who do not have all the symptoms of FASD.

Fetal alcohol spectrum disorders (FASD): An umbrella term describing the range of effects that can occur in an individual whose mother consumed alcohol during pregnancy.

Fine motor development: The development and coordination of smaller muscles of the body, including those of the hands and face.

Fragile X syndrome: A genetic disorder caused by changes in a gene called Fragile X Messenger Ribonucleoprotein 1 (FMR1) characterized by specific physical, psychological, and behavioral symptoms.

General and specific feedback: Strategy through which the service provider responds to and comments on the child's behavior or responses or in regard to the parent or caregiver's interactions, actions, and/or use of strategies with the child.

Gesture: The intentional use of an action, including any hand and body movements, as well as facial expressions, to communicate.

Gross motor development: The development of skills that require coordination of the large muscle groups (e.g., sitting, walking, rolling, standing).

Guided practice: Technique in early intervention through which the caregiver takes a turn (or multiple turns) to practice using a strategy with the child, as the service provider makes suggestions during or following the interaction.

Hand-over-hand guidance: Approach in which one moves closer to the child, gets down on their level, and gently touches and physically guides them to redirect their attention to the intended task.

Hand-under-hand prompting: Physical prompting in which an adult guides a child's hands from underneath (rather than over the top of) their hands.

Hard of hearing: Any degree of hearing loss, mild to severe, that can occur when there is a problem with a part of the ear, including the inner, middle, and outer ears, or the nerves needed for hearing.

Head rotation: Strategy in which the child's head is turned to either the left or the right to direct the bolus toward the stronger side.

Head tilt: Strategy in which the child's head is tilted toward their stronger side to keep the food on the chewing surface.

IDEA Part C: The component of IDEA that addresses early intervention services (birth through 36 months of age), primarily focused on support for children with disabilities and their families.

Immediate echolalia: The repetition of words or phrases that occur immediately or very soon after the original words are spoken.

Incidental teaching: A strategy in which everyday activities and routines are used as the foundation on which intervention is supported.

Inclusion: Providing appropriate accommodations and support for each child, regardless of ability, to participate in a broad range of activities and contexts as full members of families, communities, and society.

Individualized Family Service Plan (ISFP): A written plan developed by a team of early intervention professionals that utilizes the multidisciplinary evaluations and assessments of the child to outline the supports and services necessary to enhance the development of a child who has been determined eligible, and the capacity of the family to meet the special needs of the child.

Individuals with Disabilities Education Act (IDEA): The federal law that ensures eligible children receive a free appropriate public education, special education, and related services. IDEA governs how states and public agencies provide early intervention, special education, and related services to eligible infants, toddlers, children, and youth with disabilities.

Information sharing: Exchange of information with the parent or caregiver related to the child's and family's IFSP and outcomes.

Instrumental evaluation: The process utilized within a feeding or swallowing assessment that provides specific information about a child's anatomy and physiology that might not otherwise be accessible; helps determine if a child's swallow safety can be improved by modifying food textures, liquid consistencies, positioning, or the implementation of treatment strategies.

Intake: The step in early intervention services and supports pathway that involves meeting with the family, either in person or via telephone, to explain what early intervention is, and complete all initial steps required prior to beginning the evaluation and eligibility process.

Intellectual disability: A disability that affects the acquisition of knowledge and skills, particularly those related to cognitive development, educational attainment, and the acquisition of skills needed for independent living and social functioning.

Intelligibility: Speech clarity or the percentage of a speaker's output that a listener can readily understand.

Interdisciplinary team approach: When providers from various disciplines work collaboratively, with a common purpose, to set goals, make decisions, and share resources and responsibilities; in early intervention, this involves individual services providers conducting their evaluation or assessment with the child and family independently, followed by communication among the team members to integrate their findings to determine the needs, recommendations, and services for the child and their family.

Interprofessional collaborative practice (IPP): Service that occurs when multiple providers from different professional backgrounds administer comprehensive health care or educational services by working with individuals and their families, caregivers, and communities to deliver the highest quality of care across settings.

Interprofessional education (IPE): An activity that occurs when students or professionals from two or more professions learn about, from, and with each other to enable effective collaboration and improve outcomes for the individuals and families served.

Joint attention: When two people share a common interest in an object or event, and there is an understanding between them that they are both interested in the same object or event.

Language expansion: A language facilitation strategy in which the adult attends to a child's action and/or utterance, repeats the action and/or utterance, and adds either missing words or one or two additional gestures or words.

Late language emergence: A delay in language onset with no other diagnosed disabilities or developmental delays in other cognitive or motor domains.

Linguistic diversity: The different ways people speak and communicate with each other.

Linguistic mapping: A responsive behavior in which the service provider interprets a child's interest in something they do not have the vocabulary to verbalize, based on either a nonverbal act or their attempt to communicate, and the provider uses a word or phrase to describe the child's interest.

Mand-model approach: An approach in intervention in which the provider relies on and waits for a child to express interest in an object or activity and then verbally requests (demands) a response from them.

Manner: The way in which the air is pushed through the vocal tract, and the degree or type of closure of the vocal tract when a sound is produced.

Means of communication: Ways in which an individual communicates; may include vocalizations, gestures, eye gaze, sentences, combinations of two or more prelinguistic means (e.g., eye gaze and gesture, gesture and vocalization), word approximations, words or signs, word combinations, and sentences.

Milieu teaching: An evidence-based approach in which the service provider, parent, or caregiver manipulates or arranges stimuli in a young child's natural environment to create a situation or setting that encourages the child to engage in a targeted behavior.

Mixed hearing loss: Difficulty hearing in both the middle or outer ear (i.e. conductive hearing loss) and the inner ear (i.e. sensorineural hearing loss).

Multidisciplinary approach: An approach in which service providers from different disciplines (i.e., physical therapy, occupational therapy, and audiology) provide their diverse perspectives, assess, and implement intervention to the family and child separately.

Native language: The language typically used by an individual or by the parents/caregivers.

Natural environment: Settings that are natural or normal for the child's same age peers who have no disabilities; these can include the home and community settings.

Norm-referenced tests: Standardized tools designed to compare test takers in relation to one another.

Number Sense: The development of the concept of numbers and the relationships among numbers.

Observation: The process through which a service provider observes, gathers information, and shares feedback, as a family interacts with their child within a routine or activity.

Object permanence: The recognition by a young child that an object still exists even though they can no longer see, hear, or smell it.

Ongoing assessment: The process in early intervention through which the team observes the child engaged in everyday activities with parents and caregivers who are typically present in these activities to address current IFSP outcomes or determine the need for a new IFSP outcome; this process also includes the review of the strategies and supports that promote the child's participation in natural settings to achieve their IFSP outcomes.

Oral motor skills: The ability to use and coordinate the lips, tongue, jaw, teeth, and hard and soft palates.

Oral-motor therapy: The stimulation and exercise of the oral musculature with the aim to improve the strength, control, and coordination of the oral muscles.

Oral preparatory phase: A volitional swallowing phase during which food or liquid is manipulated in the mouth to form a cohesive bolus, and includes sucking liquids, manipulating soft boluses, and chewing solid food.

Oral transit phase: A voluntary swallowing phase that begins with the posterior propulsion of the bolus by the tongue and ends with the initiation of the pharyngeal swallow.

Pacing: The practice of moderating a child's intake by controlling the rate of presentation of food or liquid and the time between their bites or swallows.

Parallel talk: An early intervention strategy in which an individual describes or narrates the child's actions with a toy or when engaged in a routine.

Participation-based outcome: An outcome statement that reflects how the behavior supports the child's engagement and participation in their natural environment and settings in which everyday activities and routines occur.

Pediatric feeding disorder: Impaired oral intake of a child associated with medical, nutritional, feeding skill, and/or psychosocial dysfunction.

Pharyngeal phase: The swallowing phase that begins with a voluntary pharyngeal swallow that, in turn, propels the bolus through the pharynx via an involuntary contraction of the pharyngeal constrictor muscles.

Phonological disorder: A speech sound disorder characterized by predictable, rule-based errors that affect more than one sound.

Phonology: The study of the individual sounds of a language (the phonemes), their patterns, how they are learned (i.e. phonological development), and how they work together.

Physical development: Physical changes throughout childhood, including gross and fine motor skills, the degree or quality of a child's motor and sensory development, health status, and physical skills.

Place: Refers to the location in the oral cavity where a sound is produced.

Plan, Act, and Reflect (PAR): A coaching strategy utilized in early intervention through which the service provider collaborates with caregivers to identify goals for the child and family and develop a plan to achieve these goals, observes the parents or caregivers as they interact with the child and demonstrate the identified strategy, and provides supportive feedback and reflection with parents about what went well, and how they might engage more effectively with their child.

Play-based assessment: An evaluation and/or assessment technique used to assess the functioning of a young child through observation and engagement in play; play serves as the primary context for observation and documentation of a child's behavior as they interact with toys and people.

Postural and positioning techniques: Adjusting the child's posture or position to establish central alignment and stability for safe feeding.

Practice-based coaching: An evidence-based approach in early intervention that builds the capacities of the families by supporting them to learn, develop, and use their own knowledge and skills to enhance their child's development in a wide range of areas.

Prelinguistic communication: Behaviors, including those that are both intentional and unintentional, used by infants and toddlers to communicate their wants and needs.

Primary referral source: An individual (e.g., parent, pediatrician, or health department representative) who identifies and refers a young child who may have a possible developmental delay or who might need further assessment to the early intervention system.

Primary service provider (PSP) approach: An evidence-based process in early intervention in which a full team supports and is available, while one service provider functions as the primary support, to the family.

Problem solving: The step in practice-based coaching in which the service provider and parent or caregiver consider and discuss strategies to improve routines and activities, outcomes, and strategies with, and for the entire family.

Professional boundaries: Recognizing and understanding what is appropriate to share, how much, and how to handle situations when engaging and building rapport with families.

Recasting: A strategy used by a service provider in which they respond to a child by providing the correct speech or language model in a way that encourages the child to continue communicating, while also facilitating the development of the targeted skill.

Receptive language: Encompasses our ability to understand and comprehend spoken language.

Reflection: The step in practice-based coaching during which the service provider communicates with the parent or caregiver to reflect on a particular routine, home visit, strategy, or behavior by the child.

Remote service delivery: The provision of services and supports to young children and families through the use of technology-based platforms.

Responsive feeding therapy: Practices that prioritize a child's autonomy and empower the parent or caregiver as the primary mealtime partner to facilitate their child's emerging self-regulation, development, and growth.

Routine-based Assessment: The process of engaging families as partners in their child's assessment; this may include gathering information from families about their child's strengths, interests, needs, and the ways in which they participate within daily routines.

Routines-based intervention: An approach that builds the capacity of the family to address the child's strengths and needs by embedding instruction within the context of their everyday activities and routines.

Screening: The process of identifying children who might need further evaluation to determine the presence of a developmental delay or disability.

Self-talk: An early intervention strategy in which an individual describes their own use of or action when engaged with a toy or within a routine.

Sensorineural hearing loss: Any cause of hearing loss due to a pathology of the cochlear, auditory nerve, or central nervous system.

Sensory stimulation: Could target any of the relevant oral structures involved in feeding, including a child's lips, jaw, tongue, soft palate, pharynx, larynx, and respiratory muscles. Oral motor strategies can range from passive (e.g., tapping, stroking, and vibration) to active (e.g., range-of-motion activities, resistance exercises, or chewing and swallowing exercises).

Service coordination: An active, ongoing process through which a service provider assists and enables families to access services, and ensures their rights and procedural safeguards.

Shaken baby syndrome: Serious brain injury resulting from forcefully shaking an infant or toddler.

Simultaneous bilingualism: When an individual is exposed to two languages from birth and lives in a home in which two languages are spoken on a daily basis.

Social development: Involves learning to form and value relationships with others, feelings about self, and social adjustment to a variety of interactions over time.

Social-emotional development: The way children relate to their social world and their ability to understand and express emotions, including both their own and those of other individuals.

Social play: A type of play through which children develop social-emotional, communication, language, and physical skills.

Spastic diplegia/Diparesis: Type of cerebral palsy in which muscle stiffness is mainly in the legs; the arms are either less affected or not affected at all.

Spastic hemiplegia/Hemiparesis: Type of cerebral palsy in which only one side of the individual's body is affected; the arm is usually more affected than the leg.

Spastic quadriplegia/Quadriparesis: The most severe form of spastic cerebral palsy in which all four limbs, the trunk, and the face are affected.

Speech-Language Pathologist: A professional who engages in professional practice in the areas of communication and swallowing across the lifespan.

Speech Sound Disorders: Any difficulty or combination of difficulties a child might have with perception, motor production, or phonological representation of speech sounds, speech segments, or both.

Standardized Assessments: Tools and tests that have been developed based on empirical data with established statistical reliability and validity.

Strengths-based Approach: Strategy utilized in early intervention to identify what works well for a child and their family, what they know, what they can do, and how to use this information for further development; the focus is on the strengths of the child and family rather than on the child's delays and/or deficits.

Strengths-based assessment: The inclusion of the strengths-based approach to evaluate the child's learning and development, including the collection of data about the skills the child presents, the activities in which the child likes to engage, and the social and physical contexts within which the child's and family's learning and development occurs.

Submucosal cleft palate: Type of cleft palate that results from a congenital condition associated with abnormal development in muscle tissue of the soft palate.

Supports and services pathway: A coordinated process in early intervention to support families of eligible infants and toddlers, ages birth to 36 months, who have developmental differences including delays, disabilities, or atypical development; the pathway begins with referral for assessment and includes implementation of all levels of supports while a child and family receive services through the IDEA Part C program.

Swallowing: The complex process during which saliva, liquids, and foods are transferred from the mouth to the stomach, all while the airway is protected.

Swallowing disorder (also known as Dysphagia): A disorder in which an individual experiences difficulty with one or more of the four phases of swallowing; can result in aspiration, in which food, liquid, or saliva passes into the trachea, or the retrograde flow of food into the nasal cavity.

Symbolic play: When a child uses objects or actions to represent other objects or actions.

Teach-Model-Coach-Review (TMCR): An approach that incorporates the practice-based coaching practice to teach families and caregivers support strategies, particularly within the context of play, to facilitate and expand their children's receptive and expressive language skills, and to teach them how to use enhanced milieu teaching.

Telehealth: The provision of healthcare remotely by means of telecommunications technology.

Tethered oral tissues (TOTs): Tight, restrictive connective tissue between oral structures.

Tie: Connective tissue that is thick, tight, and restrictive of typical movement, and can affect a young child's feeding skills, proper facial structure development, breathing, sleeping, and/or speech and language development.

Transdisciplinary team model: An approach in which a group of professionals work in a collaborative model to share the responsibilities of evaluating, planning for, and implementing EI services for infants and toddlers.

Transition: The process of change within or between services that involves children, families, other caregivers, and service providers.

Trauma: Any intense event that threatens or causes harm to an individual's emotional and/or physical well-being.

Tube feeding: Alternative avenues of nutrition and/or food intake such as a nasogastric tube; transpyloric tube; gastrostomy tube; gastrostomy–jejunostomy tube.

Voice: Refers to whether a phoneme requires voice (e.g., /b/ or /g/), or is voiceless (e.g., /p/ or /k/).

www.ingramcontent.com/pod-product-compliance
Lightning Source LLC
Chambersburg PA
CBHW080516030426
42337CB00023B/4542